Beauty, Health, and Happiness

A Way of Life

Lily

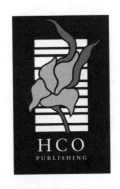

HCO
PUBLISHING

For more information on Lily of Colorado products or to mail order products, call (800) 333-LILY (5459) or write P.O. Box 12471, Denver, Colorado 80212, or visit us at www.lilyofcolorado.com. Or simply ask for our products at your local health food store.

The author and publisher have researched to provide complete accuracy. We assume no responsibility for errors, inaccuracies, omissions, or any inconsistencies herein. Readers should consult a physician before taking any new remedies.

Copyright 2000.

For book orders, comments, and questions, please contact:

HCO Publishing, Inc.
P.O. Box 437
Henderson, CO 80640
(303) 455-4194

ISBN 0-9669383-0-5
LCN 99-091823

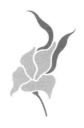

Dedication

This book is dedicated to my family. To my mother for all the artwork and help with writing this book, for raising me to know anything is possible, and for encouraging me when I was unsure of myself. To my father for giving me the determination and power to work hard and accomplish much. To my sister Theresa for giving me so many insights and life experiences. To my brother John for giving me so much joy and fun in my life. To my brothers Joe and Bill. To my nephews Jason, for just being himself, and J. R., for being the "hub" of the family. To Bob for being the best friend I ever had.

To the Lily of Colorado employees for all their hard work: Shirley, Joann, Sharon, Joyce, and Dorothy. And to our hard working reps: Laurie, Stephanie, Jane, Louise, Sue, Judith, Susan, and Carolyn.

To all my friends and customers at health food stores in Colorado, to name a few: Lisa Shapiro at Wild Oats, Sharon at Alfalfa's, Marilyn at Nutri-foods, Jill at Zerbos, Tena and Christine at Vitamin Cottage, Dawn at Wild Oats Market in Boulder, Kristina at Alfalfa's in Denver, Darcy at Whole Foods in Boulder, Suzanne at Arbor Farms in Ann Arbor, and Veronica at Whole Foods in Chicago. To all my friends in Denver and Boulder, Colorado, and Grand Rapids, Michigan.

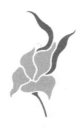

Contents

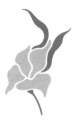

Preface

I am not a medical doctor, or a doctor of any kind. I am not a biochemist, or a chemist of any kind. I am not a cosmetologist. I am not a naturopath, or a nutritionist. Neither am I a great writer. As a matter of fact, when I entered college and took the test to decide if I should be placed in English 100 or 101, they put me in English 99. I then flunked English 101 and 102, twice each. But my writing, like my skin, has improved with my determination that I could be better. I have worked as hard to write well as I have for clear skin. Both have taken decades.

This book is a sharing of myself with you. It is simply an introduction to a way of life.

I am an average American woman who has suffered greatly with problem skin and out of desperation, much searching, and the process of elimination come to these conclusions:

* Mother Nature is the best cure for Father Time.

* A product cannot perform better than its ingredients.

* Ingredients are everything.

* Apply externally what you do internally (where appropriate).

* There are no easy answers in life.

* Always bring positive habits into your life.

* Take responsibility for your own beauty, health, and happiness.

Please check with your physician before trying any new way of life.

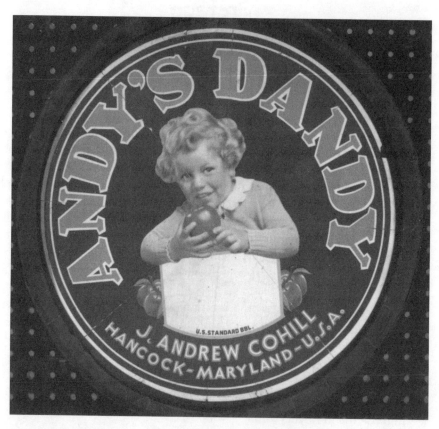

My dad pictured on the family farm apple barrel my grandfather used to ship his apples around the world.

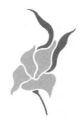

My Story

I am a farmer's daughter. My dad was a farmer's son, and his father was a farmer's son, going back at least six generations to before the American Revolution. My great-great-great-grandfather who served in the Revolutionary War was a farmer. I am not sure how many more generations farmed before him. My father even studied farming in college. He was a graduate pomologist and horticulturist.

It was interesting growing up with my father's farm. Oh, how he loved his apple trees! In the spring, if we were expecting a killing frost, he would get us up in the middle of the night to light heaters under the trees. If a tree had a limb that was too heavy from the fruit, he'd climb up a ladder and tape it—like someone would wrap and support a sprained arm. There was only one mortal sin on the farm: throwing an apple. Apples were representative of everything my father worked for, honored, and loved. They were his little babies, and he treated them and protected them as such.

Our orchard was beautiful. Dad insisted on that. During apple blossom season, there was not a prettier sight—the blossoms in full bloom, the lush green orchard grass, consistently well mowed by us, the gentle slope of the ground. It was lovelier than any park.

I have to agree with my dad: There is something almost magical about farming. To have a quality crop—and he would raise nothing else—you have to have deep respect for the land, plant the right seed (or in fruit growing, the varieties and rootstock), labor with love, and protect your trees.

It is primarily from my father's reverence for the land that I gained a respect for botanicals. My sister, however, was a parallel influence in this process. My father's deep-seated respect for the land and fruit did not transfer over to animals. One day when my sister was five or six years old, my dad cut the heads off our pet chickens. Unbeknownst to him, she witnessed this and, making the connection between live animals and meat on the table, never ate meat again.

Back in the sixties and seventies, it was logistically very difficult to be a vegetarian. My mom would make spaghetti or lasagna or whatever, and we would have the one with meat in it and my sister would get her own little vegetarian version of the dish.

In addition, whenever we were on vacation or in a nearby town, my sister would drag me into health food stores. As a young teenager, I was not too interested and would rather wait outside. But when I developed acne at age fourteen, I became interested. I would go into stores, look at the skin care products, and ask, "What is this lavender stuff?" "Why are these flowers in these products?" I was developing a serious condition called *acne vulgaris*, which is cyst acne, very unattractive and painful. This kind of acne shades one's entire existence; it affects your well-being and self-esteem. I was desperate, and I would have spent any amount of money or done anything to clear up my complexion.

About this time, I began seeing a dermatologist. "Avoid potato chips, fried foods, and chocolate," he told me. His prescribing topical ointment offered hope, but not much more. He also prescribed tetracycline. Tetracycline permanently yellows your teeth. Luckily, my parents could not afford it, so I never took this antibiotic. For ten solid years, I did not eat one potato chip, french fry, or chocolate bar—but I still had acne.

I would go to the cosmetic counter at the department store, examine all the labels, and try to figure out why the astringent there was $30 while the astringent at the grocery store was only $3. "What ingredient made these products perform?" I wondered. I concluded that there was no difference in the ingredients in the products from the department store versus the grocery store. Furthermore, there was no ingredient I could find in the products that by chemical definition would clear up skin. I discovered, however, the products in the health food stores were very different. Often they had botanical ingredients like witch hazel, calendula, and chamomile, which by *chemical constituency* are astringent, anti-inflammatory, pore tightening, and healing.

Years ago, I was at a friend's house where I spotted a department store brand of toner. The ingredients were water, SD alcohol, acetone, and fragrance—all this for over $30. I told her to save her money; if this was the kind of product she wanted to use she could make it herself for almost no cost. Take one quart of water, add two tablespoons isopropyl alcohol, a few drops of fingernail polish, and a dash of your favorite perfume on hand. Of course, I am not recommending this, but this would give you the basic product for which many people now pay up to $45.

My parents raised me to be an extremely independent-natured and strong-minded individual, but at sixteen I became more independent and strong-minded than they intended! I decided to drop out of high school to pursue my passions—mainly traveling. I had places to go and people to meet. I wanted to traverse the globe via car, plane, motorcycle, train, bus, rickshaw, and any other mode of transportation available, including hitchhiking. My goal in life was to see the seven continents by the time I was twenty-one. I made it to five. After peeling shrimp in Miami, living in my car in Daytona, Florida, picking fruit in Oregon, cleaning hotel rooms in Tennessee, serving food in Vail, Colorado, and sewing ski parkas in Boulder to support my travels, college seemed like a really good idea.

My parents thought that college was imperative, and of course I intended to attend college, but my dad had this adage: "You kids are on your own. I put myself through college. You can, too." He had lots of interesting adages: "It's a cruel world out there; you better get used to it." His favorite one was something about "snow water in hell." He wanted us to be tough and for the most part, it worked. I was on my own.

I worked two to three jobs at a time and took out national student loans that took me ten years to pay off, and I graduated with a bachelor of science degree after four years of college. Then running a non-profit organization I started in Denver made me realize just how much education I did not have, so I began graduate school at the University of Colorado at Denver. I had to work full time while going to school, but I received my master's degree six years later.

I had traveled to five continents, been to college, founded a non-profit organization—and I still had acne. It had cleared up considerably since my teenage years, but was still with me. I had continued to study skin care, still reading all the labels and ingredients, but by now I knew what most of them were: synthetic or petroleum-based.

My search for a cure for problem skin continued. I'm sure having bad skin is much like being chronically overweight. You try everything, do anything, and spend any amount of money to relieve the problem. It is emotionally painful and requires constant attention. I am often curious

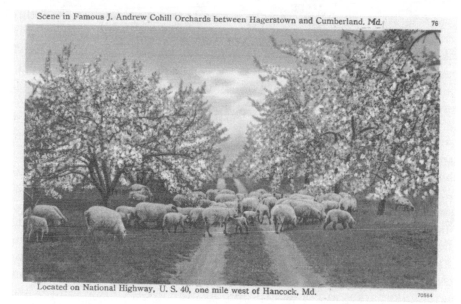

Located on National Highway, U. S. 40, one mile west of Hancock, Md. 70564

A postcard of my grandfather's farm from the 1940s

why so many people in the skin-care business appear to have never had a blemish. If you never had bad skin, why would you ever be interested in skin care? If you did not have to spend your lifetime trying to find the answer, why would you know much about it?

For example, I have never had a weight problem, and I don't know a Jenny Craig diet from Weight Watchers. Why should I? I have never had to care, mostly for the grace of God and a very healthy diet from a young age. My parents did not believe in buying food that they could grow, so we ate tons of fresh vegetables and, of course, fruit. In addition, my mother was into healthy eating and a healthy lifestyle before these became popular.

Being raised farming, we were very active kids, always running (mostly from my dad when he suspected we were not working). We had to work on the farm almost every weekend. Plus my dad literally thought the purpose of legal holidays was so we could get out of school to work. My mother would not allow us to watch much television and when our old TV broke down when I was twelve or thirteen, my dad refused to buy another one. Because we went a year or two without a TV, we had to find our own methods of amusement.

I have always been hyper and extremely physical. I am at the point in my life now where I love to work out, walk, and do yoga or even my morning crunches. All these exercises make me feel good. So I know I am blessed in the weight department. I never had to give it much thought, but not so in the skin department. The process of discovering how to have healthy skin was steady, but slow. Over the years I made lots of my own applesauce masks, mashed strawberry cleansers, witch hazel and chamomile toners, and glycerin and rosewater moisturizers.

In my mid-twenties, I made a ghastly discovery: Fine lines were developing and I still had acne! I redoubled my efforts and was completely determined to find the answers. My sister took me to see Hanna Kroeger, a gifted and well-known herbalist in Boulder, Colorado. Hanna recommended herbs for my kidneys to aid in cleansing toxins from my system.

Slowly but surely, I began the path that cleared up my skin. I decided I had some bad habits, but more important, I needed good ones. My sister said that you should not beat yourself up for eating a candy bar or having a beer, but if you're going to do it, enjoy every morsel, every drop. I thought that was good advice. I decided I was going to gradually bring positive things, people, and habits into my life.

Over the next several years, I tried several liver and kidney-cleansing herbs that seemed to really help. I started going into health food stores and picking up new products all the time. I began drinking chamomile tea every night to calm myself, something I truly needed. I really started studying herbs. Buying every book available, I began experimenting with herbs both internally and externally. I attended the Colorado Herbal College in Boulder and learned a great deal about herbs I had not used before. I started making a wonderful concoction of spirulina, wheat grass, alfalfa, brewer's yeast, and apple juice, fondly referred to as "pond scum" by those of us who drink it daily.

I gave up beef soon after my sister explained to me why cows are sacred in India: "Cows are kind and harmless. Beyond that they provide milk, yogurt, butter, cream, and cheese. Why would you kill your golden goose?" It made so much sense, and those cows are cute!

About the same time, I became almost frantic; my acne had cleared up but I had deep pox-mark scars. After speaking to five or six dermatologists, I chose one to do dermabrasion. The first time was rather traumatic. The dermatologist takes a very small wire brush to tear off the first layer of your skin. Other people have told me that they thought it was extremely painful. I didn't think so. I was so happy to get the scars removed from my face, no pain would have been too great. I didn't even think about the pain.

I remember lying there, after being given two Valiums and pain-killing shots in the face, and the area frozen before the doctor would take the high-speed wire brush to it. He was doing a part on the left side of my chin where I had particularly nasty scars, and I could feel the skin and blood splattering everywhere. I kept thinking, "Yeah, there it goes, those scars are going to be gone, my skin is going to be smooth." I was never happier. I was so pleased.

People often ask me if I recommend dermabrasion, and I do, absolutely. The price is determined by the size of the area that needs the treatment. It can easily be several thousand dollars. But it can be much less, if you only need a small area done. The greatest hardship for me was the doctor demanding that I take two weeks off work.

Why do I recommend it? Once you have finally overcome the acne, you do not want to continue to be burdened with the scars, the permanent recollection of such a difficult time. You want to be completely free from any reminder in the mirror. (You must be free from any acne before you can remove the scars.) You want to look as good as you can possibly look. It makes you feel better about yourself. It helps build your self-confidence. There is a direct correlation between your perception of how you look and how you feel. This cannot be denied. Dermabrasion is a permanent solution. And it is a natural procedure. Nothing foreign goes into your body, such as collagen. It is usually done just once, unless your acne scars are severe like mine were. I had it done three times.

After that, I was looking and feeling much better. I began a morning ritual of drinking a vinegar, apple, garlic, horseradish, and ginseng drink, plus taking handfuls of different herbal capsules and vitamin supplements. I was really having fun with the herbs. In addition to all the internal treatments, I was enjoying making pineapple astringents, honey and papaya masks, putting essential oil of lavender in my bath, and almond, primrose, rosemary, and kukui oil in my hair.

I made a wonderful herbal moisturizer for oily skin, for people who needed a moisturizer but wanted something light and oil free. It had the benefits of nineteen different healing herbs, including lily and aloe that help reduce scars, comfrey root, which is a cell proliferate and helps collagen re-knit itself, and seaweeds that are anti-inflammatory. I blended them in a kosher vegetable glycerin and aloe vera base. It was perfect. It improved the very texture of my skin. I could even apply it over makeup when I felt dryness around my eyes and mouth. It just seemed to make my skin more elastic, the pores a little smaller. It made my skin crack less and wrinkle less when I smiled. I thought everybody and their brother (or sister) would want to have it.

I was so enthusiastic about my herbal moisturizer that I spoke to my mom and sister about marketing it. They told me the name of my company should be Lily of Colorado, although I wanted to go with something else. (I can't remember what.) They were adamant. "The name should be Lily," they insisted. "We know; we are your target customers. We have been shopping in health food stores a lot longer than you. Trust us; we know what we are talking about." I said, "Okay. Okay."

I paid an artist to do a logo. It took much longer and cost a lot more than I thought it should, but I really liked it, and thank goodness, so did my mom and sister. I ordered bottles, ingredients, and labels. I put the product together and showed it to Alfalfa's, a large health food store in Colorado. The purchaser at the time told me I had two herbs spelled wrong on the label. OOPS! I should have run *that* by my mom and sister. I had to redo all the labels!

I went to Wild Oats, another large health food store in Colorado. Nobody was too excited. I kept trying to tell them all how exceptionally wonderful it was and that they just needed to try it. I tried to convince them to look at how clean the ingredients were—no parabens, no propylene glycol, no urea, nothing but God-given botanical ingredients. Nobody really cared.

I went to a nutritional foods show in Las Vegas. I didn't get a booth but just walked around with my product in my purse. I showed it to several people and gave out samples. No one was interested. I could not understand it. I had this terrific little product. It was purely botanical™. People who worked in health food stores would really like that. I shop in health food stores. I liked the idea of a high-performing skin care product made with only purely botanical™ ingredients.

Someone once told me that I had more tenacity than brains. Maybe, because I just kept on plugging away. Before I could even sell the first product, I was driven to develop the next three. From the beginning, I knew what I was going to do. I was young and this was what I wanted to do for the rest of my life, along with directing the non-profit organization that I had founded and still love. I had a fifty-year plan. I wasn't going anywhere; I had decades.

Tens of thousands of dollars later, things still looked pretty bleak. No, I am not a trust-fund baby. All the money invested in the company I made the old-fashioned hard way—work. I think I have such an ingrained, hard-core work ethic, that the lack of money has never been an insurmountable problem for me. I know how to get more—just work more. I also have very simple needs. I live in a small house, enjoy inexpensive foods such as burritos, tostados, beans, and rice, and drive an older car.

Meanwhile, more and more stores were not interested and turned me down. Finally, though, I got the product in two stores, one in Nevada and one in the Midwest. I shipped out the product and was "happy as a pig in mud." A few weeks later, both stores phoned to tell me that some of the product had gone bad and what was I going to do about it? They were not very cheerful. Of course, I would stand by the product and replace it, but I had a much larger fundamental problem. The product was deteriorating because I didn't want to have harsh chemical preservatives in it.

The first time this happened to a customer I had in California, she was almost delighted. I was listening to her tell me about the different shades of the mold and preparing for the worst when she surprised me by saying, "You know, I'm almost glad this product went bad because now I know for sure it's clean," meaning free of harsh chemical preservatives.

I had preserved the products with essential oils and grapefruit seed extract and could not figure out what was going wrong. I was determined to get this right. I ran hundreds of tests, putting this ingredient first, that one last, heating this one, chilling that one, mixing two first before mixing them with the rest of the batch. I incubated them, and on and on. Years later, I finally figured it out!

In the meantime, Wild Oats, in Boulder had finally brought my line in. Interestingly enough, one of the first buyers I sold to there, Sunny, is now the owner of Herbs for Kids. The product was placed in Wild Oats when I had only one product and Wild Oats had only one store. It was rough; nothing much sold. I don't know how I made it through those days. Today you could never survive with your product not moving. It moves, or you are off the shelf. Things were a lot calmer then, a lot more laid back.

Lisa, another health and beauty manager at Wild Oats, noticed that my product was clean, made fresh-to-order weekly, and she cared. We still had some spoilage problems then, too, but she was patient waiting for me to "get it together." It was difficult having products go bad on the shelf. I was so relieved when I got past that.

Lisa is probably the best friend that Lily of Colorado has had. I loved Lisa's kind words of support. She also had many good ideas for the company, but sometimes I didn't want to hear them, only because if anything was going to happen in the company, guess who was going to have to make it happen? Lisa suggested we shrink-wrap all the bottles and jars, come out with more vegan products, and do demonstrations. I must have spent a hundred hours in that store. Most of the time, I enjoyed chasing people down the aisles so I could stop them and ask them to try my product. Every once in a while, however, it took everything I had to go into the store, and then to smile. It was just too much. I was just too tired.

Sometimes in a store where I knew my product wasn't selling and the clerks in the store were not supportive, I would have to sit out in my car until I convinced myself to be positive. It is surprising how it worked. I would be as down as a beaten dog, but I would put on a smile and go in a store, and in an hour or two I would meet some really wonderful people while doing a demo. They would not necessarily buy the product, but they would be so kind, saying how nice it was, and I would find myself really enjoying working there.

I had to eat and breathe those positive comments from my customers and consumers for nearly ten years. I had nothing else. Continuously, every year, I had to take money from my full-time job and pour it into the company. The company took a much greater share of my income than I did to live!

One of the things that kept me going was that every time I would even momentarily entertain the brief thought of quitting, someone would call me on the phone at the same time. They'd say they were from California or Georgia and they had vacationed in Aspen or Boulder this summer and had gone to a health food store and purchased my product and they absolutely had to have more; could they order directly from me? Or someone local would call and leave a message to tell me how much they loved the product and they just wanted to thank me for making products so clean and wonderful. This continues today. Whenever I get even a little down, someone calls and makes all the trouble worthwhile.

One time, a woman phoned while I was pretty upset about the company. She said she had been using the products and just adored them and asked what else was I going to come out with. I shared with her how I was feeling and she sternly asked, "You're not thinking of stopping the manufacturing of your products, are you?" She was really upset. "Please, don't even consider it. Your products are the only products I can use without my face breaking out. Please, don't stop making them!" God bless my customers; they have got to be some of the nicest people on earth.

The most memorable conversation I ever had with a Lily of Colorado customer took place several years ago. The product had really started to take off and develop a following. With a wonderful sales representative here in Colorado and reps in other states, it was getting a lot of placement. The conversation I'm referring to was preceded by one of the most traumatic events of my life. I still look back on it as a message from God when I most needed it.

It was Halloween night and I was sitting at my kitchen table when the phone rang. I answered it but I could not understand the woman on the other end of the line. I knew I must know her because she was screaming my name. I finally figured out it was my sister screaming, but I could not understand what she was saying. My brother-in-law took the receiver and said, "Lil, are you sitting down?" I said yes. "Your parents were in a car accident in Michigan. Your dad is dead and your mom is in intensive care. They don't know if she is going to make it." Details of the accident did not matter so I did not ask. I was on the next flight out.

That two weeks in Michigan with my siblings could fill volumes about love, emotional stress, scars, sibling relationships, dealing with death, hardship, life lessons, priorities, friendship, loyalty, honesty, and soul searching.

We had my dad's body flown to his family plot in Maryland where members of his family had been buried for the last 200 years. Half of my siblings went to my dad's burial and half of us stayed with my mother. After two weeks dealing with insurance companies, police reports, lawyers, coroners, accountants, banks, and visiting my mother in the hospital across town twice a day, I had to get home.

A couple of months later, a memorial was held for my father in Maryland. It was especially important I be there because I had not been at the burial. Just before starting my drive across the country, the Federal Food and Drug Administration phoned. To make a long story short, they wanted me to recall a product. It was an Irish moss eye gel and mask. The product was wonderful, but because all the ingredients were botanical and the grapefruit seed extract and essential oil preservatives would not preserve it, it had a propensity to go bad. The FDA wanted this product off every shelf in America, yesterday! The FDA also wanted two of their agents to come out and visit my laboratory for a day. I told them they could do the site visit upon my return. They agreed, and I set off for Maryland.

I barely remember the 1600-mile drive. I was numb.

The night before the memorial, the phone rang at my sister's house. My assistant called to say the FDA phoned from their headquarters in Washington, D.C. They were putting out a national press release stating the eye gel had a strain of bacteria that they said could be potentially harmful. There was nothing I could do. It was past 5 P.M. on a Friday night. It was then that my memorable conversation took place.

When I called my voice mail to get messages, I learned a woman had called with a question about another product. Out of habit, I returned her call. For some crazy reason, I told her what was going on. Amazingly, she told me, "Honey, don't worry, everything is going to be fine for you. You'll tell stories about this overwhelming craziness in your life someday. Just try to relax. You are going to get through this. Now, if it gets too tough, you call me back. I'll be here." I could not believe her kindness and support, and the best thing is that I believed her. I was almost relaxed for a moment—I knew she was right. I had to have faith in God, in myself, and in my fledgling company.

Following the memorial service, I arrived back home and prepared for the FDA's visit, finishing the paperwork on the recall of the eye gel for them. The day they were to arrive, I was watching out the window for them an hour early. While pacing, I talked to my dad: "Dad, please help me out here. You know how much I love this little company. Help me. I know you can do it. You can help me." I switched periodically between this and chanting "Om," trying either to convince my father to help me out or at least to be calm enough to deal effectively with the federal agents.

Two FDA agents spent about six hours in my lab. They took samples of every herb, every oil, everything. I was sweating the entire time. All I could think was one way or another, this nightmare was going to be over soon, and whatever happened, I could handle it, I could accept it. I had been through so much over the last couple of months. Keeping my Zen book close by provided me with my only sanity. It is *Everyday Zen* by Joko Beck, an American who really understands the way we get too caught up in our whirling thoughts, and reinforces the notion that everything is just life; therefore, we do not have to attach a good or bad label to the event. The most important thing is just to live each moment with awareness. This book and the support of my customers were immensely helpful through this difficult time.

The federal agents were quite nice, particularly the woman agent. She said it is the luck of the draw what agent you get and that some are much more pleasant than others. I had heard and read many horror stories about the FDA busting down doors, toting automatic weapons, seizing products, and shutting operations down. I have to say the agents I dealt with were professional and I really appreciated it. When they were finished, they got up to leave and said that everything looked in order.

Again, I learned I just had to have faith in God, in myself, and in my company.

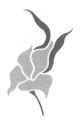

Introduction

This book is intended as an exploration of beauty, health, and happiness. It is for the American woman who is interested in, although maybe not yet completely committed to, learning new ways to acquire beauty, health, and happiness through herbs, essential oils, natural skin care, and other alternative methods. My intention is to help you look and feel better through the methods outlined here.

A gradual approach

This book and my method invite you to continue to live your life as you see fit, complete with your bad habits, while slowly bringing positive practices into your life. Probably 90% of American women do at least one of the following: eat red meat, don't exercise, but do smoke, drink alcohol, eat too much, drink coffee, and are overweight. I say that's okay, start where you are. You're perfect where you are now. Accept and love yourself complete with your flaws.

Intention: fun

This book and the practices outlined in it are intended to enhance your appearance, overall health, and therefore, your happiness. It is intended to be fun. I hope I will convince you to slowly bring into practice one or two of the recommendations I have tried, researched, and found helpful. Maybe you could start by wearing an essential oil instead of a synthetic perfume, or by bathing with lavender oil added to your bath one night a week. You could start by using a natural body care product instead of one full of harsh chemicals.

How about just eating one apple each day or adding one salad? Or start by drinking a cup of cleavers tea instead of black tea. Try substituting carrot juice for a soft drink occasionally or listing three things you're grateful for each day for a week. Maybe plan to meet a friend at the gym instead of for lunch, then treat yourself to a full body massage.

Try *one* thing

My point is just take one thing, try it, and see the results. If you feel better, make a commitment to it. You will receive two major benefits: First, you are going to look better, and second, feel better. As an added bonus, you are going to feel confident and good about the self-discipline you have brought into your life. This will create more health, which will create more beauty, which will create more confidence, which will create more happiness. To be happy you need not only to look good but to feel good and to feel confident about controlling your life. This consists of no more than controlling your habits—what you do everyday.

This book is about basic fundamental self-discipline. In other words, to have beauty, health, and happiness requires self-discipline. So begin today. Just bring one positive thing into your life. Try it for a while. Try it for one week. If it benefits you, make it a part of your daily routine—create a daily ritual. If it doesn't suit you or make you feel better or improve your life in some way, drop it and try another practice. Don't push yourself; don't beat yourself up. Just have fun trying new things and bringing positive additions into your life. If nothing else, this will make your life more interesting.

A natural method

The Lily Method asks you to just keep trying new things and committing to those that work for you. As you become more comfortable and confident, feel and look better, not only will you continue to bring positive things to your life, you will naturally lose the old bad habits. So for the time being, keep your old habits and don't worry about them. Instead, slowly start to bring positive things into your life. It's way too hard to be perfect anyway, plus it's not that much fun and nobody likes you for it. So try my method. Plan on being a little more beautiful, a little healthier, and a little happier.

Is this book for you?

This book is for people who want to be introduced to a lifestyle of beauty, health, and happiness. Benefiting from this book does not require that you change everything in your life, but rather that you be interested in a serene yet fundamental transformation to beauty, health, and happiness that many people are striving for in their lives. This book is an introduction to a way of life that is enjoyable, productive, and full of ideas you may want to employ in your life.

More and more people today are interested in making changes in themselves to live a better life. Perhaps you are among them. If so, welcome to this way of life.

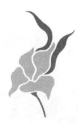

My Photo Album

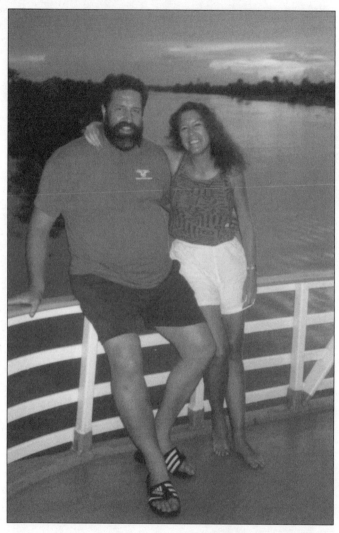

My brother John and me on the Amazon

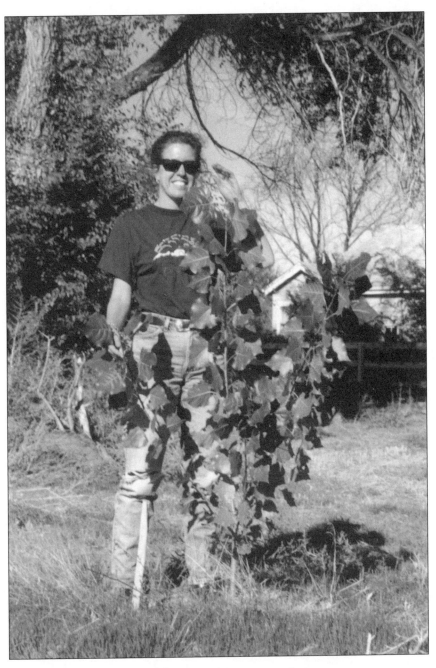

Cottonwood tree on my farm

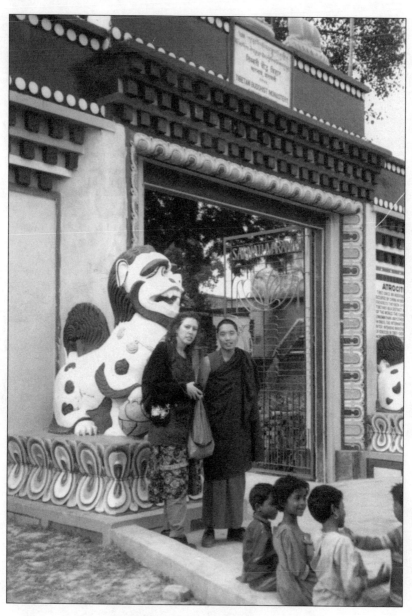

*Standing with a Buddhist monk outside a
Tibetan monastery in Sarnath, India.*

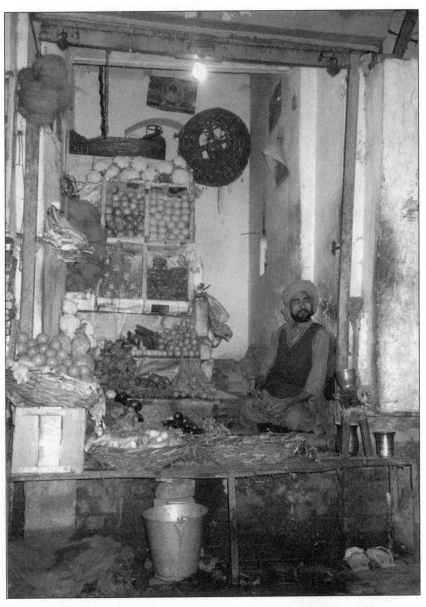

A vendor sits tranquilly among the dirt and noise of India

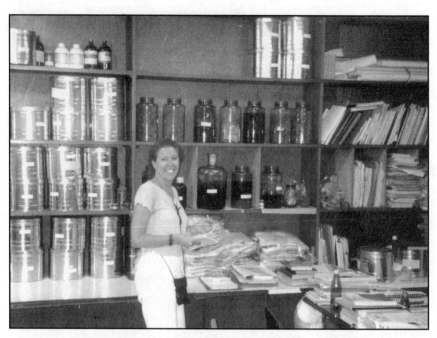

The Amazon Research Center in Manaus, Brazil

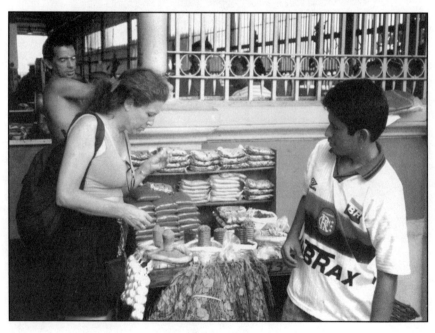

Buying herbs in Manaus, Brazil

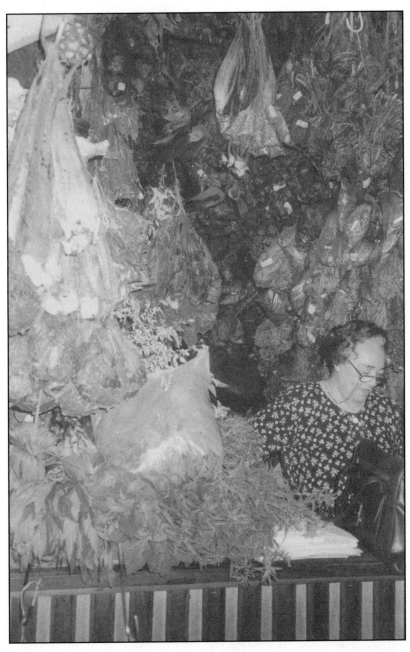

Woman selling herbs at the market in Manaus, Brazil

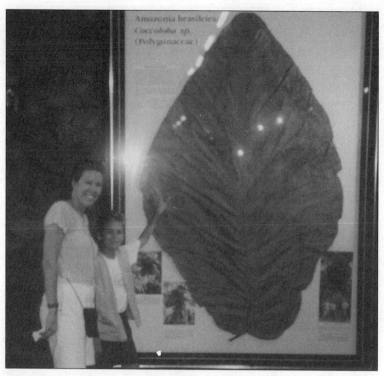

The largest leaf found on the planet, at the Amazon Research Center in Manaus, Brazil

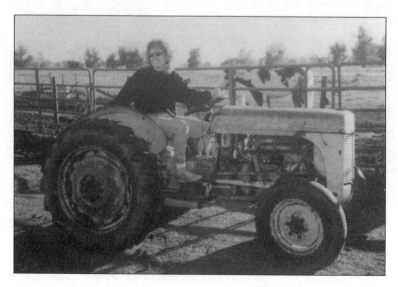

My tractor on my organic farm

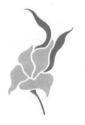

PART ONE

Introduction to Happiness

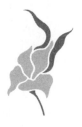

Happiness

We begin with happiness . . .

You were made for happiness.

—Dalai Lama

He made you that he might shower his gifts upon you.

—Sri Dada

*I am come that they might have life, and that they might have it
more abundantly.*

—John 10:10

Happiness, gift-receiving, abundant life, we are told (on good authority!), are our inheritance, our legacy, our very purpose. Thus it was in
the beginning. Thus it is today. Thus it was, too, at the time of the
founding of our nation.

Life, liberty, and the pursuit of happiness

"Life, liberty and the pursuit of happiness" is the highest American
ideal. It was so important to our founding fathers that they boldly pro-
claimed it in our Declaration of Independence. When Thomas Jefferson
came up with this thought, it was considered a radical idea. Life expectancy at that time was about thirty years. So to even have the time to
consider such a possibility was a blessing.

In America today, we seem to see the supreme ideal more as "life, liberty, and the *purchase* of happiness." We live in a culture that celebrates affluence. Many Americans really think that a bigger car or a more elaborate house will provide the fulfillment they seek.

Most people in Third World countries don't really contemplate or ponder the concept of happiness. But Americans even test themselves on the subject. According to one poll, average Americans rate themselves as seven on a happiness scale from one to ten, one being the least happy and ten being the most happy.

Only one thing will attract love, and that is love.

—Napoleon Hill

Loving yourself

First, to be happy it is important to love yourself. Love is a verb, so just like loving someone else has to be full of action so does loving yourself. The art of appreciating yourself involves action. Action includes participating in your own well-being, your own beauty, and your own health—doing what you know is good for you.

For instance, fueling yourself with the best foods, taking the needed time to get sunshine and exercise, telling yourself good things, knowing you are worth the struggle to keep a positive attitude no matter how dark things can look. We must develop the art of accepting ourselves. Doing things we know are good for ourselves. Physically applying beneficial ointments, creams, and lotions. Exercising. Taking long, warm, soothing baths. Going to hot springs. Putting a hot oil treatment in our hair. Brushing our hair. Walking around the block or the lake. Meditating. Doing yoga. Going to a steam room. Working out at a recreation center.

True self-love

The art of appreciating yourself should not lead to arrogance. Here's the best way I have heard it expressed. Nelson Mandela said this in his 1994 inaugural speech when he became president of South Africa:

Our deepest fear is not that we are inadequate. Our deepest fear is that we are powerful beyond measure. It is our light, not our darkness that most frightens us. We ask ourselves, who am I to be brilliant, gorgeous, talented, and fabulous? Actually, who are you not to be? You are a child of God.

Your playing small does not serve the world. There is nothing enlightened about shrinking so that other people won't feel insecure around you. We were born to make manifest the glory of God that is within us. It is not just in some of us: It is in everyone.

And as we let our own light shine, we unconsciously give other people permission to do the same. As we are liberated from our own fears, our presence automatically liberates others.

A good practice might be to read this quote each day as a constant reminder of who we really are, what we are really like, and what our basic calling in life is.

Affirmations versus negative self-talk

Most people, if not all of us to some degree, are caught in a web of negative self-talk. There is a way to combat this: affirmations. Affirmations are positive statements we can repeat to ourselves as many times as we find helpful. Initially, we need to listen to our self-talk to be aware of the negative mental conversation we are involved in. Affirmations give us the power to replace this negative self-talk with positive self-talk, resulting in greater happiness. You can make up your own positive affirmations, or take quotes, for example, from Nelson Mandela's speech.

Consider, discern, prioritize, choose

An effective method of figuring out what is important to us is prioritization. Stop and ask yourself what is important to me, my life; what do I want to accomplish before I die? A good way to find out what is working and what is not working in your life is journal writing. Every day, write down what is on your mind. A great book to help you with journaling is called *The Artist's Way* by Julia Cameron.

We need to take the time to ponder, to discern, to prioritize, and to choose. I know what you're thinking. That's easy for her to say, but I have a husband, three kids, and a full-time job. I understand. My advice? Choose your priorities. Are you working so you can afford a more expensive car and a larger house than you need? How much do you spend on clothes and furniture that don't bring you lasting joy? How much do you spend on fast foods that may not be healthful? What is really important to you? Take time to consider these questions, then align your life with your priorities and be happy with them.

Remember, you aren't locked in for life with these new decisions. You can change your priorities and actions if, after due consideration, other ideas work better for you.

Working as an essential of happiness

My own personal, nonscientific research among my eclectic collection of friends, which includes vegans, Buddhists, trendsetters, bikers, home-makers, college professors, incarcerated inmates, factory workers, and lawyers, has led me to conclude that happiness comes from the act of working toward whatever *you decide* is important in life. For example, herbalists working with herbs, farmers farming, healers healing, lawyers winning difficult but important cases. *You determine for you* what pursuit will bring you happiness. To be happy, *work* on that pursuit with all your energy, creativity, and insight.

In my opinion, work, your effort at accomplishing your goals, is a major foundation for happiness. Other aspects of life play a part, too. Take time to be playful! Try to learn something from every negative situation. Learn to take responsibility.

The hidden gift in responsibility: empowerment

Many people think responsibility is a burden and therefore to be avoided. Not so! Taking responsibility is taking control. If you blame others for your problems, then you are handing them your power. Furthermore, claiming responsibility means you have the power to make changes. Taking responsibility for yourself is empowering.

You could avoid the thinking, the discernment, and the choosing what is important in your life. Perhaps you're afraid of criticism. Napoleon states: "One way to avoid criticism is to do nothing and be a nobody. The world will then not bother you." True, but my bet is you won't find happiness that way.

Money

Money is only really valuable when you don't have any!

Once you get over the poverty line, the more money you have, the less importance it has in your life. It takes acquiring everything you need plus a couple of extra dollars in the bank to be convinced of this fact. Having just a little extra money leaves you more time to ponder and prioritize about what would make you happy—*if* you don't get caught in the squirrel cage of always "needing" more. People who think having money will make them happy often invest their whole lives in that goal, only to be disappointed in the end. They are often no happier than poor people.

Research studies suggest that some lottery winners are less happy a year after winning large sums of money than before they won. The same old emptiness returns, but bigger and more burdensome.

Further proof of the lack of correlation between money and happiness can be found in a study of many on the Forbes 400 list, which identifies the 400 richest people in America. The study showed that the superrich rate themselves less happy on the happiness scale than the average American.

Acquisition: a plus or minus?

Forget the current American ideal of happiness—more money, nicer cars, bigger houses, greater prestige, fancy vacations, flashy clothes, expensive furniture and appliances. Forget the American way of acquisition for acquisition's sake. You prioritize; you choose. What is it *you* want? Identify it. Focus, then move the rest out of the way. Figure you have 24 hours in each day. How do you want to invest them? Do what's important to you.

If you decide having a beautiful, big house will make you happy, then go for it. But don't buy someone else's dream if it doesn't suit you. Never mind what the proverbial Joneses are buying. You determine for yourself what will bring you happiness.

Less is more?

Even many financially successful people are finding that "less is more." They are opting for less. Having accumulated all the material goods that they were told they needed for happiness, they reached a point where they discovered material possessions didn't bring the anticipated joy.

What did they do? They chose simplicity. "Voluntary simplicity" is the name of the movement, and it's taken hold in Europe as well as the

United States. These people pondered and prioritized. Out went the extra cars. In came a smaller home. Out went the prestigious, all-consuming job. In came more time for family, volunteerism, and other activities they decided were important. These people invested the money from the sale of large homes, expensive cars, and other recently judged unimportant items and now live off the interest. They chose voluntary simplicity as their way to happiness.

Simplification

Simplification is both a process and a state of mind. The process of simplification is empowering because it cleanses you of a lot of excess baggage in your life. I highly recommend the book *Simplify Your Life* by Elaine St. James. It is a very small, uncomplicated book with many helpful ideas.

An initial part of the process is determining what is important in your life and what is not. It includes everything from your relationships to enjoying a sunset to freeing yourself from all those dishes and pots and pans you haven't used in years. We humans seem to hang onto stuff in our closets the same way we cling to our emotional stuff.

St. James's recommendations free you from the stuff you don't need in your life, the stuff you have been tripping over, and the stuff you haven't recognized as impediments in your life.

The search for sanity

How do we find the path to sanity? I feel there are several areas we must each explore to find sanity and happiness:

Control

There seems to be a direct correlation between how much control we have over our own lives and how happy we are. People in authoritarian countries seem to be much less happy than those in free countries. Employees who have some control over their time on the job are much happier. So personal control is an important aspect of feeling good. Running your own life as you see fit brings happiness. Being free to make good decisions for yourself and finding the value even in decisions that don't have positive outcomes can bring happiness.

Optimism

Optimism creates opportunities. Despair creates despondency. People who expect the best are happiest and are then better prepared to overcome obstacles. Defeat spurs optimists on. Optimism is a fundamental, rock-solid belief that everything is going to be okay.

Faith

The happiest people not only have faith that all things will work out, but a spiritual faith as well. People who say they are actively religious are happier. Faith not only gives people a sense of purpose, but often a clear code of ethics to live by, and something larger than themselves to believe in.

Activity

Much happiness is derived in life by testing our skills through meaningful activity. We enjoy getting into the rhythm of life. We like being caught up in the flow and losing ourselves in total involvement. People want to feel useful, that they are investing their time, talents, and energies in something worthwhile. Those who believe that happiness is a side effect of doing things rather than searching for happiness are right.

There is a rule in sailing that the more maneuverable ship should give way to the less maneuverable. I think this is sometimes a good rule to follow in human relations as well.
—Dr. Joyce Brothers

Relationships

Feeling connected to the people you love can bring great joy. Open yourself up so your own innate happiness can blossom. The Amish seem to be very happy. They attribute their happiness to having a clear purpose and working together to benefit the entire community. Extroverts are said to be happier, possibly because they may create relationships more easily.

Humor

Look for the humor in life. Humor lurks everywhere just waiting to be discovered, even in otherwise negative situations. Search for it. Lighten up! Smile! Laugh!

People who are happy experience a happy life. Others are drawn to them, which can add more happiness. They have more friends and loved ones. Importantly, they have a larger support system when things go wrong. It is said that happy people have at least four people they could call on a down day. However, they experience less down time.

Some people seek happiness through diversions like drugs, alcohol, shopping, fame, applause, or food. But these are temporary, at best. At worst, they can be negative, even destructive.

Wisdom from Tibet: the Dalai Lama

The Dalai Lama told me: "The purpose of our life is happiness . . . you need self-confidence, determination, a warm heart, and to overcome your suffering."

The Dalai Lama spoke at Denver's McNichols Sports Arena to me and thousands of other people, but his words were so meaningful I felt he was talking specifically to me. As a result, I have made a decision to listen to this brilliant, simple, humble man who has dedicated his entire life to spreading his message around the planet.

With fervor, I told someone that the purpose of our life is happiness. The person responded deprecatingly that this is like someone saying, "Check the oil in your car." I said, "Yes! Exactly! Brilliant in its simplicity!" Yes, checking the oil in your car is brilliant advice, too. Take five minutes to save yourself a potentially tremendous amount of damage. It really is the same thing, in automobiles and in life—damage control.

I truly believe the Dalai Lama said everything we need to know about happiness in his statement, "The purpose of your life is happiness." Let's take it under study. "*The purpose of your life is happiness.*" First of all, no one at any time in my life, in any religion, in any book I have ever read, had told me that happiness is the reason God put me on Earth. Nobody had ever given me an adequate explanation as to why I was put on this planet.

When the Dalai Lama said this, I thought, "Wow! How great! I knew God had a plan for me, but I never thought it was this cool, this good." Not only had no one ever given me an adequate explanation, but I also really liked this one. It suited me, my life, where I was at that time, and my disposition.

Being happy

So the purpose of your life is happiness. What does that mean? I think it means *be happy*, be appreciative, be kind, be nice, be lovable, be loved, be grateful to God for all of the wonderful gifts he has provided you. Thank your Creator for the sight to see nature in the trees and flowers, the mobility to move, walk, run, in-line skate, swim, ski, and enjoy all the activities that bring you happiness, even work. Being happy means appreciating the people you love. Indulge yourself in the awareness of the happiness they provide you, the way you smile when they walk in a room or call you on the phone. Open yourself up to all the love and beauty of the world. Be open to all, their ideas, their lifestyles. You might just learn one of life's most valuable lessons. As my sister says, "Everybody is our teacher."

Being appreciative for all you already have is one of the keys to happiness. Appreciate your loved ones, nature, *huevos rancheros*, your morning coffee or tea, your home, the sunshine, the flora, your continued presence on Earth, your intelligence, your beauty, your health, your humor, and all the people around you.

This means taking a daily inventory of all the gifts that God has given us. We cannot do this enough. This means constantly looking for the good in *all* situations, even in death.

Insights into death

When my dad died and we did not know whether my mom would make it, I fortunately had a tremendous amount of work to keep me busy. I had to fly to where she was, meet my brothers and sister, answer constant phone calls from concerned friends, relatives, and neighbors regarding my parents, deal with insurance companies, lawyers, and accountants, visit my mom in the hospital, and more. I say "fortunately" because activity is the enemy of depression. Even though all these negative events had occurred, I was busy trying to make them all better. To me, trying to better a situation is another key to happiness.

Events will occur that we do not like. The key is to do what we can to limit the damage and enhance the outcome. For example, my dad was dead, but he would want us to handle his affairs carefully. We tried our best to follow his wishes. We still could control that, and we did so to the best of our ability. My dad wanted us to take good care of my mother and we did. So controlling what we could and making things the best possible lessened our pain.

Even in death there are benefits if we search for them. I can appreciate the fact that I had a great dad for 35 years. And I learned that losing one family member gives you the opportunity to start appreciating the remaining ones more.

A surprising benefit

At first, I didn't believe that the dead can help us from the other side, but now I am convinced. I feel our dead loved ones can help us live better lives if we ask them. I think they are always with us, like many tribal people believe. We don't need to feel their physical presence to know they are near us in spirit.

Ways to find happiness

There are as many ways to find happiness in life as there are people on Earth. And it is a wonderful journey. As a friend of mine said, "It's not the destination; it's the road trip." There is so much wonder in the world, and it's our job to find it and appreciate it. Happiness takes thought and effort, but achieving it is a beautiful thing.

The last words uttered by Buddha were: "Be a lamp unto yourself." This means to make yourself happy; it is your responsibility, your job, your purpose. You must provide the light for your own life.

Openness

In a book by Pema Chodron entitled *The Wisdom of No Escape,* Trungpa Rinpoche makes the statement: "The everyday practice is simply to develop a complete acceptance and openness to all situations and emotions and all people. Experiencing everything totally without reservations or blockages, so that one never withdraws or centralizes into oneself." Pema says in the same book, "Working with obstacles is life's journey." [*]

About heaven and hell

In the same book there is a story about heaven and hell, life and death, good and bad. It's a story about how those things don't really exist except as a creation of our own minds. It goes like this:

A big burly samurai comes to the wise man and says, "Tell me the nature of heaven and hell." The roshi looks him in the face and says: "Why should I tell a scruffy, disgusting, miserable slob like you?" The

---

[*] Pema Chodron, *The Wisdon of No Escape and the Path of Loving Kindness,* Boston, MA: Shambhala Publications, Inc., 1991.

samurai starts to get purple in the face, his hair starts to stand up, but the roshi won't stop. He keeps saying, "A miserable worm like you, do you think I should tell you anything?" Consumed by rage, the samurai draws his sword, and he's just about to cut off the head of the roshi. Then the roshi says, "That's hell." The samurai, who is in fact a sensitive person, instantly gets it, that he just created his own hell; he was deep in hell. It was black and hot, filled with hatred, self-protection, anger, and resentment, so much so that he was going to kill this man. Tears fill his eyes and the samurai starts to cry and he puts his palms together and the roshi says, "That's heaven. There isn't any hell or heaven except for how we relate to our world. Hell is just resistance to life."

Me-first attitude: selfish?

Some people may criticize you for putting your own happiness first, but they don't get the concept and, frankly, that is their problem, not yours. In case of an emergency in an airplane, we're told to put our own oxygen mask on first before helping another put his or hers on; it is the same concept. If you help yourself, you are in a position to help others. You can't pour milk from an empty pitcher. If you're not happy, you cannot help others achieve happiness. If you haven't achieved things that are important to you, you cannot teach others how to achieve things that are important to them. If you don't have any money, you can't help a friend pay his rent. If you haven't taken the time to learn compassion, handle frustration, and interpret your own emotions, how are you going to understand and relate well with others?

Taking responsibility is taking control. For example, if you discern you are responsible for your last relationship not working out, then you can improve the next one and make it work. Taking responsibility is empowering.

Increasing the amount of happiness

My mother says that if you are truly involved in being happy for other people when good things happen to them, then you can be happy a lot more of the time. I like that. And if you have taken the time to like, love, and take care of yourself, and good things happen to you, and you are happy with yourself, you are going to be in a better place and more able to be genuinely happy for others. But if you never did the inventories of what you appreciate in your life and haven't done the planning to achieve what you think is important in your life, you are much more likely to end up regretful, resentful, bitter, and jealous.

We're still on the sentence, "Your purpose in life is happiness." If it is your purpose, then it's very important. If it is your purpose, you better put a lot of time and energy into it. If it is your purpose, it's everything. So the Dalai Lama is saying, "For God's sake, go make yourself happy, first." First and foremost in your life, make yourself happy. Do what is going to bring you happiness and do it now. Take the time to develop a plan. Meditate. Make happiness happen. Do what is going to bring you great joy.

If you really want to do something, you'll find a way; if you don't, you'll find an excuse.

—Anonymous

Avoid confusion

You have to be careful not to confuse the above with the things that could ultimately bring you great sadness. For example, using drugs may bring you momentary gratification, but in the long run they may bring you great pain. On the other hand, you may not want to go visit a sick friend today, but you know that in the long run you will feel better about yourself if you do.

Feeling good about yourself is the road to happiness; doing things that make you feel better about yourself is a key to happiness. Exercising discipline produces long-term happiness.

Happiness: your life purpose

The greatest thing about the statement, "Your purpose in life is happiness," is that it lets you feel good about spending the time, energy, and resources to produce this happiness. It's okay to focus on yourself and make yourself happy. As a matter of fact, it is your responsibility, your purpose in life, why you are here.

Why would a man as altruistic and giving and selfless as the Dalai Lama make what could be construed as such a selfish and self-centered statement? Because unhappy people are a very negative force on the planet. They produce negative vibrations and events. It's that simple. Unhappy people are mean, ill-mannered, angry, and fill themselves and the world we live in with violence, ugliness, and destruction.

Perpetuating happiness

Happy people emanate and perpetuate the same happiness they feel. They produce positive energy that stays around long after their physical presence is gone. For example, how elevated do you feel when a friend notices you have lost ten pounds, genuinely comments how much better you look, and recognizes what it took for you to accomplish this? When she voices appreciation of you by saying positive things, it uplifts your spirits. Both of you are then positive forces on the planet.

When your confiding in a friend about your plan to write a book is met with kind words of encouragement, it fills you with the energy you need to help fuel the project. Later that day, you are driving your car down the highway still filled with that energy. You are thinking, "Yeah, she's right. I do have the skills, talent, brains, ability, and something important to share with the world. I'm going to write that book." Her good influence lingers long after she's gone.

Maybe weeks or months later when you have jumped into the project and are going through your first big obstacle, her words ring back to you: "You have something important to share with the world. You will do well." This gives you more positive energy to complete the project.

The Dalai Lama said you need self-confidence, determination, and a warm heart. You need self-confidence to achieve happiness, which is doing what you think is important in life. You need determination to produce self-confidence; nothing happens without effort. It takes determination to make the things happen that are going to produce your self-confidence. A warm heart is what makes you like yourself and causes others to like you and you to like them.

Note

I want everyone who reads this book to understand that I am not a perfect model of what I preach in these chapters. These principles are still very much a part of what I desire to become. What I have learned intellectually may not have spilled over into my daily life the way I have hoped. But I think it is important to know, as Joko Beck states: "Where you are now is perfect."

Where you are now is perfect for you now! Overall love and acceptance of yourself is the first step. Where you are now is where you are and it is perfect. As I've said before, there is no need to beat yourself up for anything you do now or have ever done. The beauty of not beating yourself up is that not only do you give yourself a break, but you start giving others a break, too. As you forgive yourself for not being perfect, you also forgive others.

If you think changes are necessary in your life to make yourself happy, here are some ideas to brighten up the challenges and revitalize your life:

* Learn new things: learn Spanish, take up painting or gardening.

* Create a project: make a quilt, write a poem or a novel.

* Do fun things: go to the art museum or the theatre.

* Do self-exploration; meditate, do yoga, get your astrological chart done, get your handwriting analyzed, plan a trip alone, write a journal, explore who you are, go to a Zen center or church.

* Volunteer your time: work with troubled kids.

* Hang out with a different crowd: join a club.

* Practice diversity, not only culturally, but also in how you spend your time: if you work in an office, try to get outside on the weekends.

Bringing balance into our lives can add to our happiness

The Chinese claim they have been using herbal medicine for 10,000 years. They believe great health means balancing the five humors: fire, metal, earth, water, and wood. Historically, many cultures looked at disease as "dis-ease" in the body, that is, an imbalance, a basic problem with a lack of equilibrium in one's life. We must try to ensure balance in the following areas:

* *Love.* We need to try to keep our relationships positive and worthwhile. Love must be given and received. Anger must be acknowledged and dealt with in a positive way.

* *Environment.* We need to help keep our environment clean, in our homes, our offices, our towns, our countries, and our planet.

* *Hormone balance.* Having your hormones in balance is imperative to good health, happiness, and a sense of well-being.

* *Nourishment.* Your body must have high-quality fuel to operate most effectively.

✳ *Spiritual life.* To enjoy true happiness, it is important to have a belief that there are forces operating that we may not see, that there is operating in the universe something bigger and better than we are. One has to have a code of ethics and a way to deal with unpleasant things like death in a positive way, to have mechanisms and a support system in place to rely on in the darkest days.

If you are feeling down, try using these essential oils: ylang ylang, jasmine, clove, neroli, orange, or cinnamon. Try St. John's wort. This ancient traditional herb has been rediscovered and found valuable even by modern medicine.

—⊰•⊱—

Desiderata

Go placidly amid the noise and haste, and remember what peace there may be in silence. As far as possible without surrender be on good terms with all persons. Speak your truth quietly and clearly; and listen to others, even the dull and ignorant; they too have their story. Avoid loud and aggressive persons, they are vexations to the spirit. If you compare yourself with others, you may become vain and bitter; for always there will be greater and lesser persons than yourself. Enjoy your achievements as well as your plans. Keep interested in your own career, however humble; it is a real possession in the changing fortunes of time. Exercise caution in your business affairs; for the world is full of trickery. But let this not blind you to what virtue there is; many persons strive for high ideals; and everywhere life is full of heroism. Be yourself. Especially, do not feign affection. Neither be cynical about love; for in the face of all aridity and disenchantment it is perennial as the grass. Take kindly the counsel of the years, gracefully surrendering the things of youth. Nurture strength of spirit to shield you in sudden misfortune. But do not distress yourself with imaginings. Many fears are born of fatigue and loneliness. Beyond a wholesome discipline, be gentle with yourself. You are a child of the universe, no less than the trees and the stars; you have a right to be here. And whether or not it is clear to you, no doubt the universe is unfolding as it should. Therefore be at peace with God, whatever you conceive Him to be, and whatever your labors and aspirations, in the noisy confusion of life keep peace with your soul. With all its sham, drudgery and broken dreams, it is still a beautiful world. Be careful. Strive to be happy.

—————

Remember: your visit on this planet is temporary, so whatever it is you want to be doing in life, you better be doing it.

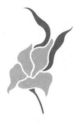

Discover a New Way of Life

A new lifestyle

Embarking on the rejuvenation therapy trail is exciting. There is so much to try, to experience and to learn about from chiropractic, massage, colonic hydrotherapy, psychological therapy—so many treatments, theories, ways of life to delve into and try out—Zen centers, yoga, meditation.

Rejuvenating yourself through an improved way of life is delving into yourself and your relationship to the rest of the universe; it's honoring the body God gave you, the planet you live on, and your rightful space in it all.

A healthy commitment to self

It's a commitment to taking better care of ourselves. It's really a lifestyle—like bikers, yuppies, or jocks have—except we hang out at health food store juice bars, shop for wheat- and dairy-free products, read the magazines and browse the books, talk to the well-informed staff, buy the latest herb we have investigated along with our organic fruit. It's our way of life. We want to talk to people who are demonstrating a new product in the store; we're interested in the newest supplements or skin-care lines. We are always open to new ideas and new products and new ways of doing things.

Compare

We think life on earth can be a positive continuous learning experience. This lifestyle is a statement against the bourgeois, mediocre, mundane, middle-class, suburban, frazzled, work nine-to-five, fifty weeks out of the year for two weeks vacation, typical sedentary American lifestyle.

We don't need big cars and houses. We need time each day to walk, do our yoga, meditate, prepare whole foods, have our tarot cards read, ride our bikes, visit the people we love, see our many alternative health care professionals, and time to just simply be.

Best models of this new way of life

These are life choices, most exemplified by health food store employees. They are the ones on the front lines and the ones that epitomize these life choices through their chosen lifestyles. These are many of the people I have learned from. As a group, they are highly educated, not only formally at the universities, but self-educated, astonishingly well-read, well-traveled, and open-minded. Their lifestyles truly represent this emerging yet unnamed, inspirational lifestyle.

They in-line skate, walk, dance, or run, drink tons of green drinks and purified water, own their own juicers, but go to the health food store to get their shots of wheat grass. They hang out together at smoke-free parties and events.

Characteristics of this new way of life

Many of us who practice this new lifestyle don't buy anything from China or other countries that oppress their people. We recycle. We get the mercury taken out of our teeth. We seek psychics and have our astrological charts done. We're into taking control of ourselves and exerting our power over our bodies and minds in a big way. We're positive and active. We try to be sensitive to others without a lot of judgment. We're open and accepting of alternative lifestyles of all kinds.

I think this way of life makes life more interesting and is one of the things that attracted me to it; feeling good and learning new ways to deal with old problems is what kept me in it. Read on to discover descriptions of and my personal experiences in several rejuvenation therapies and alternative health modalities.

Using the body's own wisdom

All the modalities of healing I discuss in this book are based on the belief that the body is already comprised of the inherent wisdom to heal itself. Your skin, your cells, and your organs are each capable of healing themselves, regenerating and even reproducing.

Acupuncture

Ancient healing art

Acupuncture has been a healing method for over 2000 years and is based on the Taoist philosophy of natural balance, harmony, growth, and change. It recognizes that the body has the capacity to heal itself.

According to the book by Peter Firebrace and Sandra Hill, *Acupuncture: How It Works, How It Cures:* "Acupuncture is a system of medicine which seeks to aid these natural processes, helping the body to correct itself by a realignment or redirection of energy, which the Chinese call *Qi* [pronounced 'chee'].*" Qi is essentially your vital energy or vital force.

My experience in Belize

I first experienced acupuncture in Central America in Placencia, Belize. I was vacationing there with my family over the year-end holidays.

A quiet sandy spot by the sea, Placencia is a wonderful place just to hang out. It is a very small village that only recently acquired electricity, and its first and only road was built in the last ten years. There are no fences and no concept of private property. The whole village is community property. Only with the influx of Americans moving in has the matter of private property ever been discussed. Everyone helps watch everyone else's kids, and no one ever has any occasion to wear shoes.

The people are, for the most part, of African descent rather than Spanish. They have beautiful English accents and are some of the kindest and most open people I have ever met in my life. They are warm, friendly, and always smiling. My family and I felt like we made many friends while we were there.

One morning after we had been there a few days, during my morning walk around the village, I saw a small cabana painted blue with a sign that read "acupuncture." I inquired within and met the acupuncturist, an

---

* Peter Firebrace and Sandra Hill, *Acupuncture: How it Works, How it Cures,* New Canaan, CT: Keats Publishing, Inc., 1994, p. 9.

American who had moved to Belize in the early 1960s during the Vietnam War. He had been living in Central America for over 35 years.

I told him I had had a lot of stress and my neck and shoulders still felt the strain, even though I was now on vacation and relaxed. He stated that the body often continues to hold stress long after your mind lets it go. My Denver chiropractor and massage therapist had told me the same thing, so I agreed. We had tea and a nice chat. He couldn't work on me that day, he said, because he had other patients coming in, and he couldn't work on me tomorrow because the village was having a dance that night and he would probably not be feeling too great the following day. I agreed we would wait until the day after next.

I returned as planned and found him up and spry. He asked questions concerning my medical history and had me lie down on the table. We chatted while he inserted the affected area with very small needles. The needles were so fine I couldn't even feel them go in, so they did not hurt in the least. He removed them after about fifteen minutes and then he had me sit in a chair. He rubbed some vegetable oil on my neck that he said also had orchid oil in it. Next, he used a Japanese soupspoon to scrape the oil off. He warned me that this would be slightly painful, but the treatment would be very effective in releasing tension and getting energy to flow back into my neck. It did hurt, but it was worth it.

Leaving his place, walking down the dirt road back to my little hotel, I realized it was the first time in months I had felt pain-free. There was no pain at all in my neck, a condition I had only experienced a few times in the last several years.

Provides relief for varied conditions

Acupuncture can benefit many ailments, including acne, cramps, and many other complaints. I have had great results for PMS and back pain from my Denver acupuncturist. If you need hormonal and energy balancing, I highly recommend acupuncture. These problems are also treated with specific herbal-blend teas.

Books

There are many good books on acupuncture available at your local health food store. Your library may carry some. I recommend the one I mentioned above, *Acupuncture: How It Works, How It Cures* by Peter Firebrace and Sandra Hill.

Locating an acupuncturist

To find an acupuncturist, ask a friend or ask at your local health food store. If you're lucky enough to live in Colorado, there are many people that work at Alfalfa's or Wild Oats who are acupuncture practitioners.

Try contacting the National Commission for the Certification of Acupuncturists, 1424 16 St. NW, Suite 501, Washington, DC 20036 and/or the American Association of Acupuncture and Oriental Medicine, 4101 Lake Boone Trail, Suite 201, Raleigh, NC 27607.

Baths

Baths' long history

Water has been used as a therapy as far back as the ancient Egyptians. Native Americans used hot springs in the treatment of disease. Water can be used beneficially in baths, steam baths, mists, footbaths, enemas, douches, and compresses. Hippocrates, the Greek physician, knew water was a type of hydrotherapy, or water cure. Historically, since man's earliest times, baths have been used as both a means of relaxation and to induce a state of healthfulness.

The Bible refers to bathing in Leviticus 16 and 17, and Numbers 19. A 3000-year-old built-in bathtub and drainage system lies in the ruins of King Nestor's palace near Pylos, Greece. The Romans had warm public baths in which they used natural mineral springs. Two famous ones were near Naples and Thermopolis. Bath, England, is still famous for its ancient baths. Native Americans congregated at the warm springs in Bath, West Virginia, now called Berkeley Springs, as did our founding fathers.

Varied purposes for baths

Baths have been used to cleanse the body, relax the mind, remove evil spirits, improve attitudes, create awareness, celebrate life, attract love, relax, produce invigoration, and aid in meditation. The infirm in hospitals and nursing homes are placed in protective seats and lowered by pulleys into warm, jetted tubs. Taking a bath can be a very pleasant, relaxing, almost ritualistic experience.

Varied temperatures

I remember on sweltering hot summer days, we would get up very early to work in our apple orchard. We had no pool or pond or creek. In the heat of the afternoon, we would climb a tall ladder to bathe in a raised

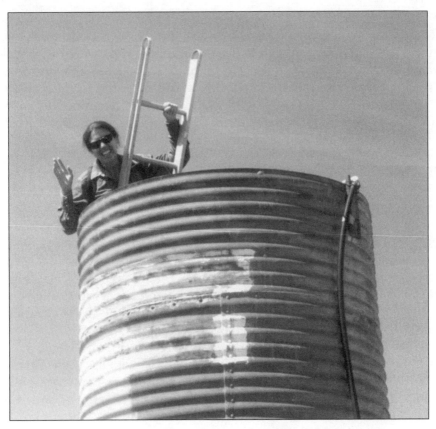

The "pork 'n beans" can on my dad's farm in Howard City, Michigan

water tank that resembled a giant "pork 'n beans" can on stilts. The water was cold and invigorating, and conducive to getting us back to work for the rest of the day and evening.

Increasing the benefits

There are many products, herbs, and essential oils you can put in your bath to heighten the experience and to make your skin soft and moisturized.

You can buy prepared bath products or you can easily make your own using an infusion, or tea, of chamomile, calendula, arnica, lily, and rose. Put any combination of these herbs in your bath. You can also put them in almond or safflower oil first and let the herbal properties impart to the oil, then put the oil in your bath. Putting essential oils in almond oil and then adding it to your bath is also a wonderful experience and a remedy for dry skin.

Persons who perspire freely and have oily skin should bathe more frequently. People with sensitive skin can bathe less often. In the winter, itching may develop with too much bathing unless creams, oils, or moisturizers are used.

Different kinds of baths

* *Milk bath.* Use one cup powdered milk with ten drops of lavender oil. Sprinkle milk into tub.

* *Vinegar bath.* For dry or itchy skin, add one-half cup organic apple cider vinegar to bath.

* *Honey bath.* Add one-fourth cup honey to bath to relieve tiredness or as sleep aid.

* *Epsom salts bath.* To reduce inflammation and chemical pollutants, draw a deep bath, add four cups of Epsom salts, and soak for at least twenty minutes.

Herbs in your bath

Today's pace of life—the pressures, the increasing tempo, the constant demands—absolutely requires us to build in small blocks of time to renew, relax, and recharge. One easy, fun, and great way to do this is to take two hours a week for yourself for a long, comforting, wonderful bath. Many herbs can have a powerful effect on the mind, some by encouraging calmness, others by stimulation.

Start by planning the time, then turn down the lights, lock the bathroom door, light a candle, and sink into a warm or hot herbal bath. Rest your head and neck on a folded towel. Let your arms float.

Easy methods

One of the easiest ways to prepare an herbal bath is to put dried herbs into a small cheesecloth or nylon-net bag, or an old nylon stocking, and hang them from the spout while running the water. When you have filled the tub, let the bag steep for awhile before removing it. Be sure to squeeze it often to release the essences of the herbs.

A second school of thought on herbal baths is to simply bring the herbs to a boil in a nonmetal pot on the stove. Let them steep for five minutes, then strain the herbs out, pouring the liquid into the bath. I do not recommend putting the herbs directly and loosely into the bath because of the mess they cause all over you and the tub!

You can also place tea bags in your bath. For example, chamomile is soothing both to mind and spirit and helps reduce aches and pains. The benefits of the herbs' essences are absorbed through the pores.

Alleviate pain

Another way to alleviate aches and pains, add a cupful of equal parts of the following herbs: agrimony, comfrey, St. John's wort, mugwort, sage, plus one tablespoon of Epsom salts to your bath water. Or take a mixture of the herbs and bring them to a light boil in a nonmetal pot for fifteen minutes. Or you can put the herbs in a small muslin bag to run under the hot water as it comes out of the faucet.

Hot baths are used to relax, warm baths to enjoy, and cold baths to stimulate. You can choose the temperature of the water, the herbs, the essential oils, the time of day, the use of candles and incense, and the thoughts in your mind—you can alter the experience.

Relieve tension

To relieve tension, try using valerian, sweet flag, lavender, and hops. For general beautifying, try lavender, rosemary, comfrey, and mint. For stiff joints and muscles, try sage, strawberry leaves, mugwort, chamomile, and comfrey. For overall toning, try lavender, parsley, comfrey, blackberry, and nettle. To aid in circulation, try calendula, bladderwrack, ginger, and nettle. And *think virtuous thoughts.*

Ritual baths were practiced in Africa and elsewhere for healing, love, success, spiritual cleansing, and any other important event in life. A love bath, for example, contained rose, cloves, cinnamon, and honey.

Relaxing herbs and oils for baths

- Elder flowers
- Lavender
- Rose
- Valerian root
- Epsom salts
- Sandalwood essential oil
- Ylang ylang essential oil
- Rose, orange blossom, geranium

General detox herbs and oils for baths

- Geranium
- Rosemary
- Juniper
- Lavender
(three drops of each to bath and soak for 30 minutes)

Invigorating ingredients for baths

- Lemon verbena
- Fennel
- Lemon peel
- Juniper
- Yarrow
- Pine
- Mustard
- Peppermint
- Nettles
- Rosemary

Skin-soothing ingredients for baths

- Chamomile
- Lily
- Calendula
- Comfrey
- Oatmeal
- Seaweeds
- Aloe vera

Tension-relieving ingredients for baths

- Valerian
- Sweet flag
- Hops

Beautifying ingredients for baths

- Lily
- Lavender
- Rosemary
- Comfrey
- Mint

Ingredients to relieve stiff joints and muscles in baths

- Sage
- Strawberry leaves
- Mugwort
- Chamomile
- Comfrey

Ingredients to increase circulation in baths

- Calendula
- Nettle
- Bladderwrack
- Ginger

Toning ingredients for baths

- Comfrey
- Parsley
- Lavender
- Nettle

Essential oils in your bath

I have always enjoyed the art of bathing. I like to feel my body immersed in water. Water is such a wonderful element. Aromatic baths can influence us in many ways through the fragrance, thus pleasing our spirit, improving us psychologically as well physiologically. Bathing cannot only drench our skin in wonderful essences and soothe the body, but also the mind. It is wonderfully therapeutic.

There are two ways to use essential oils in your bath. One is to just add a couple drops of oil in a drawn bath. Do not put the oil in sooner because the oil can dissipate while the hot water is filling the tub. Another way of using an essential oil in your bath is to mix it with a fixed oil such as almond or sunflower. Put three or four drops of the essential oil per tablespoon of fixed oil, and then put the mixture into a full tub of water.

* *Lavender.* If you have ever used any of my products, you know this is one of my favorite essential oils. It has a classic scent. In a hot bath, lavender is very relaxing and helps induce sleep, but in a cool bath, lavender can be a stimulant.

* *Ylang Ylang.* This is my favorite, and smells just wonderful. It is an anti-depressant, an aphrodisiac, and has been used as a sedative.

* *Chamomile.* Like the tea, this oil is used to calm nerves and reduce tension.

* *Rose oil.* Valued for its ability to reduce tension in women, this oil is particularly for post-natal depression and the stress that follows a broken heart.

* *Bergamot.* This oil is reputedly good for depression and helping the body fight infection.

* *Frankincense.* With its warming and soothing effect on the mind and emotions, some traditions used this to ward off evil spirits that we create (our fears, obsessions, and anxieties). It is useful to induce a meditative state, plus it is an astringent and an anti-inflammatory.

* *Neroli.* Used to reduce tension and encourage sleep, This oil calms the mind and is especially useful for those who are prone to upset themselves unnecessarily. It is said to work on a cellular level, stimulating the elimination of old cells and promoting the growth of new ones.

* *Melissa.* This oil comes from the lemon balm plant. Its soothing properties are used as an antidepressant and to remove negative thoughts.

* *Jasmine.* For promotion of emotional well-being. It is both a sedative and uplifting. It also helps to produce confidence and optimism.

* *Peppermint.* Cooling, invigorating, and refreshing, this oil is great for a summer bath.

* *Rosemary.* Useful for muscular pain and its astringent and antiseptic properties, this oil is stimulating and clean smelling.

Precautions

It's possible to overdo a good thing. Be aware of heat hydration. I'm presuming your tub has adequate handrails. Keep a bottle or cup of cool water within reach to sip or to splash yourself.

If, by chance, you feel lightheaded during one of your hot soaks, open the drain and let the hot water flow out, so your body gradually gets exposed to the cooler air. *Do not try to get up.* Sip some of your nearby cool water. Splash yourself with it. Stay put until you truly feel able to get up. If lightheadedness strikes you after you're out of the tub, find a place to sit. Lower your head until you feel okay.

I've never had this happen to me, but as I've stressed repeatedly in this book, everybody is different. In fact, even the same body can react differently at different times and under various conditions. I add these remarks so that like a good Girl Scout, you can always "be prepared."

You decide what's good for your body. You make the decisions, and then take responsibility for those decisions. Thus you become more self-determining, more self-reliant, and more and more self-actualized. And there's beauty, health, and happiness in that, too!

Natural springs

Natural springs involve the use of special waters. They may be hot, cold, carbonated, bubbly, sulfured, and/or gently flowing. We are blessed in Colorado to have a great abundance of natural hot springs. I have made it one of my personal goals to visit each and every one of them. I have not succeeded yet, but I have been to many. There is a great book out by Rick Cahill, *Hot Springs Guide of Colorado*. The issue I have is old, but it is still a great reference.

One of my commercial favorites is Hot Sulphur Springs, which was recently voted the worst hot springs in Colorado! However, it has inside caves with flowing water at all temperatures, an outside swimming pool, and outside hot springs. It is never crowded. To get there, you traverse Berthoud Pass. Hot Sulphur Springs is also the name of the adjacent unspoiled Colorado mountain town, and it is only eleven miles to Granby and Grand Lake, one of my favorite recreational areas.

Idaho Springs is the closest hot springs to Denver, with easy access from the metro Denver area. It offers massages between soaks and a darkened room where you can lie down and nap for complete relaxation. Idaho Springs has women's caves and men's caves, so the main caves are same-sex only and you must bathe nude. They also have private caves for couples and a mud bath is available.

Glenwood Springs is a very nice town right off I-70, convenient if you are traveling through and do not have much time. It's even better if you can linger.

If you ever get so wound up that you cannot relax, hot springs are for you. You cannot spend a few hours at a hot springs without relaxing; it is physically impossible. You *will be* relaxed. I think hot springs are definitely curative measures and they have a reputation of being very helpful in the treatment of rheumatic disorders, chronic fatigue, and skin, muscular, and nervous disorders.

———

Life is like stepping onto a boat which is about to sail out to sea and sink.

—Suzuki Roshi

———

Buddhism: Lust for Enlightenment

For just about as long as I can remember, my sister was a vegetarian, had a guru, and had a serious interest in all aspects of spirituality. I, however, did not. My brother John and I used to jokingly call her a "hin-bu," halfway between a Hindu and a Buddhist. Her interests in the esoteric and her vegetarianism always provided John and me with a little entertainment, except, however, when it inconvenienced me by making me eat in some off-beat vegetarian restaurant with only bean sprouts and beet juice, or making me stay too long in some spiritual bookstore. Sometimes I'd get so bored I would actually start reading some of the books.

In the early 1980s, we were in a bookstore in Ann Arbor, Michigan. Ann Arbor, Michigan, is the "hippest" place I have ever been to in the Midwest. The University of Michigan is there, and so is about every kind of ethnic food, cool coffee shop, and New Age bookstore. Ann Arbor reminds me of Boulder when I lived there in the mid-seventies.

Anyway, I was moseying around this bookstore, and I almost found some of the books interesting. We had been there for a couple of hours and browsing kept my attention. The store had a stack of Jack Kerouac's books, and I think I even picked up another copy of *On the Road*, since I hadn't seen my original copy in fifteen years. My sister, as usual, was engrossed in a particular book. "Hey, Lily," she called, holding up the book, "you may be interested in this one."

This was funny because she knew I wasn't interested in the kind of books she read, and she never tried to push her spiritual thing on me, so I was intrigued just because it was the first time she had ever said that to me.

Buddhism and sex

"What do you have there?" I asked. "Check it out," she replied. I took *Lust for Enlightenment: Buddhism and Sex* by John Stevens and thought, "Hmmmm, sounds pretty interesting. Maybe I'll figure out just what is this attraction my sister has to all this spiritual stuff." I started reading it and that was the first time my sister ever had to drag *me* out of a spiritual bookstore. I really didn't want to spend the money to buy the book, but I couldn't put it down. My sister and my mom, who was with us, wanted to eat, so I bought the book.

I began to read it back in Colorado and learned how sexually tolerant and non-repressive the people were in old Tibet, where sex and Buddhism are closely interrelated. It covered Buddha's promiscuous life as a prince before becoming enlightened and pointed out how if we put the energy into spirituality that we put into finding and securing romantic love, we would all be enlightened.

After reading that book, I sought to find out more information on Buddhism. I bought more books, talked to more people, went to India to Sarnath where Buddha gave his first lecture, and I sat under a descendant of the Bodhi tree where Buddha found enlightenment.

Meeting the Dalai Lama

My search continued. I went to ashrams in Boulder, took yoga and meditation classes, and went to the Shambhala Center. Most inspiring of all was meeting the Dalai Lama and hearing him speak both in Boulder and in Denver. What I like most about the Dalai Lama is his beautiful simplicity in such a complex world. He makes everything so simple. "What do you think we should do about disintegrating families?" he was asked. He took a moment and thoughtfully replied, "Quarrel less, smile more."

I thought this was brilliant, brilliant in its simplicity. I have told a lot of people that and they look at me like "Yeah, wow, big deal. I am that profound every day before breakfast." But I think it is the truly brilliant who can take the most complex, difficult subjects that technically you could argue back and forth about for years and put it succinctly into four words. Many people are in therapy for decades before they really come to that same basic conclusion: Quarrel less, smile more.

He was wonderful when asked a difficult question about marriage, having the wisdom to say, "I don't know" and moving swiftly on to a question he could answer. Of course, the very most impressive things about the Dalai Lama are his patience, his perseverance, and his love.

The Chinese

His actions, his stance with the Chinese who now occupy his country, his code of nonviolence, his respect for humanity no matter what form it takes, and his methodology are about the furthest thing we Americans think of in reaction to an attack. I have often thought of violent acts because someone cut me off in traffic—and the Dalai Lama is kicked out of his own country, all of his possessions gone, his people beaten, raped, imprisoned, killed, and their way of life destroyed. How does he react? Well, he doesn't really react at all to the violence, the hate, and the destruction. He makes his mission "awareness," making the rest of the world aware of what is going on in his country and to his people, and helping people become cognizant of their own awareness.

But the question I had to ask myself, as an American trying to make my daily life fruitful, productive, and to live a life that has depth and meaning is "Can I learn from this serene, short, Asian man in the orange robe?" The answer had to be "Yes." Any man that is capable of his tenacity, his clear intelligence, his compassion, his calmness, his love, and his complete lack of hate and resentment, yes, I think we can all learn a tremendous amount from him.

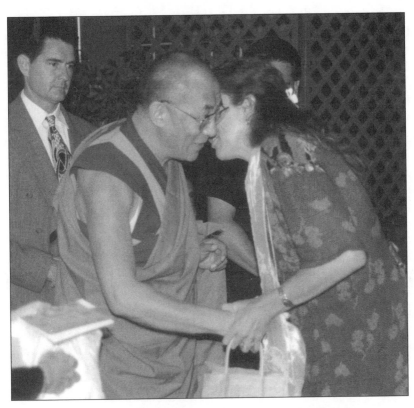

*Meeting the Dalai Lama when Lily of Colorado
helped sponsor his visit to Colorado*

I am a Buddhist

Before I met the Dalai Lama and before I heard him speak, people used to ask me, "Are you a Buddhist?" Not knowing what the criteria was in terms of the protocol, my reply was always, "Well, I am a wanna-be." I mean, how could I say I was a Buddhist, when I had never been to Buddhist school, had never met a lama, and never attended a Buddhist church or temple—not to mention the violent impulses I still felt.

In Boulder, at Macky Auditorum, someone asked the Dalai Lama, "Do you have to believe in incarnation to be a good Buddhist?" He replied, and I am paraphrasing from memory, "No, you must have only a warm heart, use your intellect, and study the teachings of Buddha."

I sat in the audience listening, and then thinking, "Damn! I *am* a Buddhist; the Dalai Lama just said so! Hey, wow, I can start telling people that according to the Dalai Lama, I really am a Buddhist. Well, who knows better than he does? It's like the Pope saying you are a Catholic. I really am a Buddhist now!"

The Dalai Lama's mission

After forty years of traversing the globe, he seems to be accomplishing his mission of informing the world of the tragic circumstances in Tibet. Hopefully, before this book is published, most of America will have a basic understanding of the cruelty and genocide occurring in his small nation, as well as a greater understanding and appreciation of the Dalai Lama's nonviolence and compassion.

Exploring Buddhism

I have found it fun and uplifting to explore Buddhism. There are many good books written on Buddhism—just a few are: *Everyday Zen* by Charlotte Joko Beck; *Shambhala: The Sacred Path of the Warrior* by Chogyam Trungpa; *Teachings of the Buddha* by Jack Kornfield; and *Transcending Madness: The Experience of the Six Bardos* by Chogyam Trungpa.

For more information contact the following:

The Shambhala Center
1345 Spruce Street
Boulder, CO 80302
(303) 444-0190

Denver Shambhala Meditation Center
718 E. 18th Avenue
Denver, CO
(303) 863-8366

International Campaign for Tibet
1825 K Street NW, Suite 520
Washington, DC 20006

Zen quotes

I have found the following quotes from Zen Buddhism to be amazingly thought provoking and elevating and wish to share them with you. I was impressed with Stephen Gaskin's *This Season's People*,[*] so many are his:

─━◆━─

Zen teaches that what you put your attention on, you get more of. Each one of us is a fountain of energy, a valve through which universal life energy is metered into the world, and we can each point our self at whatever we want to. We add life force to our surroundings—to everything we pay attention to. If you put your attention on the best, highest, finest, most beautiful thing that you can, that will be amplified.

If you know that Spirit and energy determine matter, not that matter determines that spirit and energy—then you can do things that make a difference in the world.

If you be an empty square, empty of desires, empty of prejudices, empty of heavy opinions, empty of being really attached to how it comes out—if you can be an empty square, you can be the variable in the situation, and the whole thing can change.

If you can change, you can do anything. If you change yourself, you change the world.
—Stephen Gaskin, This Season's People

We are wounded simply by participating in human life, by being children of Adam and Eve. To think that the proper or natural state is to be without wounds is an illusion. Any medicine

───────────────

* Stephen Gaskins, *This Season's People: A Book of Spiritual Teaching*, Summertown, TN: The Book Publishing Co., 1976.

motivated by the fantasy of doing away with woundedness is trying to avoid the human condition.
— Thomas Moore, *Care of the Soul**

You're supposed to be grooving as hard as you can all the time.
— Stephen Gaskin

⇒•◦•⇐

Chiropractic

Chiropractic's basic premise is that the bodily functions are controlled by the nervous system, which is surrounded by the musculoskeletal system. A chiropractor re-balances the musculoskeletal system to improve the nerve impulses and stimulate the body's natural immune system. The adjustments or spinal manipulations eliminate blockages of energy and realign the body's structure. Chiropractic can increase range of motion and relieve stiffness, tension, poor posture, and often menstrual pain and headaches.

Chiropractors mainly engage in spinal manipulation, called adjustment. They can also use electric massage units, electrical stimulation ultrasound, and trigger-point pressure. Chiropractic is a Greek derivative meaning "practical hand," as most of their work is literally "hands on."

Personal example

Some health-producing modalities are more dramatic than others. It varies with individuals. Here's an example from my life. Occasionally I noticed when driving the twenty minutes to work that I could feel my body's tension increase the closer I got to the office. My mind swirled into a frightful tizzy, spinning like a hamster running on a wheel. Jaws clamped, teeth clenched, my shoulders were pulled up to my earlobes. Thoughts about other people were negative. Annoyance bordering on anger spread through me. My neck pain was dull, yet intense; my head hurt, my back was in knots, and I hated my office, my car, and my life. On those infrequent occasions I realized if I went into the office I could really create havoc, so whenever I felt this bad, I would go directly to my chiropractor's office and just sit and wait until he had time to see me.

---

* Thomas Moore, *Care of the Soul: A Guide for Cultivating Depth and Sacredness in Everyday Life*, New York: Harper Collins, 1992.

After my adjustments and traction neck exercises, I would leave his office almost skipping down the sidewalk to my car. And I would notice for the first time that day that it was beautiful out and the sun was shining on my face. I would realize how lucky I was to be able to just slip down to the chiropractor's whenever I needed to, to enjoy that kind of freedom. I'd slide behind the wheel and drive to the office noticing what a great song was on the radio. Maybe some of the problems I was concerned about would creep back into my mind. They were still there, but I felt like I could deal with them.

My experience? Chiropractic treatment is wonderful! I love it because it gives me release from tension, frustration, and pain. It is one of the most wonderful therapies I have experienced.

Exercise

Thomas Jefferson called exercise the "sovereign invigorator of life." Since I grew up with my dad's farm, we were always running, jumping, and climbing trees. We were ruffian farm kids. We loved to be outside in the sun and breeze. I am still that way.

My dad had no appreciation for "useless" exercise, or something you might enjoy. He thought the only exercise you needed was hard manual work. Anyone who wanted a workout should go out and climb a ladder and pick apples, he figured, or grab a curved saw and loppers and prune trees, swing an ax for firewood, or weed the garden.

Get outside

On the rare occasion we didn't have to work on a nice day, my mom always had us outside. We were never allowed to watch TV, or go to the movies, or be inside if the weather was decent. I still can't sit inside on a beautiful day. I want to get out there and enjoy it. I love anything outdoors—walking, skiing, and boating. It just feels good to be outside with the sun on your skin. Even if you have been an indoors sort of person, start by just reading a book outside sitting under a tree or in the sun. Then start walking, mild exercise. It is just wonderful.

Nature has always provided us with the cure for depression, a reason to be joyful and appreciative, being connected with the plants, trees, and animals. It is estimated that the average American spends almost 93% of his time indoors. Outdoor exercise can have a powerfully positive effect on your well-being.

Find exercise you love

Exercise is a natural movement of our bodies and minds to embrace and love. If you have been having difficulty in getting yourself on a regular regime, I think the key is finding something you really like. For example, I love to walk both on my own farm and down the road where there is a beautiful lake with a mountain view. I often ride my mountain bike there. It is such a joy and pleasure to check out Mother Nature there, with the Platte River winding through the hills, the grass, and the wildflowers. I usually put on headphones and jam around the lake listening to my favorite music. It is divine. I look forward to it all day. I also walk around a couple of lakes near my office. When I need to have lengthy discussions with employees, or friends call and want to get together for a meal, I usually try to steer them to the lake instead for a long, pleasant walk.

I am lucky because my mom and her family have always exercised and been in really good shape. My aunt is 68 and has a nicer figure than most eighteen-year-olds, thanks to good old exercise. She always played basketball and jogged and enjoyed all outdoor activities. She played first string on a competitive basketball team until she was almost 60. The rest of the team members were in their 20s and 30s.

Walking

My mom has always championed those things that are beneficial and at the same time free. That's why she encourages breathing exercises and like me, walking. She says, "Nothing to buy, no dues to pay, no machines, just using the human body we're born with."

So while I have my headphones blasting to rock or blues music, my mom walks in quiet solitude and meditation. She likes to follow the idea of Thich Nhat Hanh, the Vietnamese Buddhist monk and author who founded Plum Village outside Paris. He suggests walking as if we are leaving a lotus blossom in each footprint. Mother likes that image. She happily figures she has strewn lotus blossoms all over the place.

She likes to walk "slow and easy." "I might miss something!" she says in defense of her unhurried pace. "I might miss a crocus that bravely forced itself up through the thinning layer of snow, or the leaf buds in the trees swelling in response to longer days, or any gently colored blossom in spring, or brighter ones in the summer. I like to take the time to appreciate the blazing color changes in autumn's leaves and the stark quiet beauty of winter."

Skiing

Several years ago when Mom still lived in Michigan, she announced, "I did a brilliant thing this winter. I hired a snow plow to clear the driveway and bought a pair of cross-country skis." She told me when friends drove 100 miles to get to the ski slopes, Mother put on her cross-country skis and went up and down her street. "I hate to get in a car and drive to where I can exercise," she explains.

So come on! Find something you will really love to do outside and start doing it. Exercise. It's not drudgery! It's a lifestyle! There are so many fun things to do. You just need to go out and find something that suits you. Start looking! Riding a bicycle is fun. We all loved it as kids and it hasn't changed. Get on one and go. In-line skating is a lot of fun, too. It takes a little more skill, but it's a ball. Hula-hooping is great. Sometimes I really enjoy going to the gym, and sometimes I'd rather swim. But I always do something.

Dancing

The first time I remember dancing was in middle school, somewhere around the sixth grade. We learned the do-si-do in gym class. It was so much fun I loved it.

Dancing is the love for life in motion. There is nothing I would rather do on earth than dance. It's a wonderful expression of appreciation for the body. To hear music that moves your soul and to have your body follow it is heavenly. You can go out and dance with your friends, you can just turn up the music in your living room and go crazy, or you can join in ceremonial and spiritual dances.

Goddess dances

During a stay at Shoshoni Retreat, near Nederland, Colorado, I took part in goddess dances that were halfway between country line dances and the do-si-do. I had such a good time. It was Saturday night and there were about ten of us, all women, and none of us but the ashramite knew the dances, so we had to learn as we went. Of course, we all kept forgetting our steps and screwing everything up, but it was so much fun. We laughed so hard my sides were aching. (See section on retreats.)

In the book, *The Everyday Meditator* by Osho, the author says, "Dancing came into the world as a technique of meditation. In the beginning dancing was not to dance; it was to achieve an ecstasy where the dancer was lost, only the dance remained—no ego, no body manipulating, the body flowing spontaneously."*

I feel like I have been to that place. Sometimes I have been out dancing to a rock band when a favorite song gets played, and I discover after dancing to it I almost wake up as if from a trance. It's a little scary. I'd been unconscious of everything, myself, my movements, the space I occupied, the person I was dancing with, my friends around me, the crowd, the band. It is like I disappeared and only the dance and the music remained. It's being in your own "zone." It is a wonderful, all natural moment in space and time.

Flower Essences

Flowers always make people better, happier, and more helpful; they are sunshine, food and medicine to the soul.

—Luther Burbank

Are flowers important? An old proverb notes that food nourishes the body, but flowers heal the soul. An ancient Persian proverb recommends if a man has two loaves of bread, he should sell one and buy hyacinths for his soul.

Flowers have probably been used for healing since the beginning of time. The Bible refers to them time and time again. The therapy of flower essences is founded upon the premise that flowers have a subtle and particular healing quality of energy that can cause fundamental shifts in our emotions, and are therefore used to address profound issues of well-being. It is said that flower essences can relieve feelings of insecurity, frustration, and anger, and that they can even work on a deeper level of emotions that can help you change your response to negative situations.

Flower essences differ from other healing herbs because their benefit is not from the chemical constituency of the product. Instead, they work when the "life force" of the plant is imparted into the water in which the flowers are immersed in outdoor sunshine. It is believed that the water then contains the vibrational energetic patterns of the plant. Flower essences' ability to create a place for healing to happen is not based upon chemical action with the body. "Rather, flower essences work through the various human energy fields, which in turn

---

* Osho, *The Everyday Meditator*, Rutland, VT: Charles E. Tuttle Company, Inc., 1993.

influence mental, emotional, and physical well-being,"[*] according to the book, *Flower Essence Repertory—A Comprehensive Guide to North American and English Flower Essences for Emotional and Spiritual Well-being.*

It is said that flower essences help bring emotional change through subtle insights of awareness. *Flower Essence Repertory* explains how this works: "The action of flower essences can be compared to the effects we experience from hearing a particularly moving piece of music, or seeing an inspirational work of art. The light or sound waves which reach our senses may evoke profound feelings in our soul, which indirectly affect our breathing, pulse rate, and other physical states." This occurs without impacting our bodies by direct physical or chemical intervention.

Dr. Bach's flower essences

In the 1930s, Dr. Edward Bach discovered the flower essence system we now use. He studied the effects of the plants' subtle energies on specific emotions, and came up with his system. Dr. Bach was one of the first people to understand and create a therapy based on the correlation between what we think and how we feel. A main principle was the terrible toll that negative emotional states could have on one's health, creating havoc and causing dis-ease. "Bach went further, however, in that he knew that true health is based on a connection of one's life and destiny with a larger purpose."[†]

Hanna Kroeger and flowers

In her book, *The Seven Spiritual Causes of Ill Health*, healer Hanna Kroeger states: "Flowers are messengers of the angels and are symbolic of angelic communication. They have a spiritual ministry and are signatures of the soul. Each flower has its own shape, size, color and tone, and sings in its own vibratory note. Each flower family is given its own

---

[*] Patricia Kaminski, and Richard Katz, *Flower Essence Repertory—A Comprehensive Guide to North American and English Flower Essences for Emotional and Spiritual Well-Being*, Rev. ed., Nevada City, CA: The Flower Essence Society, 1994, p. 3.

[†] Ibid., p. 13.

special work to perform for humanity. Each plant bears deeply with its heart a message to the human family."*

Flower essences contain the vibrational frequency, or essences of the flowers' healing powers, and are made by floating flowers in purified water in the sunlight outside for several hours. The flower essences receive healing power from the earth, sun, air, and water. Essences are made from flower blossoms picked at the height of their blooming cycle.

You can take three to five different flower essences at one time. However, as a function of the cure, I think every time you take a dropper of a flower essence you need to be mindful why you are taking it. The purpose is to reinforce and support yours elf in your efforts to heal.

A sampling of healing flower blossom essences

Here are a few flower essences and the particular aid they have been known to provide. Try others that appeal to you and meet your individual needs.

Moonshine yarrow helps keep emotions balanced.

Pink yarrow is used for trouble defining boundaries and for not absorbing others' negativity.

Rose helps through transitional times of growth.

Blackberry helps call in discipline when needed.

Chamomile relieves tension and has a calming effect.

Yarrow protects against negativity.

Wild oat helps with finding direction in life.

Willow helps heal resentment, a "poor me" attitude.

Larch helps with lack of self-esteem.

Holly is for feelings of hatred, jealousy, and envy.

Heather is for self-obsession.

Flower essences are available at your local health food store, or you can contact the following companies or organizations:

Flower Essence Society
P.O. Box 459
Nevada City, CA 95959
(800) 548-0075

---

* Hanna Kroeger, *The Seven Spiritual Causes of Ill Health*, Boulder, CO: Hanna Kroeger, 1988, p. 25.

Nelson Bach USA Ltd.
Wilmington Technology Park
100 Research Drive
Wilmington, MA 01887
(508) 988-3833, or for orders: call (800) 314-Bach

Flower Essences of Fox Mountain
P.O. Box 381
Worthington, MA 01098-0381
(413) 238-4291

Another book I have found helpful is *The Traditional Flower Remedies of Dr. Edward Bach A Self-Help Guide: The Famous Drugless Therapeutic System and How You Can Use It* by Leslie J. Kaslof (New Canaan, CT: Keats Publishing, Inc., 1993).

Hair

Far back into the reaches of history and across cultures, hair has been an important part of one's personal appearance. No physical feature of our bodies can be more easily changed.

Hair is a very important part of American culture. Generally, men love long hair on women and many women love men with long hair. No matter what length you prefer, people love hair and are willing to go to great lengths to enhance it, preserve it, or bring it back after it's gone. St. Paul apparently didn't approve of women's "crowning glory." He admonished women to cover their heads so as not to be a distraction.

Hairstyles

Note the variety in hairstyles. Some people wear their hair long, some short, and some shave it off entirely. We wear it in braids, bobs, bangs, ringlets, straight, curly, spiked, in poufs, pony tails, buns, French twists, Mohawks, corn rows, and in all colors. It is teased, ratted, bleached, dyed, and streaked. Some people are bald naturally and reluctantly.

The ancient Egyptians shaved their heads. To look their most ferocious, wild warriors of old spiked theirs, so twentieth-century youngsters' spiked hairstyles aren't new. Our forefathers wore powdered wigs. The broken shafts of their long clay pipes were recycled and used to make the horizontal curls on the sides of their wigs.

Fair-skinned Scandinavians wore braids, as did red-skinned Native Americans and black-skinned people. Renaissance women wore towering hairdos, bedecked with all sorts of decorations, including on occasion a complete model of a ship. Louis XIV wore a periwig of dark, cascading curls.

Enhancing your hair

Before each strand of hair is pushed through the surface of a human scalp, the cells in the shaft are already dead. Yet what we want is to keep our hair looking alive and lively! How do we do this? How do we best care for the 100,000 hairs the average person has on his or her head? What can we do to make our hair as clean, healthy, lustrous, long-lasting and lively appearing as we can? How can we enhance, preserve, and, where necessary, restore it?

Let's start with diet

Diet is, as noted throughout this book, vitally important. Hair can be one of the first areas to benefit or suffer by our choice of diet. This fact is underscored by women with anorexia who lose their hair after months of self-imposed extreme dieting which results in nutritional deficiencies. A healthy diet is essential for healthy hair.

Whole grains, brown rice, oatmeal, brewer's yeast, cold-pressed olive oil, organic vinegar, nuts, sunflower seeds, chickpeas, cauliflower, and lentils are said to be necessary for hair's health, as are biotin and essential fatty acids. Some suggest kelp and wakame, two types of seaweed, as well.

Brushing

Brushing is an easy addition to our hair-enhancing regimen. Brushing removes dirt and increases circulation. Each of your 100,000 strands of hair has its own tiny artery just beneath the scalp's surface to feed the hair follicle. Stimulate them by brushing. One hundred brush strokes per day for lustrous hair was the rule my mother followed, as did her mother before her. Brushing also spreads the natural oils of the scalp throughout your hair.

Conditioning

Dry hair seems to require a little more maintenance. I have dry hair and I often do kukui hot oil hair treatments. I use my brand of kukui oil with essential oils of lavender and lily, comfrey, and calendula. I simply oil down my hair with the oil, apply heat for five minutes with a blow dryer, put a towel over my pillow, go to sleep, and wash it the following morning. Sometimes I use our seven exotic oils, a blend of oils including primrose oil, rosehip seed oil, almond oil, kukui oil, wheat germ, vitamin E, and essential oil of lavender.

You can make your own by using all of the above; other oils such as olive oil are also perfect, as is any blend you enjoy. You can slowly and watchfully heat the oil on a very low heat (most safely done in a double-boiler), remove from heat, and put comfrey, coltsfoot, elder flowers, or horsetail in the oil. Soak for four hours and then strain the herbs out and apply the mixture to your hair. You can blend them with the essential oils of frankincense, chamomile, lavender, or rosemary. You can also simply add these essential oils to your shampoo. For dry hair, it is also beneficial to take one or two tablespoons of high-quality unrefined olive oil internally daily.

Coloring

Dyeing our hair is nothing new; people did it as early as 3000 B.C. The Babylonian women are said to have preferred to dye their hair red, while the women during the Roman Empire preferred blonde.

Dr. Paul Eck of the Eck Institute of Applied Nutrition and Bioenergetics, Ltd., theorizes that "Gray hair is a warning signal that your body is decreasing its supply of energy." Furthermore, he states that it isn't a matter of aging; it is a matter of a depletion of minerals in the body. He states, "The cause of gray hair is chronic fatigue and exhaustion. Gray hair is nature's way of warning us that we are running out of energy." Interestingly, he states, "Calcium is white. So is zinc. In fact, zinc oxide is a popular white pigment. It is used, for instance, in the white ointment that lifeguards use to protect their noses from sunburn. As these two minerals accumulate in your tissues, and therefore, in your hair, the hair then turns the same color as the minerals in it, in this case, white."[*]

Joy, a wonderful older woman who works at a Vitamin Cottage in Englewood, Colorado, has a beautiful head of long hair that is its rich, dark brown, original color. She has less gray than most thirty-five-year olds. She contributes it to fo-ti, the Chinese herb. She says taken over long periods of time, it will retain your natural hair color. My mother

---

[*] *The Healthview Newsletter,* Issue #27–29, 612 Rio Road West, Box 6670, Charlottesville, VA 22906, p. 9.

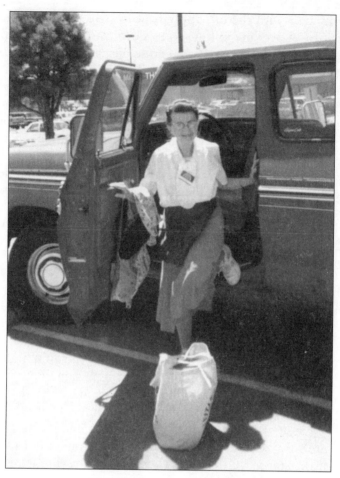

A favorite customer—Joy at Vitamin Cottage

recently said she met a woman well into her 80s with the most beautiful hair and skin; the woman said it was from drinking kombachi tea.

Aubrey Hampton, author of *What's in Your Cosmetics?*,[*] says that walnut extract from the husk of the walnut (*Juglans regia*) is superior to artificial hair-coloring chemicals. It is said to dye hair a natural deep brown color and it can be combined with henna and coffee to make a deep red-brown. Hampton further states that henna can turn hair orange unless it is mixed with indigo and logwood. For long-lasting

---

[*] Aubrey Hampton, *What's in Your Cosmetics? A Complete Consumer's Guide to Natural and Synthetic Ingredients*, Tucson, AZ: Odonian Press, 1995, p. 176.

results, a 5.5 pH must be obtained by adding citric acid. Non-coloring henna makes an excellent ingredient for shampoos and neutral rinses.

Light Mountain Henna is a company that makes 100% henna dyes in eight colors, which are available in most health food stores.

Preserving your hair

Shampooing

It's possible to wash your hair too often. I wash my hair as little as possible; if I don't have to go anywhere that day, I don't wash it, in order to preserve the natural oils as much as possible. Even the nicest shampoos can be harsh to your hair by their very nature. Use warm water and as little shampoo as possible; brush your hair first, and massage the shampoo into your scalp.

I refuse to use any shampoos that contain sodium laurel sulfate or anything that even sounds like that; so you have to be an ingredient reader to get a quality shampoo. Aubrey Organics makes clean shampoos that people with dry hair especially like.

A perfect hair-growth shampoo should contain yarrow and rosemary. Mrs. Grieve, in *A Modern Herbal* suggests that "an infusion of the dried plants (both leaves and flowers) combined with borax and used when cold, makes one of the best hair-washes known. It forms an effectual remedy for the prevention of scurf and dandruff."[*]

For a dry, quick shampoo, sprinkle cornmeal through your hair and then brush out with 100 strokes. The dry cornmeal absorbs oil and soil.

And from your kitchen

You can make a good shampoo at home. Infuse the desired herbs in water. After straining, mix with a good soap, rosehip seed oil, rosemary and lavender essential oils. It will not need a preservative if you use it within a week.

To make your own shampoo, try:

1 cup water

¼ cup horsetail, dried or fresh herb

10 drops rosemary essential oil

---

[*] Mrs. Maud Grieve, *A Modern Herbal: The Medicinal, Culinary, Cosmetic and Economic Properties, Cultivation and Folk-Lore of Herbs, Grasses, Fungi, Shrubs &Trees With All Their Modern Scientific Uses*, Vol. II, reprint, New York: Dover Publications, Inc., 1982, p. 683.

10 drops primrose oil

1/4 cup castile soap

1 teaspoon molasses

Bring the water to a boil. Add the horsetail and lower the heat, let simmer for twenty minutes. Cool and then strain the herbs out, and add the soap to the water. Stir in the rosemary, primrose oil, and molasses; use and then store in a jar in the refrigerator. Use within a week.

To make eight ounces of shampoo, add three-fourths cup of any of the above-mentioned herbs to two cups water in a nonmetal pan. Gently bring to a boil. Lower heat and simmer for ten minutes. Turn off the heat and let it sit until cool. Strain the herbs out and add one-fourth cup of soap flakes. Cook together until emulsified. Then add one tablespoon of rosehip seed oil and five drops rosemary oil. Store in the refrigerator for one week.

For a pure herbal product try:

1/2 ounce soapwort root

1 1/2 pints water

Powder the soapwort root. Pour boiling water over the soapwort root and allow to steep for one hour. Strain the soapwort out, and use the liquid as your shampoo.

Dry-hair shampoo is another item you can make at home. It can contain any or all of the following herbs: comfrey, elder flowers, calendula, aloe, chamomile, witch hazel, horsetail, and coltsfoot.

Native Americans used a member of the lily family called chlorogalum for a shampoo. Yucca was also used like the soapwort shampoo.

Rinses

For a wonderful vinegar rinse base for all hair types, add two tablespoons vinegar to one cup purified water. Simply pour this over your hair after shampooing. *Caution:* Do not use this on chemically treated hair.

Try applying aloe juice or gel directly to cleansed hair and leave in for an hour and then rinse out. Try putting ten drops rosemary oil into eight ounces of water and rinse through your hair.

Split ends
For split ends, Jessica B. Harris, author of the *World Beauty Book*,[*] recommends "scorch[ing a] corncob over a flame: then use it to brush the ends of your hair. The cob will remove split ends."

Detangling
I have long hair so I need serious detangling. Try this oregano hair detangler:

> In a small pan, heat one cup of water and one-half cup fresh oregano. Make a tea and let steep for 45 minutes. After cooling, strain out the oregano, add five drops rosemary, and put in a spray bottle. After washing and conditioning your hair, spray on your hair and don't rinse out.

A healthy scalp
I like to stand on my head every morning to increase the circulation of my scalp (among other benefits). This is only recommended for the more athletic among you and only with specific training. You can benefit from lying on a slantboard as well.

Dandruff
For dandruff, try putting warm cider vinegar all over your scalp and hair and then wrap a towel around your head, leave on for an hour and then wash. Do this twice a week until the dandruff stops.

Another interesting application for dandruff is the fresh juice from an apple applied to the hair; massage in for ten minutes and then rinse out with one tablespoon of apple cider vinegar in one cup of water. Rinse. Use this method once a week.

Some suggestions that others have found helpful:

* Take PABA supplements daily

* Take vitamin B

* Take zinc

* Take brewer's yeast daily with spirulina and wheat grass in apple juice

---

[*] Jessica B. Harris, *The World Beauty Book*, San Francisco, CA: Harper Collins Publishers, 1995.

* Take vitamin E internally

* Apply vitamin E to your scalp and leave on overnight

* When drying your hair, burn your favorite incense or dry your hair out in the warm sunshine and gentle breeze

Hair loss and baldness

Bringing your hair back after it's gone
The ancient Roman Emperor Domitian, who reigned from 81–96 A.D., wrote a book on hair, according to the History Channel's program on Roman Emperors, which aired April 13, 1998. (He was losing his.) Thus, we learn that losing one's hair has a long history of causing concern.

The cause of hair loss for men is usually a genetic predisposition, related to pattern baldness. Hair loss for women is usually diffused through the scalp, rather than concentrated in one area. The hair loss with women is usually genetic, too. A condition called *androgenic alopecia* affects most women with hair loss; the hair falls out at normal levels of 50 to 100 strands per day but does not grow back. Women are not as likely to experience early hair loss due to estrogen, which fights other hormones' negative effect on the hair. After menopause, many women have thinning hair, due to estrogen levels decreasing.

Women and hair loss
Hair loss in women can also be caused by severe stress on the body, giving birth, high fever, divorce, sickness, drug abuse, or alcoholism. Antibiotics and blood thinners are also said to cause hair loss. It is said a thyroid hormone deficiency is another reason hair may continue to thin with age.

Recommendations
Culpeper, author of *Culpeper's Complete Herbal & English Physician*, recommends taking kernels of peaches, bruising them, and boiling in vinegar. Apply to the affected area. He enthusiastically states: "It marvelously makes the hair grow again in bald paxes or where it is too thin."[*]

Alfalfa juice or tablets are said to stimulate hair growth; I have heard that anything that sprouts is good for "sprouting" hair. Many say

---

[*] Nicholas Culpeper, *Culpeper's Complete Herbal & English Physician Enlarged*, (London, 1814), reprint ed., Glenwood, IL: Meyerbooks, Publisher, 1990.

receding hairlines can be helped by eating germinating foods such as raw wheat germ or raw sunflower seeds, and by eating onions.

Some recommend rubbing the juice of an onion on your head and going out into the sun. Many aromatherapists recommend mixtures of essential oils of sandalwood, cedarwood, sage, tea tree, and rosemary with almond oil applied to the head. Lavender and rosemary oil rubbed into the hair roots stimulate growth. Other essential oils that are beneficial include birch, cedarwood, clary sage, juniper, lavender, sage, and thyme.

According to *The Complete Book of Natural Cosmetics* by Beatrice Travern, "Baldness remedies based on garlic juice have been advocated for centuries, usually mixed with bay rum and olive oil."[*] Simmer the garlic in the oil and apply to the area.

Aubrey Hampton, author of *What's in Your Cosmetics?*[†], states that products with PABA are said to help prevent hair loss and protect the hair from the sun. He also recommends combining coltsfoot and ginseng for the scalp; scalps that are low in silica acid, sulfur, and cystine reportedly have a higher hair loss.

Other remedies

❋ Castor oil applied topically

❋ Drinking licorice tea

❋ Cider vinegar mixed with sage and nettle tea applied topically

❋ Zinc, B vitamins, and supplements specifically made for hair

Hangover
The best way to avoid a hangover is not to drink alcohol. But if you are like me and enjoy imbibing from time to time, it's good to have remedies handy. Here are some suggestions to help keep the drinkers among us healthier and happier.

Folk medicine often considers heavy drinking to be a sign of potassium deficiency. Honey, a perfect source of potassium, works with the body to overcome the craving for alcohol and helps an individual sober up.

---

[*] Beatrice Travern, *The Complete Book of Natural Cosmetics*, New York, NY: Simon & Schuster, 1974, p.138.
[†] Hampton, *What's in Your Cosmetics?*, p. 127.

Acidity

Animals and humans seek food and drink high in acid. Beer has a very high acid pH of 4.5. Alcoholic beverages that are high in acid may meet an instinctive need for acid. Coffee and tea have the same pH as beer.

Steaming

Go to a steam room first thing in the morning and detox your entire body, alternating with swimming to increase your oxygen intake. When my parents lived in Michigan, I used to go out and party a lot, and then my parents would take me to their health club and I would spend hours there alternating between steaming and swimming; before we left I would feel like a million bucks. Then it helps to go for a long walk in the sun doing deep breathing.

If you are a regular casual drinker, I highly recommend you take dandelion root on an on-going basis. You may also want to take milk thistle, burdock root, yellow dock, and licorice root to keep your blood and organs detoxified. Some other helps follow:

* Drink fruit juices. They contain fructose, which helps burn the alcohol faster and helps cleanse it from your body the next day.

* Cysteine, a water-soluble amino acid, has been known to help protect against the damages of alcohol consumption.

* Take willow bark, a natural pain reliever.

* Replace the salt and potassium in your body with honey or a banana.

* Drink plenty of water before, after, and during your drinking. Three glasses of water before going to sleep will help end the dehydration, which is a major cause of a hangover.

* Really taste the drink. Savor it.

* Take evening primrose oil capsules before drinking.

* Drink only after eating.

* Take vitamin Bs before and after drinking.

* Take amino acids before and after drinking.

* Drink drinks with cranberry or orange juice. I used to carry small packets of alfalfa juice powder or spirulina with me to mix into tequila and orange juice drinks.

* Take vinegar and vitamin C.

* Guarana will make you feel better the next day and contains 3-to-5% caffeine.

* The next day, eat again to replenish nutrients.

* Don't drink beer in aluminum containers, including draft beer.

* Be sure when you are out drinking, you breathe deeply and often. If you are dancing, you are getting oxygen and exercise to help counteract the negatives. On the way, home take many very deep breaths. And don't drive or ride with anyone who has been drinking.

Homeopathy

Homeopathy was founded by German physician Samuel Hahnemann in the eighteenth century. It is based on the "law of similars," that is, the concept that "like cures like." It differs from herbal medicine in its basic healing premise. Homeopathy is a system that employs the whole body by using very small "doses" of plants, animals, or minerals to stimulate the immune system. It is similar to an immunization, which uses small amounts of the virus to get your body producing the proper antibodies against it.

Since "like cures like," it follows that a substance which would produce a symptom, for example an onion which makes your eyes water and nose run, would be employed as a remedy for colds. It is almost as if the substance reminds the body's immune system how to fight the illness. Homeopathic remedies are usually taken sublingually, or under the tongue, where they are quickly absorbed.

Difference from herbal

Homeopathy also differs from herbal medicine in its basic healing premise. Herbal medicine is action and then counteraction. And homeopathic remedies are not always composed of plant-based ingredients. They most often come in small white pellets, tiny tablets that dissolve quickly under the tongue. Many stores sell a complete home starter kit for your medicine cabinet and books to help you identify your symptoms and their various remedies, or you can purchase each remedy separately.

The first homeopathic remedy I ever used was oscillococcinum for a cold. While I was working in Aspen and Glenwood Springs (Colorado), I started getting all the classic symptoms of a cold. Before I went to bed,

I couldn't even breathe because my nose was so stuffed up. I took a couple of tiny oscillococcinum tablets and went to bed. I breathed easily. I couldn't believe how well they worked.

Hanna Kroeger

The last time I went to see her, Hanna Kroeger, with Hanna's Herb Shop and the Church of Miracles near Boulder, recommended I take some homeopathic remedies with some herbal capsules and tinctures. She said I had Epstein Barr virus. I was feeling very tired and run down. I really had to fight to get moving in the morning. I couldn't believe how much better I felt in less than a week. (For more information on Hanna Kroeger, see the chapter on alternative therapies.)

Hanna's remedies also had a slightly beneficial effect on my skin. I have not personally found a homeopathic remedy that really worked on my skin. That doesn't mean they don't work, but rather I have not yet had that fortunate experience. Some that are recommended for skin ailments are apis, nux vomica, and sulphur.

You also need to read and follow instructions when taking homeopathics. You need to let the pellets dissolve in your mouth. Avoid mint even in your toothpaste and mouthwash as it counteracts the homeopathic remedies' effects. Many essential oils and caffeine can all interrupt the process, too.

Homeopathy is used for many imbalances including, but not limited to:

- Anxiety
- Nausea
- Skin conditions
- Eczema
- Pain and swelling

- Arthritis
- Digestive disorders
- Morning sickness
- Headaches
- Sinus problems

For more information write:

National Center for Homeopathy
801 North Fairfax
Alexandria, VA 22314

They can provide you with a directory of homeopathic practitioners.

Other sources

There are plenty of great books on homeopathy at your health food store and maybe your library. Two I recommend are:

Homeopathic Medicine at Home by Maesimund Panos, M.D., and Jane Heimlich, 1980, and *The Complete Book of Homeopathy* by Michael Weiner, M.D., 1989.

For herbs, information, and Hanna's books write or visit:

Hanna's Herb Shop
5684 Valmont
Boulder, CO 80301
(303) 443-0755

Joe Lilleth operates the largest homeopathy manufacturer east of the Mississippi:

Homeopathy Works
Fairfax Street
Berkeley Springs, WV 25411

Journal Writing

If you bring forth what is within you, what you bring forth will save you. If you do not bring forth what is within you, what you do not bring forth will destroy you.

—Gospel of St. Thomas

Self-discovery

I have been keeping a journal consistently for the last five or more years, for many different reasons. One is to document events, people, and places I don't want to forget. Another is I like to keep a journal to help figure out my moods as they relate to my behavior and to help sort out my anxieties, joys, and so on. Essentially, I journal to get to know myself better. For example, why did I get so upset about that event, discussion, or comment? I want to uncover the conflicts that may really be going on.

Journal writing is a great way to self-discovery. Your feelings and insights are documented for future use. It's a learning tool. You can see how you felt a year ago about a relationship. Was it better back then, or were you suffering from the same dilemmas?

The Artist's Way

There is an outstanding book called *The Artist's Way* by Julia Cameron, published by G. P. Putnam's Sons. If you need help sorting out what is really going on in your mind and need a nudge or guidance, I highly recommend this book. You don't have to be an artist to benefit greatly from this book.

Get started

If you don't know how to get started, it's easier than you might think. I first got started in college. As I mention elsewhere in this book, I fully realize I am not a gifted writer. After flunking English a couple of times at Metropolitan State College in Denver, I was advised to attend tutoring sessions at the writing center at the school. I had a great tutor who simply sat me down with a notebook and pen and said, "Okay, write."

I asked, "Write about what?"

She said to write about whatever I wanted.

"Like what?" "Just write about whatever you want to write about."

I said, "I don't want to write about anything."

She said, "Write that."

"What?"

"Just write. It doesn't matter what you write about."

"I don't want to do this," I said. "I am really busy and have a lot to do."

"Write that," she said. "Just shut up and start writing!"

I was thinking, "That is kind of rude," and she said, "Write how you feel about that. Write about all the things you think you need to do. Write about how I am getting on your nerves. Just keep writing."

Give up your resistance

Finally, I gave up my natural resistance and just started writing how I thought I was way too busy for this writing class and how I shouldn't have to go there twice a week and how this was really a stupid exercise and how sure I was that I wasn't going to benefit from it. When I gave up my resistance, I couldn't believe how much I had to say. She could barely get me out of there when my hour was up. So if you have a problem getting started, I suggest the same thing to you—just write. You will benefit more than you could ever anticipate.

Find the best time of day for yourself to write. I find first thing in the morning very beneficial. I find that my dreams can really affect my mood when I wake up. Thus, I think it is important to do it close to waking up. Journal writing is about discovering yourself. It's about having a better understanding about yourself. Consider it an adventure. Just start writing!

The Landmark Forum

The purpose of this book is to help you (as the title states) find ways to promote beauty, health, and happiness in your life.

Beauty is both an interior and exterior state. Health begins inside and shows on the outside. Happiness is an inner condition that overflows to the outside. All three begin inside. Thus it becomes obvious that we should invest time and energy on our inner selves—who we are and what makes us tick.

Make your discoveries

People can do this in many ways. Discovering the inner self can be done alone or in groups. It can be done with or without professional assistance. It can be done at home, by a lake, in a garden, in a church or temple, on a walk, and/or at a spiritual retreat.

My sister chooses to make her discoveries alone. She meditates daily. She believes that ultimately all problems can be solved through deep meditation, by connecting with that Source of Power which holds all creation intact.

My mother, who is inspired by being surrounded by uplifting people, profits from retreats, especially those put on by Jean Foster (Team Up, Box 1115, Warrensburg, Missouri 64093).

Explore

Like so much in life, it's an individual thing. Explore all the avenues available for finding, understanding, and expanding your inner self. You'll be amazed how many there are! Find what's right for you.

The Forum

I found a very interesting organization called The Landmark Forum. The Forum forces you to take a good look at yourself and the havoc you create in your own life. It then demands you take responsibility for it. It simultaneously lets you in on a big secret: You are just human and so is everybody else around you. It plugs you into the pain of the universe and leaves you with a connection to all humanity.

The Forum is about making your life work for you. It's about taking real responsibility for your happiness, which is accomplished through taking control of your life. It helps you see that you are the one making all the drama, pain, and craziness in your life. Yes, you may have a good excuse for your story, but The Forum refuses to let you live in the domain of your "stories."

One of its prize tenets is that you do what you say you are going to do. Simple, yes; difficult, yes. Do most people do it? No. It is about maintaining your integrity at all times, not just when it suits you.

Logistics

The Forum is held three days in a row, Friday, Saturday, and Sunday, 8:00 A.M. to approximately midnight, then the following Tuesday night. It costs $325 for the first course and $700 for the advanced one. It is held throughout the country at various times. Contact information is below. Be forewarned, it's a mind blower. If you're up to it and if you want to push yourself to your emotional limits and if you want to explore all modalities of healing—go for it; it's a wild ride. And it may just get you over some of your constant complaints in life, forever.

If you are really ready to open the box that contains all of your demons and fears and see your own humanness at its core, and if you are really ready to get over your own self-deluded, problem-oriented life, and if you are starting to really bore yourself with the "poor me's" and want to see what is really possible for you on this planet and in this lifetime, I highly recommend it.

Possibility

The Landmark Forum describes in its brochure its advanced seminars the following way: "Each of us has a sense of something possible beyond the ordinary. Each of us has moments when something about our lives, our family, our community, our world awakens in us a sense of possibility. Each of us has glimpses of that most fundamental of all possibilities—that life really could be extraordinary. The Landmark Forum's advanced course is based on the premise that each of us can design that life now—an extraordinary life—a life of possibility."

History of The Forum

The Landmark Forum has an interesting story if you can get anyone in the organization to tell it to you. I have had to piece it together. Over the last 25 years, The Landmark Forum, as it is called today, developed from what was called "EST" back in the 1970s. EST stands for Erhard Seminar

Training or *est* in Latin for "it is." Nobody at the Landmark seems to deny or engage in a discussion about this without some explicit query.

EST

I, however, find it extremely interesting. I first heard about EST in a specific way from a wonderful Lily of Colorado representative I had in Michigan. I noticed how she was so dependable, so honest, so nice to be around, and always did what she said she was going to do. I was so impressed I asked her about it one day. I was with her visiting stores in the Ann Arbor area and I just came out and asked her where she got her attributes. She said it was from her EST training. I found a few clues in the November/December 1997 issue of *Nexus*, which is "Colorado's Holistic Journal," in an article entitled "Where Have All the Gurus Gone?" The founder of EST, Werner Erhard, was a car salesman in the late 1950s. "A number of lawsuits were filed against Erhard and EST claiming they were responsible for emotional distress," the article states. The article claims that Erhard is in exile, somewhere in Europe.

More information

The Forum is hard to describe for even the most educated, esoteric, and articulate, so I am not even going to try; but there is a great book that may help clarify it for you, although I really didn't understand it myself until I actually went to The Forum, as we graduates call it. So to get more on EST, read *EST: Making Life Work*, by Robert A. Hargrove. *Time* magazine did an interesting article on The Landmark Forum in its March 16, 1998, issue, which you can read for reference.

The Harvard Business School published an article on The Landmark Forum on November 3, 1997, by Daren Hopper Wruck and Mikelle Fisher Estley, which I found to be really interesting and a good source of information. In order to get copies, you can contact the Harvard Business School Publishing, Boston, MA 02163 or call (800)545-7685.

The Forum has organizations in many parts of the country. You can contact them and get further information by writing the Landmark Education Corporation, 353 Sacramento Street, Suite 200, San Francisco, CA 94111, (415) 981-8850, or go to http://www.landmark-education.com.

Massage

Massage is one of the easiest, simplest and most effective stress busters on the planet. Massage has the following benefits:

* Reduces stress

* Produces deep relaxation

* Increases circulation

* Soothes anxiety

* Provides needed human contact

* Improves healing

* Relieves tension in muscles

* Increases range of motion

* Increases awareness of where we're holding tension in our bodies

* Feels good

Massage is a wonderful way to spend an hour, or if you're lucky, two. If you cannot afford a professional massage therapist, you can get a massage from your spouse or a friend. You can also go to a massage school. I sometimes go to one in Denver where the students do massages for $20. True, they are usually not as good as paying an expert, but if the cost from a professional massage therapist is prohibitive, it is an alternative.

You can also offer to do a "trade-out" with a massage therapist, where you trade them your talent or products for their services.

Massage is a wonderful gift to give yourself or to give others. I was getting a massage once or twice a month for years. It has a perfect healing effect. You have to make sure you know what relaxation feels like so when you get uptight and out of balance you have the sense to get to a massage therapist quickly.

A few of the many different kinds of massage:

Deep Tissue Massage releases tensions in tightly held patterns to regain mobility.

Shiatsu ("Shi" = finger and "atsu" = pressure) is a Japanese method that applies precise pressure to aid the restoration of balance and energy. The therapist applies pressure with his fingers to help release blocks in the energy meridians.

Swedish Massage seems to be the most common of massage therapies, perhaps because it can be done on anybody and it is easier on the therapist. It is a very relaxing treatment in which the therapist smoothly applies different strokes to release muscle tension.

Trager Method, also called Trager Psychophysical Integration, whose namesake coined the word "mentastics" meaning "mental gymnastics," employs a series of releasing physical holding patterns by gently cradling and stretching movements.

Foot Reflexology is a therapy where the practitioner applies pressure to various areas of the feet that reflect the body's major systems and organs.

Cranio-Sacral Therapy balances the bones of the cranium.

Meditation

When face to face with oneself, there is no cop-out.
—Duke Ellington

The first time

I'll never forget the first time I ever meditated. I didn't mean to meditate, I didn't even want to, but it was that sister of mine again. It was years ago. It was some guru's birthday or some sort of spiritual holiday and she needed a ride to Gold Hill, near Boulder. I took her there and we ate a good vegetarian dinner in silence. Afterwards, I met a couple of her friends from the ashram. Then we all went over to the meditation hall. I remember she told me, "Now, if you want to leave the meditation early, just slip quietly out that side door." I thought that was kind of a funny thing for her to say to me: 1) What made her think I was going to leave early, and 2) Like, I couldn't find the door or what?

Anyway, they started chanting. I thought it was kind of weird, but harmless. Then they started meditation, just sitting there, still, without moving, for what seemed a week. I couldn't stand it, my brain was on overdrive doing the grocery list, a grant proposal I was working on . . . boy, I want a cigarette, spin, spin, spin. I couldn't stop it. I wanted to jump up and jog around the room just to move. Finally, I had to do as she had instructed, or should I say predicted, and head for the side door. Wow, was it good to get out of there and go sit in my car and get distracted by the radio. So I sat there and listened to the tunes and waited for her.

I didn't get it then, but I get it now. That is the entire point. You are supposed to sit there and see how crazy you really are, how haphazard, how obsessed, how unaware, how violent, how angry, how selfish, how neurotic, how dramatic, how insecure, how "not in the moment," how charged, how caught up, how "not directly involved," how distracted, how completely overtaken you are with your own constant chatter.

Distractions

Yet distractions are beautiful: alcohol, TV, movies, food, friends, family, conversation, cigarettes, recreation, music, shopping, travel, games, motion (trains, planes, motorcycles). They are all diversions from your true self. Meditation is a very effective way to find out who you are, not to mention, to help you get centered and get what you want out of life.

As Eddie and Debbie Shapiro sum it up in their book, *Out of Your Mind—The Only Place To Be!*, "When all the trappings are taken away there is nothing but a vast emptiness. Finally we are left with that which transcends all true phenomena, our true selves."[*]

Awareness

How much of our daily life are we aware of? What do we think about all day? How many times a day do we judge others? How many times a day do we think about sex? What percent of our life are we daydreaming or wishing we were somewhere else? How many times a day do we have negative thoughts? How many times a day do we put ourselves down? How much of our day are we really present to whom we are talking or what we are doing? How many times a day do we lie to other people because we do not have the personal courage or integrity to simply tell them the truth? How many times a day are we inauthentic? What is our life force really spent doing?

Different methods

There are as many ways to meditate as there are religions. In fact, almost all religions engage in some sort of meditation, because their founders know that you really don't know what is going on until you stand still and take a quiet look. "Be still, and know that I Am God," says the Old Testament. Some meditations are like positive affirmations, some are like those in *The Artist's Way*, writing and investigating what is going on; some mimic the statues of the meditating Buddha where the goal is to empty your mind.

Definition

Meditation is defined often as a state of focused attention through which one emerges into an ever-increasingly clear awareness of reality.

---

[*] Eddie and Debbie Shapiro, *Out of Your Mind—The Only Place To Be!*, Rockport, MA: Element, Inc., 1992, p. 53.

Different sects of religions use different techniques, including imagery, breath control, observation, and mantras.

Great meditation authors

Osho, in his great book entitled *The Everyday Meditator,* states, "Stopping the world is the whole art of meditation. And to live in the moment is to live in eternity. To taste the moment with no idea, with no mind, is to taste immortality."[*] This has fifty or so different meditations for different things from laughing, dancing, working, loving, and whirling. It is a really fun book.

Joko Beck recommends in *Everyday Zen* that you just sit still and be aware of all your thoughts, like a witness: "I am thinking about my car not starting. Now, I am starting to think about how my neighbor made me mad this morning." She says that if you label your thoughts and be aware of them, sooner or later you will tire of your old worn-out thoughts like a movie you have sat through 500 times.

It works, not quickly, not easily, and not without severe pain, because what you have to do is "*be* the pain." That means face it, feel it—cry, scream, yell (without lashing out at others, a hard one). So if something very painful occurs in your life such as divorce, death, or some other sort of loss, you need to feel all that pain, for as long as it takes. That is the only way to get past it. I highly recommend Beck's book.

A great master

I recently attended a lecture in Boulder by His Holiness, Orgyen Kusum Lingpa. The flyer from the Shambhala Center described him as "a preeminent Dzogchen meditation master and treasure revealer from the Golok region of Tibet, where he is an abbot of three major monasteries. He is distinguished in his ability to receive and transmit teachings that have been hidden for generations. This will be a unique opportunity to hear a qualified master present the Dzogchen view of Buddhist meditation."

It was a very small gathering of people held at a Boulder woman's home. He stated that just sitting in the meditation position of legs crossed and hands in one's lap is very beneficial to "bind the body, help[ing] bind the mind. The mind which is under the power of constant thought activity is like the Sun and the Moon being controlled by the constant rolling of clouds."

---

[*] Osho, *The Everyday Meditator,* p. 31.

Meditation practice, he said, is to help abate powerful mental disturbances and provide even the most miserly, coarse, intense minds a greater ease, happiness, comfort, and calm state. Trying to tame the mind is like a parent trying to get a child that doesn't listen to follow directions.

Before His Holiness began his lecture and while we were waiting for the interpreter to arrive, we briefly meditated with him. It was one of the most powerful meditation sessions I have ever had.

I sit down and sort of meditate everyday, but really it is more like a really nice quiet space and time every morning when I get to write down who and what is getting on my nerves, and then plan my daily activities. His Holiness stated that this sort of practice may help organize your day, although it is not going to bring you any lasting peace or get you closer to anything meaningful.

I have read many of the great meditation books, and I always know what they are talking about intellectually, but this was the first time I ever practiced with a great master, and it was powerful. They say in many of the books how important it is to practice with a master and with a group of like-minded people. I thought this was simply to remind you to meditate, but I see now that the great masters really can transmit information or energy via their very presence.

The Tibetan Buddhists have a meditation in which you think about your body being a corpse. The purpose is for you to accept and get used to your body decomposing and decaying because that is the truth, and if you can accept it, then you can get beyond it and start living.

"The object of walking is to relax the mind," Thomas Jefferson said, adding that "you should, therefore, not permit yourself even to think while you walk; but divert yourself by the objects that surround you."[*] Sounds to me like a Buddhist walking meditation.

Benefits

Some of the benefits of meditation include healing of the body, quieting of the mind, stimulating creativity and balance, and calmness. Many people find an enhanced sense of efficiency.

A Catholic nun I have worked with years ago gave me the book, *Miracle of Mindfulness,* by Thich Nhat Hanh. "Mindfulness is the miracle by which we master and restore ourselves," the author states. He

---

[*] Young, Dr. Tim. *The Way to Christ Technique of Meditation.* p. 126.

continues, "Mindfulness frees us of forgetfulness and dispersion and makes it possible to live fully each minute of life. Mindfulness enables us to live."[*]

How can one get started in meditation?

I would get a good book recommended below, or choose among many others. Just browse in your bookstore, health food store, or library. I would pick a type of meditation that suits you. Then just follow the directions as well as you can. Many meditation classes are offered through night schools, Hare Krishnas, and Buddhist centers. Look up meditation in your phone book or ask around.

Or just go ahead and try it on your own. Kathleen McDonald, an ordained Tibetan Buddhist nun, in her book, *How to Meditate: A Practical Guide*, has the following advice for beginners:

* In order to experience the benefits of meditation it is necessary to practice regularly.

* It is best to reserve a room or corner especially for your meditation sessions.

* It is good to start with one of the breathing meditations.

* In the beginning it is best to meditate for short periods—ten to thirty minutes, and end your sessions while mind and body are still comfortable and fresh.

* Mind and body should be relaxed and comfortable throughout the session.

* Have no expectations.

* You need a teacher.

* Don't advertise, referring to your breakthroughs. Meditation is to be practiced, not talked about.[†]

This is a really great book for the beginner and includes many meditations.

---

[*] Thich Nhat Hanh, *The Miracle of Mindfulness*, Boston, MA: Beacon Press, 1987, pp. 14, 15.
[†] Kathleen McDonald, *How to Meditate: A Practical Guide*. Boston, MA: Wisdom Publications, 1984.

One last thought: "It is through meditation that the bridge of communication is built between the unfolding human soul and the inner guide, the transpersonal self." *

Other suggested reading:

The Art of Meditation by Joel Goldsmith

Theory and Practice of Meditation, edited by Rudolph Ballentine

The Experience of Insight by Joseph Goldstein

Everyday Zen by Joko Beck

The Wisdom of No Escape by Pema Chodron

Cassette tapes
Write to the MA Center, P.O. Box 613, San Ramon, CA 94583 for a catalog. They have wonderful tapes including the *MA on Meditation* tape.

More Fun

The lifestyle I'm describing in this book—this way of life that I find is most fully exemplified by health food store employees—is fun and makes your life more interesting in every possible way. I cannot believe how much better I look, how much happier I am, and how much better I feel. First, I'm stopping at Wild Oats to get some soup makings and the next thing I know I am having my palms and eyes read, getting a massage, putting a pendulum over my fruit, and standing on my head every morning. I often have the most interesting conversation in the aisles with people with whom I otherwise would not know I have so much in common.

Many things can change and transform your life: a positive attitude, yoga, beneficial herbs, aromatherapy, bodywork, supplements, super foods, and meditation; now we are going to talk about a few more offbeat fun things you may want to investigate. There are many, many more, but I am limiting the list to things I have personally tried.

Astrology

This is a really fun way to gain insight into your innate qualities. I had my chart done by an astrologer in Boulder. Essentially, astrology uses a birth chart as a map of the positions of the planets, in relation to where

---

* Kroeger, *The Seven Spiritual Causes of Ill Health*, p. 126.

you were born, and the exact time. The chart uses the angular relationships of the planets and the different signs of the zodiac, where they fall in accordance to the chart, to decipher indicators to see different potentials in you as an individual.

It helps you to explore your own potentials and innate traits, and to see how the different facets of your personality are integrated. When I had mine done, I could more clearly see some of the quirks of my personality and the relationship between them and my life. It cost $80, but that was Boulder and the astrologer I saw is widely known and respected. It can be done for as little as $10 through the mail.

Palm reading

This was a lot of fun too. I had it done a few years ago out of the back of a coffee shop in North Denver. The guy was really good. I was in my mid-thirties at the time and he said my life was really going to start in my early forties. That was fun to think about and look forward to.

Tarot

I had this done quite recently and it wasn't that much fun for me because it scared me. It was the same guy who read my palm years ago. I had to go to the bookstore three times and ask different people about him in order to find him. I knew he did astrology and tarot, too, and I wanted to check out what the cards had in store for me.

I don't know if it was my age, 39, which makes people somewhat predictable in terms of the kind of things they are thinking about, such as life evaluation: Am I happy with my life? Where have I been for the entire first half of my life? Did I accomplish what I thought I might? What are my regrets? What are my hopes for the future? What changes do I need to make the difference? Forty is a big milestone, and no matter who you are, you are going to be asking yourself these kinds of questions.

The tarot reader knew my birthdate, and his best friend for the last twenty years, a woman, was born two days before me. So he may have just had me pegged. Even the things he may have been wrong about, he seemed so sure of that I tended to believe him instead of my own instinct. And let's not underestimate the obviousness of someone going to have their cards read anyway; it clearly states you are questioning things in your life.

But self-knowledge is an adventure. I intend to try more. How about you?

Positive Thinking

> Persistence is what makes the impossible possible, the possible likely, and the likely definite.
>
> —Robert Half

From Joe Griffith, *Speaker's Library of Business Stories, Anecdotes and Humor* (Englewood Cliffs, NJ: Prentice-Hall), comes the following information:

✳ R. H. Macy failed seven times before his store in New York succeeded.

✳ Novelist John Creasey got 753 rejection slips before he published the first of his 564 books.

✳ Thomas Edison was thrown out of school in the early grades when the teachers decided he could not do the work.

✳ Harry S. Truman failed as a haberdasher.

✳ When Bob Dylan performed at a high school talent show, his classmates booed him off the stage. [I don't find that one so hard to believe.]

✳ W. Clement Stone, successful insurance company executive and founder of *Success* magazine, was a high school dropout.

I was kicked out of high school so many times that I was too embarrassed to return.

Inspirational writer Charles Swindoll tells us, "Courage is not limited to the battlefield or the Indianapolis 500 or bravely catching a thief in your house. The real tests of courage are much quieter. They are the inner tests, like remaining faithful when nobody's looking, like enduring pain when the room is empty, like standing alone when you're misunderstood."

Billy Wilder recommends that you "trust your instincts. Your mistakes might as well be your own, instead of someone else's."

You will not succeed at anything in life without a positive attitude. Pessimists may be right more of the time, but optimists enjoy life more of the time. Maybe I am just blessed or lucky, but I just can't stand to be miserable. If something sad happens to me, I get depressed and cry, but then I try to find a method or mechanism to deal with it. Because I can't stand to be unhappy, I am not that much of the time. When something goes wrong, no matter how badly, I keep working to find the silver lining.

When my parents were in the automobile accident in which my dad died, I was sitting in the airport, waiting for my connecting plane. There were several airport employees just getting off work having a beer, laughing, carrying on, and telling jokes. They were all young men in their early twenties, and at first I thought to myself, "What the hell are you all so happy about? What is there to laugh and giggle about? I hate life."

I continued in my misery giving them all an unnoticed dirty look. After observing about five minutes of their constant good humor, it dawned on me that half of them probably didn't even have a father, or one that lived in the home when they were children. I know several kids in their twenties who have never even met their fathers. I thought that despite my dad's shortcomings, he was there; he did love me very much, and I knew him like the back of my hand. Even though I never applauded my dad's methods of parenting, he had taught me most of the important lessons in life.

Then I thought that I had my dad until I was 35 years old. Averaging out how many years I had him, I was doing better than most people in America. So I started to focus on how lucky I was to have a father at all, much less one who truly loved me. My whole attitude changed. I am going to miss him, but I am damn lucky to have ever had him at all.

There are so many great books and classes in positive thinking I don't think I have to elaborate. I recommend Dale Carnegie's public speaking class as well as all of his books. Check your library and bookstore for others.

Quitting Smoking

If you are interested in quitting smoking, I will share with you what worked for me. I smoked for a long time, first with my friends on the railroad tracks that we would walk down to get to our junior high school, and then until my late thirties.

I know and understand your plight. One of my customers said, "Smoking is like romancing yourself." It's true. It's taking time out several times a day to be with yourself. There is a certain charm to that. However, taking a few minutes to meditate, read, or get up and get a clean, cool glass of water is also very satisfying. My biggest problem with giving cigarettes up was that it was like they were my little friends. They were always there when I needed them. But then I figured out I don't have time for them anymore with all the positive things I have going in my life.

Smokers have it really rough right now in America; it is perfectly acceptable in most people's minds to be rude and comment on your smoking even if you never light up in front of them. I find it amazing that people who usually try to be kind and considerate think it's perfectly okay to go right up to a perfect stranger and reprimand him or her on this habit. Someone once said to me, "It is such a bad habit." And I thought to myself, smoking is not nearly as bad a habit as the need to tell other people how to conduct their lives.

How to quit

Step one

Begin right now to forgive yourself for this habit. If you catch yourself reprimanding yourself for smoking, just say, "I am going to enjoy this cigarette, every puff." Inhale and enjoy. I know this sounds a little like you may start enjoying your cigarettes more, and therefore start smoking more, but that is not the case. What it does do is improve your relationship with yourself, help you feel better about yourself, and allow you to be more accepting of yourself. Just try it; you've probably tried everything else.

Step two

Stop smoking in one domain of your life that will be fairly easy for you not to smoke. For example, I first stopped smoking in my office years ago. If I wanted a cigarette, I just went out and smoked one, but I broke the habit of smoking wherever or whenever I wanted.

Step three

Employ the Lily Method. Look over the list of fun and positive things to do and start bringing them into your life: yoga, walking, swimming, hot springs, baths, herbal teas, etc. As one becomes a natural part of your life, pick another one.

Step four

Whenever you want a cigarette, instead of just reaching for one, first take five deep breaths; hold them each for five seconds, and then blow them out.

Step five
Eat a piece of fruit to replace one important cigarette in your day; for example, if you smoke everyday on your way home from work, eat an apple instead.

Step six
Hang out in health food stores. Do shots of wheat grass and try smoothies. Check out all the homeopathic and herbal tinctures to quit smoking. Buy some teas to help your cravings. Buy some licorice root sticks and start chewing on them. Buy some herbal cigarettes and start replacing your old cigarettes with those. Talk to the people in the natural living department to get more ideas. Drink eight glasses of purified water a day.

Step seven
After you have stopped smoking in one place for at least a month, pick another place not to smoke; for example only smoke in one room in your house or go outside. Or quit smoking in your car entirely.

Step eight
Go for a short walk after all meals.

Step nine
Begin working out, walking, or doing yoga and meditation daily, even if only for ten minutes.

How I quit

One day at home, very soon after my return from a vacation in Belize, I was doing my daily yoga first thing in the morning. When I went to take a deep breath, I had a little trouble. Now that had happened a thousand times before, but it just came to me in the middle of a yoga pose that I was no longer going to smoke.

It's funny; all of a sudden after over twenty years, no more! Now I say it was all of a sudden, but in reality I had been taking the positive steps for a very long time. I had quit smoking in my office several years ago, I had quit smoking in my car, I had quit smoking with my morning coffee, and I had brought all the positive things into my life that I describe throughout this book.

I never said to anyone that I was going to quit. I never sat there and took a drag and said how I really need to quit. I either smoked and enjoyed it or put more positive things in its place; finally, the positive things took precedence.

That is really the bottom line for you, too. Simply put so many positive things in your life that you no longer have the time or desire to smoke.

Yes, I still think about taking a puff here and there, but essentially my desire not to smoke is stronger than my desire to smoke. It would be very difficult to do everything I do in a day and still find the time to smoke.

A friend of mine who stopped smoking before I did said, "I don't look at not smoking as a sacrifice, or as something I can no longer have, or as a desire I don't get to fulfill. I look at it as a gift to myself, my lungs, and my health."

I often still think of that comment she made if I ever feel like having a cigarette. The desire to be healthy outweighs my desire to smoke.

All in time

To quit smoking, your overall desire to love and take care of yourself must override your temporary desire for instant gratification, and this takes time to develop. When I smoked, I really was hurt by and resented people telling me I should quit. If you really want to help someone quit, love them unconditionally and give up your need to tell them what to do. Smoking is an addiction. Cigarettes, the little friends the smoker can always count on to be there, are hard to give up. So let your friends smoke without the extra burden and stress of your judgments. People need to do what they need to do. Everybody is doing the best they can. To add more negativity to the smoking experience is truly causing the smoker more damage and anxiety that just reinforces their dependency on the cigarette.

I really appreciated my family for never nagging at me for my smoking. Thanks, Mom. Nobody really smoked in my family. My dad had given up cigars years ago, and his pipe long before that. One of my brothers would smoke occasionally. Even though my mom and sister were seriously into healthy lifestyles, when we dined out they would always tell the hostess to seat us in the smoking section so I could smoke. My sister would always warn, "Don't suck any negativity down with that cigarette."

My dad had pulmonary problems the last decade of his life, and because of his sort of sad reaction to my smoking, I just couldn't bring myself to light up in front of him. If did light up, he wouldn't say anything, but he would look at me and lower his eyes with a sorrowful expression on his face. I could read his mind; he wanted to reach out and help me avoid the physical pain that he was suffering from long-term smoking, but he would never really say anything. I knew what he was thinking and I couldn't bear to see that look on his face, so I stopped smoking in front of him years before I ever totally quit, to ease his pain and my guilt.

Preventing mood swings

I quit smoking for five days about a year before I really quit for good. I noticed how much emotional upheaval it caused. I was mad at a lot of people, and everything upset me. I don't think it was only the withdrawal; it was not having those little friends to light up. Not smoking had left a space where I could see the unrest and the anxiety that was underneath the surface of my life.

Joko Beck says in her book, *Nothing Special,*[*] that if any of us looks beyond the surface of our life, we find discontent, unrest, and anxiety. She says we keep ourselves busy with work, friends, drinking, exercise, travel, food, drama, drugs, and smoking, and just about anything not to have to face that unrest below what appears to be our lives.

This is why meditation and mindfulness are so fundamentally important. Do we have any idea who we are? Do we know why we do what we do? Do we dare face ourselves? Our lives are made up of our thoughts and our thoughts manifest our lives. Therefore, it is pretty important to witness and understand what goes on in our heads.

My mom states that there only two motivations in life, love and fear, so if you're not operating from one, you are operating from the other. I understand we are still talking about smoking. Smoking is deep-seated. It is a beautiful little vacation from your life twenty times a day. To really quit and not replace smoking with another addiction like food, we need to look deeply inside ourselves.

The most effective way to quit smoking forever and not to gain weight is to quit logically, mindfully, to look into why you smoke to begin with, and to implement positive lifestyle changes to ensure your success. I did not gain one pound when I quit. Instead, I lost weight because I was working out and walking instead of sitting around puffing. I was busy riding my bike, doing yoga, and journal writing. I didn't give up anything; I gained great health, breath, and freedom from an addiction.

If you start the Lily Method of bringing these healthful things into your life—yoga, meditation, reaching for a refreshingly crisp apple,

---

[*] Charlotte Joko Beck, *Nothing Special: Living Zen*, New York: Harper San Francisco Publishers, 1993.

hanging out in health food stores, going for long walks—sooner or later you will no longer need the cigarettes in your life.

Be good to yourself and good luck.

Further information
You can call the American Lung Association at (800) 586-4872 to get further information on quitting smoking.

Relaxing

What's missing in an overly stressful life is peace. Here are some words of wisdom to guide us:

> *Peace is a quality of the soul. It fills the pure heart. Peace is in the heart of a desireless person who has controlled the senses and the mind.*
>
> —Swami Sivananda

> *Touch the earth, love the earth, honor the earth, her plains, her valleys, her hills, and her seas; rest your spirit in her solitary places.*
>
> —Henry Beston

> *Earth laughs in flowers.*
>
> —Ralph Waldo Emerson

> *O, see a world in a grain of sand, and heaven in a wild flower.*
>
> —William Blake

> *Why are wildflowers so important to those of us who care at all for flowers? For me, anyway, it is because they come like gifts from God (or Nature), and to encounter them in their natural habitat is an extraordinary aesthetic pleasure.*
>
> —Katharine S. White

Natural de-stressers
Many herbs are natural de-stressers which can help you relax. I prefer a couple cups of chamomile tea, but you can also try any of these herbs in tea, tincture, or capsule form to relax: valerian, kava kava, St. John's wort, or lemon balm.

Personal de-stressing techniques

When driving around the Denver-Metro area, which has become increasingly more stressful, I first of all recognize that it is going to take me twice as long to get to my destination as I think. Therefore, I always give myself plenty of time to get to where I am going, allowing time for accidents, traffic jams, overturned tractor trailers, police-blocked areas, and the like.

Second, I acknowledge that I am going to be sitting for some time, so I plan to meditate (not too deeply) or give an idea thoughtful consideration during that time.

Third, I carry gum, our Lily moisture mist to spritz myself, lip balm, and an herbal moisturizer to apply during down time.

Fourth, I have a set of prayer beads that were made by Buddhist monks in Sarnath, India, which I purchased while I was there. They dangle from my rearview mirror, always reminding me not to get upset. They really seem to work. When a friend of mine was recently driving my car he said, "Do you mind if I take down these beads?" I said, "Oh, no, they must be there." Ever since I have placed them there, I have not been upset while driving, nor have I been in a car accident. One year I was in four, so I feel like they are bringing me the added bonus of good luck, as well as the benefit of mindfulness.

I used to be one of those persons who, if you pulled out in front of me, would yell swear words at you, loud enough so you could hear them. My new gauge of unacceptable stress and frustration is if I ever start swearing when I am driving my car, I know I am too uptight and need to do some serious relaxing.

To reduce stress

If you feel stressed, mix one or all of these essential oils in almond oil and inhale often: bergamot, jasmine, lavender, marjoram, melissa, patchouli, rosemary, sandalwood, and ylang ylang.

When you are emotionally weary, add these to your bath: lavender, neroli, rose, rosemary, sandalwood, ylang ylang, and thyme.

Homespa

Try the Lily Homespa also known as the Lily Goddess Kit (see below).

Creator of all,
Who made me for happiness,
Let my cares drain from me.
Let me spend these moments luxuriating
In the awareness of Your Divine Love.

My mother wrote this prayer for our Lily of Colorado Homespa. The Homespa is a wonderful pre-packaged, everything-you-need-to-do-at-home-spa product. It includes very specific, step-by-step instructions to take a two-hour retreat of relaxation in your own home. You can do the same thing at home with your own freshly made products. (Recipes are included in this book.)

At the time of this writing, to my knowledge, no one else has ever come up with or copied this idea. I must say it is one of my best ones ever. I love it! It is so needed in our crazy, hectic world. After completing our Homespa, you will feel like a different person—calm, relaxed, elevated. I cannot believe the life-changing effect this two-hour program can have on your life. If you fall into any of the following categories, I urge you to take a two-hour retreat in your own home. Just make sure you have everything below to go through every step, and remember to do it mindfully.

The Homespa is for people who are:

- Stressed
- Overworked
- Getting married
- Getting divorced
- Needing balance
- Needing to slow down
- Expectant mothers

- New mothers
- Suffering a loss
- Enduring PMS
- Chronically fatigued
- Starting a new job
- Still stuck at the old job
- In need of life improvement

Preparing for your homespa

First, gather the products you will need for the spa. Our Homespa includes:

- Cleanser
- Toner
- Cotton balls
- Lotion
- Cream
- Incense
- Bath oil
- Candle

- Herbal moisturizer
- Herbs for facial steam
- Herbal eye toning pads
- Hot-oil hair treatment
- Botanical enzyme exfoliant mask
- Relaxing tea
- Meditations

Then, just follow this step-by-step process, which is a copy of the instructions my mom wrote for our Lily of Colorado Homespa:

Step one
Block out a minimum of two hours where you can be completely alone and undisturbed. Lock the doors. Disconnect the phone. Play soft, soothing music—begin to recognize the healing power of silence.

Step two
Cleanse your face with Lily Facial Cleanser (also great for all over your body in place of soap). Treasure the silence, knowing wonderful things happen in silence—seeds germinate, flowers bloom, the body repairs itself.

Step three
Apply Lily Astringent/Toner with a cotton ball to remove any residue of soap or cosmetics.

Step four
Apply Herbal Moisturizer to dry areas of your face, around eyes and mouth. Smile happily as you work around your mouth, knowing that simply by smiling you relax hundreds of facial muscles.

Step five
Boil two quarts of distilled water in a non-aluminum pan. Take one cup of boiling water to steep one tea bag. Use the rest of the water to steep the herbs for your steam facial. Put the herbs in the pan and heat for five minutes. Turn off the heat. Place a towel over your head so it covers the pan also. Breathe in, completely relaxing your whole body. As you inhale, mentally bless the plants which are now imparting to you their healing essences. Use Toner/Astringent again on a cotton ball to remove residue from the steaming. Strain herbs and add the remaining water to your bath.

Step six
Choose a pleasant spot and sit comfortably with your cup of tea. Relax and be mindful of drinking your tea. Allow everything to flow from your mind, setting it adrift. If any concerns or cares intrude, let them float off like wispy clouds, out of your consciousness.

Step seven
Prepare for your bath. Apply Oil of Kukui lightly to your dry hair and wrap in a heated towel.

Step eight
Put Seven Exotic Oils in the running bathwater. See the rushing water as blessings being showered your way.

Step nine
Step mindfully into your bath. Apply Botanical Exfoliant Mask to your face and neck, while asking for—and expecting—greater wisdom in handling your everyday life situations.

Step ten
Hold the two remaining tea bags briefly under cold water. Lie back in the tub and apply them to your closed eyes. As you relax in the warm water, repeatedly bless these eyes that give you the gift of sight: the ability to see a star-studded sky, an orchard in full bloom, the majesty of mountains, the face of a loved one.

Step eleven
Sit back and relax for at least thirty glorious minutes. Enjoy each moment of the gift of silence and solitude you are giving yourself. Take pleasure in seeing yourself in your mind's eye as the perfection you are meant to be. Silently, within, you might ask:

———⊱•⊰———

Creator of all,
Who made me for happiness,
Let my cares drain from me.
Let me spend these moments luxuriating
In the awareness of Your Divine Love.

———⊱•⊰———

Step twelve
Gently rinse off. Wash your hair with shampoo and conditioner as usual. Towel dry. While you gently dry yourself, observe the water draining out of the tub, seeing in your mind's eye the stresses, concerns, and negativity being carried down the drain and out of your life.

Step thirteen
Lovingly apply Lily Facial Lotion to your moist face. In this quietude, in this serenity that you are creating, know that ideas, inspirations, and solutions come through to you more easily.

Step fourteen
Apply Lily Moisturizing Cream to your entire body, caressingly. As you spread the cream over your skin, consider this largest of the body's organs. Give thought to the muscles, nerves, bones, and blood vessels hidden beneath it which silently, constantly work so effectively to serve you.

Step fifteen
Quietly and comfortably enjoy another cup of tea, realizing how much pleasure there can be in simple things. Make a mental note of the way you feel so that in the future, whenever you wish, you can recapture this sense of well-being.

Step sixteen
Light the candle and the incense. Consider the flame and ponder the many meanings of light: inspiration, ideas, and understanding. Consider the sense of smell and how seldom we think of what a gift it is. Become more grateful for the gifts in your life, and for the gift of life itself.

Step seventeen
When it is comfortable for you, bring yourself back to "reality." Ask your body and brain to step up the tempo (but not too much!), to sharpen your awareness, to prepare you to step back into your "normal world," but in a better space, a quieter, more confident place, allowing you to live more mindfully in each present moment. Welcome back to your world this kinder you, this stronger you, this refreshed, rejuvenated, more patient, wiser, more loving and more mindful you.

Respite from an over-busy world
If you gather these items and follow these instructions you are going to benefit greatly; I personally guarantee it. It is only two hours. I urge you to give yourself this small, yet powerful gift.

So many women say they do not have time, and I understand. People in this country are running their lives at such a frantic pace, many because they have to; it takes moving quickly and swiftly all day every day to get it all done. But you know as well as I do that if you are not having some quiet time, some balance, you start operating on two out of eight cylinders. Like a car, you become inefficient, ineffective, and often times, stall or even go in reverse.

When you don't take a little time for your own peace of mind, you can become irritable and downright mean-spirited, harming yourself and others, even wreaking havoc. Think about it. You make bad decisions and poor judgments that can cost you weeks or months of time, all because you didn't give yourself a two-hour break. Truly think about it. Now mark down the two hours in your daytimer, call your husband, sister, neighbor, or friend to take the kids, gather the needed items, and give yourself a happy break.

Stress

A great deal has been written about stress because it is now recognized not only as a cause of illness and dis-ease, but as an actual killer. That being the case, I'll just make a list of helpful suggestions. You can read more in depth elsewhere.

* Change your attitude—it's not what happens as much as the way we react.

* Avoid being too attached to an outcome, or too determined to produce a particular one.

* Think positive.

* Recall a success and go over it in your mind.

* Use affirmations.

* Take slow, deep breaths.

* Stretch.

* Get a massage.

* Meditate.

* Chant.

* Pray.

* Massage your temples.

* Move around, go for a walk.

* Listen to music, dance.

* Listen to relaxation tapes.

* Lie down and stare at the ceiling or at the sky.

* Kiss someone you love.

* Write an old friend.

* Turn off your TV.

* Sit by a lake.

* Sit under a beautiful tree.

* Write in your journal the problem and solution.

* Have a cup of kava kava or chamomile tea.

Many have found the following essential oils to be helpful in reducing stress:

* Eucalyptus
* Yarrow
* Nutmeg
* Lemon
* Sandalwood
* Frankincense

* Lavender
* Melissa
* Ylang ylang
* Jasmine
* Bergamot
* Geranium

Ylang ylang is my favorite anti-depressant. I use it in my mist, cream for dry skin, and lotion for combination skin. When I put it on, I literally see nearby people's faces light up. My second favorite is lavender, and I like to blend equal parts of the two of them.

Use these two essential oils, diluted with almond oil, and apply directly to the skin or put in a bath.

Retreats

My mom's definition of a retreat is to "get away from your ordinary life and seek the importance of things of the soul."

She used to take us to retreats when we were kids. They always included "hootenannies," enthusiastic group singing, and guitar playing. Of course, I thought they were goofy, but there were often other kids my age, 11–14, that thought the same thing so we could stand around outside and hang out. The retreats were usually in conjunction with the Catholic Church.

Mom had many other fun-filled ideas for our entertainment. She coined the word "hootabanny," which referred to a hootenanny plus making banners in a group for the church.

My mom has been going to retreats most of my life. Now, she goes more than ever, traveling at the drop of a hat to attend weekend retreats from God-Mind Connection to Native American prophesy retreats where non–Native Americans are welcome.

My retreat experience—Shoshoni Yoga Retreat

Living in Colorado so close to Boulder makes going to retreats an easy affair. However, I have only been on one real retreat. It was at the Shoshoni Yoga Retreat Center in Rollinsville, Colorado, near Nederland, which is just above Boulder.

The Shoshoni Center is very comfortable, although the housing is in log cabins. It has 210 acres of beautiful, tree-covered mountain land. There is a meditation hall, a main lodge that includes a family-style dining room, a sauna, and a wonderful large deck with a hot tub.

I went up in the middle of winter when the entire ground was covered in snow. Once there, I was welcomed by a hospitable and kind woman. The first thing I noticed after she showed me my quarters was how quiet it was. There is absolutely no sound. That in itself is refreshing; along with the cold, clean, crisp mountain air, it was heavenly.

I was only there 24 hours attending yoga and meditation classes, but I was completely relaxed afterward. Shoshoni has a daily schedule of meditation and yoga classes, but you can go to as many or as few as you want. Also, it serves gourmet vegetarian food that is truly a delight to the palate.

On Sunday afternoons from 1:30 to 4:30 P.M., you can go to Shoshoni for a free afternoon program that includes chanting and meditation followed by refreshments and a question and answer period.

Shambhava School of Yoga

The same group that runs Shoshoni runs the Shambhava School of Yoga, which offers a teacher training program and the Eldorado Mountain Yoga Ashram, and also has yoga and meditation classes. The ashram has a Community Night every Monday that includes chanting, meditation, satsang (a spiritual lecture), and dinner from 6:30 to 8:30 P.M. It also offers a Saturday retreat that includes yoga, meditation, devotional chanting, and a delicious vegetarian lunch for $20. The guru writes a newsletter and has written many books. You can reach these ashrams by contacting:

Shoshoni Retreat Center
P.O. Box 410
Rollinsville, CO 80474
(303) 642-0116

or

Eldorado Mountain Yoga Ashram
P.O. Box 306
Eldorado Springs, CO 80025
(303) 494-3051

Rocky Mountain Shambhala Center

The Rocky Mountain Shambhala Center—which is part of the Shambhala Center in Boulder, founded by Chogyam Trungpa Rinpoche, and is now run by Sakyong Mipham Rinpoche—is located near Fort Collins, Colorado.

It has a more individualistic approach to retreats "in which you individually conduct your practice according to techniques you have already learned." It also hosts many meditation teachers for specific programs.

There are isolated cabins where you bring and cook your own food, or the retreat has what it calls "in-house" retreats where you eat meals in the main dining room with the rest of the guests and staff. The cost is only $25 to $30 a day. The Shambhala requires that you practice meditation at least six hours a day. Contact:

Rocky Mountain Shambhala Center
4921 County Road 68C
Red Feather Lakes, CO 80545-9505
(970) 881-2184
fax (970) 881-2909
Denver/Boulder Metro line (303) 466-1897
email 75347.52@compuserve.com

Sivananda Yoga Retreat

One of the retreats I have wanted to do for a long time is the Sivananda Ashram Yoga Retreat on Paradise Island, Nassau, Bahamas. It is on the beach, has a strict schedule beginning at 4:30 A.M., and includes two meditations, chanting, yoga, and breathing classes per day, plus a lecture, free time, and three vegetarian meals—all for about $35 each day.

Other retreats

Some other interesting retreats I have heard about include:

Mind/Body Caribbean Cruise. They have lectures on board and gourmet vegan cuisine. Call the Inner Voyage at (800) 546-7871.

Plum Village, Meyrac, Loubes-Bernac
47120 Duras, France
Tel: 010 33 53 947540

San Francisco Zen Center
300 Page Street
San Francisco, CA 94102
(415) 863-3136

The following places offer many classes, workshops and retreats. To get their catalogs contact them directly:

Omega Institute
260 Lake Drive
Rhinebeck, NY 12572
(914) 266-4444

Lama Foundation
P.O. Box 240
San Cristobal, NM 87564
(505) 586-1269

Breitenbush Hot Springs Retreat Center
P.O. Box 578
Detroit, OR 97342

Harbin Hot Springs
P.O. Box 782
Middletown, CA 95461
(707) 987-2477

Recommended sources

The best book I have found on the subject is *Retreat: Time Apart for Silence and Solitude* by Roger Housden. It gives clear descriptions of many different kinds of retreats divided into categories from Buddhist to Christian to wilderness to art retreats. It's wonderful, complete with photographs.

Another reference is:

Jean K. Foster
Team Up (The God-Mind Connection)
Box 1115
Warrensburg, MO 64093

Ask for information on retreats and her several books.

Rolfing

Rolfing can be defined as structural integration. A central premise is that the aligned body can balance itself better against gravity and is therefore more efficient. Human functions such as flexibility, coordination, and physiological conditions are improved when each individual segment of the body is aligned. This can be compared to a child's tower of blocks, which is more stable when each block is placed squarely upon the one below it. Rolfing re-establishes this vital balance by stretching the fascia tissue, which is a thin elastic membrane that covers muscles, bones, organs, and nerves.

This structural integration, or rolfing, is systematic in its approach; you go for a series of ten weekly, progressive treatments. The realigning of the body is through manipulation of the connective tissues. Working these connective tissues, known as the myofascial system, the support system of the body, benefits the entire body.

Tension-releasing

A major theory in rolfing is that everything you have ever done, thought, felt, or lived is stored in the tissues of the body. This includes every trauma, negative event, and injury. Patterns of stress and strain are kept in the tissues and cause them to be hard and weak, blocking the energy flow through the body. This can cause chronic fatigue, pain, and stiffness. Rolfing attempts to release the muscles or tissues that hold tensions.

Negative emotions are stored in the very cells of the body. Because each cell has its own intelligence and stores emotional trauma, rolfing can release each cell's memory. Rolfing opens up the areas where life experiences have accumulated, allowing the body to let them go and heal.

My personal experience

I had read and thought about rolfing for a very long time. After seeing a chiropractor almost weekly and massage therapists once a month for years, I thought I'd try rolfing. I was hoping for a treatment that might provide me with longer-lasting effects.

I called the Rolfing Institute in Boulder and was faxed a list of rolfers. I called several and mostly got voice mail or answering machines, but a nice receptionist at the Wellness Center explained rolfing to me as well as different traumas and situations it could help. She told me the Center had a great rolfer named Teresa.

Teresa promptly phoned me back and we spoke for quite some time. I asked her what rolfing was and how it differed from massage. Massage was a wonderful experience, she said, but rolfing provided better results for recurring problems. She used to be a massage therapist but found rolfing much more rewarding for her patients. Rolfing, she continued, could give me more flexibility, increased energy flow, relief from chronic pain, and make me look and feel better about myself. "I'm sold," I told her. "I wouldn't be devoting my life to this if I didn't think it could truly heal and help people," she replied.

Emotions

"There is an emotional side to rolfing," she warned. As the rolfer touches certain spots that may harbor pain from particular events, those events often come up and to mind. Teresa said it was important to fully recognize and acknowledge the pain, let go, and release that particular tension. Psychotherapists recommend rolfing because people can get things intellectually, and intellectually they know they should let things go, but because they hold this tension in the very cells of their bodies, they need the actual physical release to aid in complete closure and healing.

Teresa has a sincere healing quality in her practice. She was genuinely concerned and wanted to be helpful without being intrusive or judgmental. She also wanted to make sure the therapy was working for me and that I had the direct benefits of the treatment.

I immediately felt good in her hands. I felt her very capable and knowledgeable. We talked a lot during the first treatment, mostly about my troubles of the week. Twice I'd said, "Oh, let's talk about something more positive than car and motorcycle accidents, cancer and cramps, incarceration of friends and frustration," but negative subjects and events kept coming up. Not in a negative way though; it was just a discussion and sharing about our lives.

The first treatment went very well. While she was working on my back and shoulders, opening up my lungs, it felt like a massage. I wasn't sure, though, that it was going to be what she had promised. After I left her office, I noticed I felt pretty good and that it stayed with me through the evening. My breathing seemed a little deeper, a little better.

The next morning, however, I felt really good doing my yoga. Two years earlier, I had stopped doing the plow position daily because I was concerned it was hurting my neck. But I could do the plow better than ever. I couldn't believe it! I just slid right into it, perfectly. I was definitely a fan of rolfing.

Teresa and I engaged in such interesting conversations during the next several sessions that I sometimes was paying almost no attention to what was really going on specifically in my body. After the third or fourth session, I was driving my car to work down a country road by my house, and all of a sudden a couple things I did 30 years ago came to my mind. They were painful memories: two different events where I had hurt others. Both incidents came to my mind all of a sudden, apparently out of nowhere, simultaneously. The mere thought of these two events caused me discomfort and discontent. I knew they had resurfaced from the rolfing, but I also knew I had to take another look at them before I could forgive myself and let them go for good.

The pain

Over my ten weeks of rolfing, I cried a lot, and easily. I cried for my own pain, and for the pain I had caused others. After the belly and stomach session, I felt like I had a direct connection with and could tap into all the pain of the universe. This came after a friend at Ambrosia Health Foods in Pueblo, Colorado (one of my all-time favorite health food stores) was asking me about the rolfing. I told him I was preparing for the stomach area session. "Wow, that's going to be powerful," he said, "since your belly is your connection to the universe, because of the umbilical cord." I thought that made sense. I don't know if it was the power of suggestion or what, but I felt that powerful link for quite a while.

Two of my first four sessions, I walked into my rolfer's office very uptight, very stressed, and the two other times I had terrible pain in my neck and back. One session, she just worked on my feet and legs, but when she was finished my whole body felt better. Every time I left her office, I would walk to my car thinking, "Yes, life is good," feeling free, easy, and relaxed.

I am not sure if I felt good because I liked Teresa, the benefits of our stimulating yet therapeutic discussions, or the physical rolfing itself, but I knew I was going through something and was going to be better off when I reached the other end.

The sixth session

The sixth session was euphoric. She did my lower and middle back, and the back of my feet and legs. Again we talked about me, my problems, and what was surfacing emotionally during the sessions. I have a scar on my left thigh where I had 60 stitches from a bike accident when I was eleven or twelve years old. I can never stand for anyone to even whisk by it, let alone to touch it. Teresa touched it gently and immediately I braced myself. My whole body tightened up. The accident, the stitches, my mom and Aunt Helene rushing me to the hospital, the recollection of my mom having said to me for years, "Always wear your nicest underwear; you never know when you'll be in an accident," meeting the good-looking doctor in the emergency room—all these thoughts came rushing into my mind. I became convinced: every tissue in your body *does* hold memories, physical and emotional pain. When those tissues are touched, the memories arise.

I left the sixth session giddy. I was in such a good mood that I was walking on air. By the tenth session, not only was I feeling great, I felt like a lot of junk had been purged, and even a lot of the more confusing things that are an inherent part of my emotional makeup had been dealt with. Teresa and I celebrated at an Indian restaurant.

A high recommendation

Yes, I highly recommend rolfing. A lot of the benefit may come from a skilled practitioner, or it may come from the sense of security you feel from building a trusting relationship with a person you can dump your emotional baggage on. It is an emotional process and a rolfer should encourage you to talk about what comes up when he or she touches those places that do seem, indeed, to hold emotional trauma.

The fact that rolfing is ten weeks in a row may be an important reason why it is so life changing. I thought it beneficial to set the same time every week, making it a part of my cycle. It also saved me the hassle of scheduling. Plus I find I don't need to go to my chiropractor nearly as often.

For further information contact:

The Rolf Institute
205 Canyon Blvd
Boulder, CO 80302
(303) 449-5903
www.rolf.org

Sleep

> Sleep that knits up the ravell'd sleave of care. . . .
> —William Shakespeare, *MacBeth*

To look and feel good, consistent, restful, and sound sleep is essential. Sleep has many benefits not only for your looks, but for your overall health, not to mention disposition. But you already know that, so I am not going to elaborate about it.

To have optimum health, I believe you need a good night's sleep every night of your life, but I must admit, I have spent many a night not sleeping at all. In those cases, I always make a deliberate decision that staying up all night is worth more than the cost. But 355 days of the year, I go to bed and get six to eight hours of sleep. Six out of seven nights a week, I go to bed at the same time.

Benefits of sleep

Sleep is absolutely necessary for you to feel rejuvenated. It is necessary for maintaining emotional balance, good health, and to look good. You must have sleep for harmony in your body. Physical exercise, essentially physical exhaustion, is a good remedy for sleeplessness. Walk, ride a bicycle, run, work out. It's important to tire yourself out physically, especially if your mind is "working out" and spinning full time. Stress is held in the large muscles, and one must first *use* the muscles to be able to release the tension in them.

I never had trouble sleeping until I started my own businesses. Ever since, I have problems off and on. When I first started the nonprofit charitable organization to assist Denver's elderly in need, I began to have sleepless nights filled with worry of how I could keep the doors open and make payroll. I'd put my head on the pillow, and my mind would start whirling with all the problems of that day and the next.

A remedy for sleeplessness

So I thought, "I'll start reading before I go to bed." Thomas Jefferson said he never went to bed without the "reading of something moral, whereon to ruminate in the intervals of sleep." Reading really helped refocus my mind, but I read interesting books and novels on subjects I really enjoyed, so I stayed up late and missed sleep from reading, too!

Then I bought a copy of Dostoyevsky's *Crime and Punishment*. That did the trick, unless I was *really* stressed. Two pages maximum and I would be out. It takes so long to try to figure out those Russian names and follow who is whom, that between the confusion and then boredom it was easy to fall asleep.

Inviting sleep

Rituals are important. Try meditating, yoga, reading, herb teas, and tinctures when time for sleep approaches. Following a regular bedtime routine gives your body and mind a gentle alert that soon it will be time to completely relax and slip into slumber.

Make a tea of:

$1/2$ ounce peppermint leaves

$1/2$ ounce rosemary leaves

$1/2$ ounce sage leaves.

Add honey; sip and relax.

Dancing Willow Herbs, a company in Durango, Colorado, (888) 247-1654, puts out a catalog of products including a tea called Peaceful Slumber that you may want to try. It contains hops, chamomile, lemon balm, passion flower, and valerian.

Sleep pillows

Make a sleep pillow of lavender, hops, and mugwort. The lavender is relaxing and smells wonderful. The hops are a sedative, and mugwort helps you remember your dreams. You should only make your own or only use one made by a good friend, because just like food (see next paragraph), negative "vibes" can be transferred into the herbs and then into the pillow and ultimately into your body and psyche. Vibrations are everywhere and they can be transferred.

The first time I ever heard of the transfer of vibes was from my sister. Years ago, she was going to the ashram to do volunteer work. I asked her what she did there and she said she cooked. She stated how she was privileged to be chosen to be one of the cooks. My brother and I laughed and thought, "Yeah, well, we'll honor you and allow you to cook for us, too." But like so many other things I used to laugh about, I understand now and do believe.

You know vibrations exist. You cannot deny it. When you walk into a room or a party, you pick up on the tone of the place through the vibrations. Choose then, through herbs and oils, which kinds of vibes you desire in your sleep pillow. Take two pieces of three to six-inch square cloths, sew together, and fill with the herb(s) of your choice.

Face up

Sleep face up and save your good looks. Sleeping night after night with your face squished against the pillow can really make you look older. When your skin is smashed against the pillow, it can give you early, undeserved lines. Also, fluids can accumulate in the under-eye area, making you look puffy and tired in the morning.

Other thoughts on sleep

* Insomnia can be related to or a direct cause of an emotional problem, indicating an imbalance.

* Alcohol can interrupt sleep.

* Long hot baths with essential oils of lavender and ylang ylang promote relaxation and sleep.

* Homeopathic remedies can help relieve sleeplessness.

* Herbs such as valerian, skullcap, chamomile, hops, blue vervain, wild lettuce, and passion flower have long traditions for inducing sleep.

* Calcium, magnesium, inositol, niacinamide, and biotin have all been recommended for sleep.

* Biofeedback, visualizations, meditation, hypnotherapy, and acupuncture can all help.

* Essential oils to aid sleep include bergamot, lavender, neroli, marjoram, chamomile, rose, sandalwood, verbena, and ylang ylang.

Richard Shane, author of several books about sleep, believes that falling asleep is a spiritual process and that we must let go with trust to go to a place we don't know. Give this a thought at the end of your sleep-inviting routine or ritual. Sleep well!

The Sun and Sunscreens

The sun is my almighty physician.

—Thomas Jefferson

Have we Americans got it backwards? Is it possible that natural sunlight is good for us and that chemical sunscreens and avoidance of the sun are bad for us? You decide.

The energy of plants and all life depends on the absorption of sunlight. Jacob Liberman, in his book, *Light—Medicine of the Future*, states that not only is the sun good for you, it is downright therapeutic. He further points out that it is the chemical sunscreens, fluorescent lighting, and indoor lifestyle that could be detrimental to our health.

According to Dr. Liberman, ultraviolet or UV light lowers blood pressure, activates the synthesis of vitamin D, which is needed for the absorption of many minerals from the diet, increases the efficiency of the heart, reduces cholesterol, assists in weight loss, is an effective treatment for psoriasis, increases the level of sex hormones, and makes an important skin hormone active. Light is a nutrient, he says.

The real cause of skin cancer

Regarding the effects of UV light and skin cancer he writes: "One of the major researchers, Dr. Helen Shaw, found that the people who had the lowest risk of developing skin cancer were those whose main outdoor activity was sunbathing! Twice the risk of developing melanomas was found in office workers who had to work indoors all day under fluorescent lights. Additional research by Dr. Shaw has shown that fluorescent office lights can cause mutations in cultures of animal cells. Dr. Shaw concludes that 'in both Australia and Great Britain, melanoma rates were high among professional and office workers, and lower in people working outdoors.' " [*]

---

[*] Jacob Liberman, *Light—Medicine of the Future*, Santa Fe, NM: Bear & Company Publishing, Inc., 1991, p. 151.

A *mood brightener*

I think being out in the sun for part of each day is a great, healthful thing, especially if you're walking, skating, swimming, or doing some other wonderful, invigorating exercise. I agree completely with Dr. Liberman and Thomas Jefferson; the sun is a great healer and a source of nutrients that we desperately need. What makes you feel better than being outside on a sunny day? If you are concerned about your face, wear a wide-brimmed hat and avoid that part of the day when the sun's rays are their strongest.

I used to have a little, dingy, dark office. Now I have more than twenty square feet of window. It has enhanced my quality of life immensely. As I write, I am sitting in front of ten feet of southern-exposure sunlight, which is the most direct kind in Colorado, being in the Northern Hemisphere. Speaking of sunny Colorado, people here seem to be happier than my friends in cloudier climates. If we don't see the sun for three days in a row, people get irritable and crabby. I know I do. When you think about it, and let yourself answer truthfully, I daresay you intuitively know the sun is good for you. Give yourself permission, for health's sake, to bask in the sun's radiance.

Skin damage

I have seen a few people with severely sun-damaged skin, but they really overdid it every day, every summer for years. Too much sun *can* have a negative effect like too much oxygen, too much vitamin A, or too much horsetail tea. Or too much sunscreen.

It's a fact that many of the sunscreens on the market contain chemicals that can be toxic. To sell their sunscreens, companies must give you a good reason to buy it. But I think that instinctively we know what is right for us. I think we get so caught up in the fear-induced advertising and shallow reporting that bombards us constantly that we lose trust in our inherent wisdom.

Instead of using sunscreen, you can avoid sun exposure between 10:00 A.M. and 3:00 P.M. when the UVB rays are the strongest. If needed, use natural plant oil sunscreens such as sesame and avocado oil, and herbs such as yarrow, lily, and rosemary. Drink lots of water to hydrate your skin. Natural sunscreens such as sesame oil and vitamin E blend can be applied directly to your skin. You can also apply a topical ascorbyl palmitate, which is vitamin C that is fat-soluble and has recently been found to be successful; however, it is synthetic.

Homemade sunscreen

For a light, natural sunscreen, try mixing equal parts of olive oil and vinegar and apply to your skin.

Detoxing your body and being in general good health is also essential to combating any negativity in ultraviolet light. Widely discussed recently is the discovery that taking antioxidants internally, vitamins A, C, and E, combats the sun's negative effects. The theory is that plants have to produce the same substances to protect themselves from the sun. I think these ingredients have a great future in the sunscreen business.

Be careful that the sunscreens you are applying to your skin are not more harmful than the rays of the sun. We do not at this time make a sunscreen, because the only natural SPF sunscreen is PABA and it makes about 20% of the population's skin break out.

Your skin was originally designed to deal with the effects of the sun, so what you want to do is reinforce the natural defense system your body already has. People at high altitudes *do* need to be careful. For every 1,000 feet above sea level, the intensity of the UV radiation increases by about 4%. Vail, Colorado, for example, is at 9,000 feet, making the sun about 36% stronger there.

So chuck the sunscreen, put on a wide-brimmed hat, and go have some fun in the sun!

Twenty-five things to do before you die

> People need three things to be happy: someone to love,
> something to do, and something to look forward to.
> —Anonymous

Having things to look forward to is definitely an asset in both the health and happiness categories. And a healthy, happy person expresses greater beauty. What do *you* want to do for fun or to accomplish before you die? What would bring you increased happiness? Perhaps you want to assist new moms or the elderly, sail around the Caribbean, or learn to play a musical instrument.

A couple of ideas on my list follow, with some suggestions for you. Free your imagination. Create your own list.

✳ Volunteer to work with troubled kids.

✳ Tell everybody you love just that.

* Take three months off work and see what you would do with yourself without plans.

* Hike down the Grand Canyon.

* Ride a bicycle or motorcycle somewhere far away (or ride in a sidecar, if you're like my mom).

* Learn another language.

* Live abroad.

* Fast for one day.

* Make a list of what you are really afraid to do and one by one go do them; overcome your fears a step at a time.

* Be silent for one full day.

* Travel out of the country alone.

* Take a road trip with your best friend.

* Start a business.

* Buy an expensive pair of boots and wear them everyday.

* Enter an arm-wrestling contest.

* Try to learn something from everyone you meet.

* Teach a class.

* Plant a garden.

* Dance on a bar.

* Read the classics.

* Forgive someone for something terrible.

* Go to the greatest music festival.

* Decide to love at least one person unconditionally.

* Throw a big birthday party to celebrate your continued life.

* Go to the Carnival in Rio.

Twenty things to do everyday

* Do yoga—mild for some, vigorous for others—discover what's right for you.

* Drink fresh juice, pulp and all.

* Take supplements.

* Thank God for all the blessings bestowed on you.

* Tell your kids you love them.

* Read, including some spiritual reading.

* Pray to whatever being or power you believe in.

* Meditate, starting with three minutes a day.

* Laugh often—tell jokes.

* Work—accomplish something, no matter how small, remembering that *all* work that is moral and legal has dignity.

* In traffic, let someone in front of you.

* Compliment something you really appreciate in someone.

* Lose your judgments and preconceptions.

* Accept people for who and what they are.

* Don't listen to people's negative opinions of other people; tell them you don't want to hear them and that you'll make up your own mind.

* Turn up your radio and dance in your living room, in your kitchen, or on your deck.

* Focus on fun.

* Be positive.

* Go for a walk, even a short one around the block.

* Celebrate your life.

Vegetarianism

> Nothing will benefit human health and increase the chances for survival of life on Earth as much as the evolution to a vegetarian diet.
>
> —Albert Einstein

The concept of vegetarianism is not new. Plato, Leonardo da Vinci, George Bernard Shaw, Charles Darwin, and Albert Einstein were all vegetarians. There are many reasons why people decide to become vegetarians. My sister's: "I always knew the animals were my friends."

Many people don't eat meat because of religious beliefs. Others are vegetarians simply because they lack access to meat. For example, the average person in India consumes only two pounds of meat a year. I am a semi-vegetarian. I try to eat lots of fruits and vegetables, so I will look and feel good. I find my body just operates better the less meat I eat. I try to make 90% of my food intake fresh fruits and vegetables, legumes, and whole grains.

A lot of information is out there on becoming a vegetarian for health, ethical or political reasons. I am not going to discuss it for the latter reasons; but I'll share with you a few personal ones that may get you thinking about it. By eating more fruits and vegetables you may:

❋ Look and feel better.

❋ Try all kinds of new dishes, making your life more interesting.

❋ Start shopping at fun health food stores, such as Wild Oats, Whole Foods, Vitamin Cottage, and Alfalfa's if you live near one.

❋ Think health in every way, every day.

❋ Build your strength.

❋ Enjoy more energy and body efficiency.

❋ Learn to be in touch with the food you digest, putting you more in touch with your body, yourself, and your world.

❋ Make the transition to beauty, health and happiness.

❋ Be able to stop smoking.

Definitions of vegetarianism

There is a lot of confusion about vegetarians and vegetarianism. In Boulder, the definition of being a vegetarian is someone who never eats anything "that ever had, or would have had a face." So being a vegetarian here means you don't eat any kind of animal protein, including fish and eggs.

Meanwhile, in Grand Rapids, Michigan, many friends of mine think if you don't eat beef you are a vegetarian. So there are many varying degrees and concepts of vegetarianism. Here are some general definitions:

Transitional vegetarian refers to a person who is beginning to adopt a more vegetarian diet.

Semi-vegetarian diet includes poultry, fish, eggs, and dairy foods.

Pesco-vegetarian diet includes fish, eggs, and dairy foods.

Ovo-vegetarian includes eggs.

Lact-ovo-vegetarian includes dairy products.

Vegetarian refers to one who doesn't eat any of the above.

Vegan diet excludes animal-derived foods of all types, including honey.

Ethical vegans do not *use* any products produced from any animals, including honey, leather, silk, soaps made from animal fats, etc.

Combinations for increased protein

Combining foods can be important for vegetarians. Grains like wheat, rice, corn, and oats with beans or legumes complement each other, resulting in proteins when eaten together. Eating nuts with dairy foods also helps create complementary proteins. Corn and beans, like a bean tostada, make a complementary protein, as do beans and rice.

Your local health food store is your best resource. Go and browse, try the samples. There are many vegetarian cookbooks available, and the staff at most health food stores are so bright, educated, and helpful, they will be an invaluable resource for you as you make your transition. Eat at a few vegetarian restaurants; you'll be surprised how great the food can be!

If you live in a town with a Hare Krishna temple, find out if it serves a free vegetarian feast on Sunday that you can attend. We are lucky in Denver, as there is also a great restaurant called Govindas adjacent to the temple. It has a daily buffet. It is one of my favorite restaurants, and I have also been to the ones in San Diego and Detroit. I strongly recommend them. They are very inexpensive, too.

To learn more about vegetarianism, contact the following:

Council for Responsible Nutrition at (202) 872-1488

North American Vegetarian Society at (518) 568-7970

Earth Save at (800) 362-3648

A Woman's Cycle

The most interesting book I have ever seen dealing with menstruation is *Red Flower: Rethinking Menstruation* by Dena Taylor. Her goal is to "show that women do celebrate and honor menstruation." She continues, "I want to help dispel the idea that menstruation is shameful, that it should be kept hidden. We need to recognize this part of our cycle—to be aware of its subtle and powerful effects on us, and to use these in a way that enriches our lives." [*]

Taylor makes a stand that I have to admit I never heard before picking up her book. Menstruation is a wonderful, healing, healthy, creative, and powerful influence on us that connects us not only to Mother Earth, but the moon and the complete cycle of birth and death. Therefore, we need to develop a new attitude regarding its monthly visit. Her book states: "It is the force of life. It is the gift of being female. It is more than we know or understand in this day and age. I believe it to be held in honor in our past ages—we've only forgotten." [†]

If you are interested in the sisterhood of the goddesses, I highly suggest this book. It is positive, witty, innovative, helpful, healing, and fun.

There are many good books available to help you on the important subject of a woman's cycle. Because I've found a direct correlation between unbalanced hormones and acne, I want to include some general information for you to get started on balancing yourself. I don't have any scientific data or college degrees in this field. This is strictly based on my own struggles and solutions and talking to thousands of women. The main question I ask is: "Do you see a correlation between your cycle and your acne?" More than 90% in my informal, unscientific, broad survey say, "Yes." So if you are suffering from period-related acne, I suggest you really delve into this subject much further than these pages. I am just outlining some basic information.

---

[*] Dena Taylor, *Red Flower: Rethinking Menstruation*, Freedom, CA: The Crossing Press, 1988, p. 1.

[†] Ibid., p. 32.

PMS

Premenstrual syndrome (PMS) is a collection of symptoms caused by hormonal imbalances that have been recorded since Hippocrates. Symptoms include irritability, bloating, headaches, craving for sweets, fatigue, confusion, and lethargy.

Many of us simply dismiss the extra stress and tension, the arguments with loved ones, the snapping at co-workers, or the swearing at the car that just pulled out in front of us as "just PMS." Yet it can also be useful and insightful to look at what else is going on in your life. Your mood swings may be reflective of things that have been bothering you all month, but you are expressing your anger at this time of the month. Is the problem "moodiness" or is it an inequity that you have not adequately addressed in your life?

Menstrual cramps

Menstrual cramps or dysmenorrhea are thought to be a chemical problem. According to Dr. Penny Wise Budoff, director of the Women's Medical Center in Bethpage, New York, "Each month, the lining of a woman's uterus produces chemicals called prostaglandins, which help the uterine muscles contract and expel tissue and fluids during menstruation. High levels of prostaglandins cause uterine muscle contractions or cramps."[*]

The following are suggestions many have found helpful to balance hormones and ease pain:

* Keep track of your cycle and schedule your work accordingly—go easy on yourself.

* Eat fresh fruits and vegetables.

* Get a ton of sleep.

* Go to a chiropractor to obtain relief.

* Do yoga, particularly the triangle pose.

* Try acupuncture.

* Go for a walk.

---

[*] Debora Tkac, ed., *The Doctors Book of Home Remedies*, Emmaus, PA: Rodale Press, 1990, p. 419.

* Add sea salt, baking soda, and essential oil of lavender to your bath water.

* Make love.

* Drink herbal teas with willow bark or chamomile.

* Take a nap with a hops and lavender pillow.

* Make a tincture of any of the herbs mentioned.

* Inhale fennel seed essential oil to reduce pain from the cramps.

* Take all the vitamin Bs.

* Take brewer's yeast daily.

* Get your minerals checked to see if you need to take iron, calcium, magnesium, and/or zinc.

* Take alfalfa tablets daily.

* Try vitamins A and E.

* Drink cramp bark tea.

* Try pennyroyal or dandelion for cramps (used by Native Americans).

* Take primrose oil daily.

* Take vitex.

* Take omega-6 oil.

* Take flaxseed oil.

* Get a massage.

* Get rolfed.

* Take the amino acid threonine.

* Keep a journal of your cycle and feelings.

* Take dong quai.

* Drink chicory tea.

* Take white willow bark for pain and as an anti-inflammatory.

* Exercise daily, though not too strenuously.

* Lie in the sunshine.

* Do deep breathing.

* Drink lots of water.

* Apply a heating pad.

* Increase potassium through fresh bananas, orange juice, and peanut butter.

* Meditate using relaxation techniques and imagery.

Herbs

In a class I attended at the Center for Botanical Studies in Boulder, Christopher Hobbs, a noted author of books on herbs, recommended wild carrot seeds as a hormone regulator. Black cohosh has been used historically to help balance hormones. For very heavy periods accompanied by blood clots, try a tea made of a combination of pasque flower, chamomile, blue cohosh, wild yam, and motherwort.

Vitex, commonly known as chaste tree berry, was first recorded by Hippocrates in the fourth century B.C. He stated: "If blood flows from the womb, let the woman drink dark wine in which the leaves of the vitex have been steeped." Later, Dioscordides suggested vitex to promote menstruation. It is widely thought today that vitex promotes the homeostasis in the estrogen-progesterone relationship, the imbalance of which not only causes pain for women, but acne, as well. Some believe that vitex helps the pituitary gland put out more progesterone, which helps balance the estrogen. PMS is usually associated with high estrogen levels.

Yohimbe, an herb from South America, has been used traditionally as an aphrodisiac, and to treat impotence, frigidity, and painful menstruation. It is said to be able to reduce irritability, hyperactivity, and water retention.

Dancing Willow Herbs in Durango, Colorado, sells a premixed tea containing oatstraw, red raspberry, dandelion, vitex, nettle, licorice, and sarsaparilla that the company says is a "wonderful tea as a daily general tonic for women. A balancing tonic for women's hormonal system." Three ounces is $6.75. Call (888) 247-1654. Or simply blend your own.

Acupuncture

Acupuncture can help with PMS and period-related disorders within three or four menstrual cycles. One acupuncturist told me that the goal of the therapy is to teach the woman what foods to avoid and what lifestyle choices to make to end the symptoms for good. The theory is to rebalance the entire body's mechanism so it regains vibrant good health. This therapy positively affects each of the major organs and the bowels, as well as a woman's energy levels, blood, and body fluids. While Western doctors deal with PMS in terms of prostaglandin and hormones, the Chinese methods deal with the whole body and all the organs. A really good acupuncturist can prescribe teas of herbs that can balance your system. I have had great success from my acupuncturist's treatments and teas.

Essential oils

My favorite essential oil for any female problem is fennel. Simply inhale it. A great blend of essential oils for mood swings is geranium, lavender, cedarwood, and cypress; you can also add cardamom or coriander.

Try using one or more of the following essential oils blended with almond oil and applied to your wrists, then inhaled often: bergamot, clary sage, fennel, juniper, lavender, peppermint, rose, rosemary, sandalwood, or jasmine.

To balance your hormones on a regular basis, try clary sage, fennel sage, and geranium. For mood swings, also try bergamot, eucalyptus, fennel, and peppermint. For irritability, try frankincense, lavender, chamomile, rose, and ylang ylang.

Relax

Like a good Girl Scout, "Be prepared." Make yourself a PMS kit. Gather and put together in a container the following:

- Your favorite PMS tea
- Your favorite essential oils for PMS (see above)
- Your favorite body oil
- Your favorite bath herbs for PMS
- Your favorite steam herbs
- Your favorite sleep essential oils
- Your favorite meditation
- Your favorite prayer
- Your favorite candle
- Your favorite book

Follow the basic instructions for relaxation from the Lily of Colorado Homespa in the Relaxing section of this book.

Ask questions and investigate more

There are many books on the subject of a woman's cycle available at your health food store, bookstore, and library. All are jam-packed with detailed information. The people who work in the natural living section of your health food store are usually extremely knowledgeable on this topic and can be a great resource. I have personally learned much from these folks. Many of the women that work in the health food stores have worked for years finding solutions to normalizing their own cycles naturally, so have tried just about every remedy available.

An excellent book on the subject is *Menstrual Cramps Self-Help Book* by Susan M. Lark, M.D. If you are suffering from any monthly menstrual symptoms, get this book. It outlines what distinguishes a normal menstrual cycle from one out of balance, and includes chapters on everything from evaluating your own symptoms, including charts for you to track your cycles, to finding solutions through all kinds of therapies. It even includes menus, meal plans, and recipes.

Yoga

Health is wealth. Peace of mind is happiness.
Yoga shows the way.

—Swami Vishnudevananda

Yoga is a Sanskrit word meaning "yoking," that is, yoking together mind and spirit. Many say the intention of yoga is to bring you closer to your Creator. It is a philosophical system with a matrix of different kinds of yoga and paths.

Hatha Yoga

I am going to focus on hatha yoga, which is the most popular here in the Western Hemisphere and relates more to the physical poses. Except when I am traveling, I do my yoga fairly regularly. I need it more then ever when I am traveling, but it is difficult to do on hotel room floors, particularly in Third World countries where the cleanliness standards leave much to be desired.

When I am at home, however, I have my morning yoga ritual. It's not a big deal: four to eight sun salutations, where I keep some of the poses for up to one minute each time. I especially love the bow, cobra, downward-facing dog, and shoulder stand pose. The stretching and facing the earth is especially grounding and a delicious way to introduce yourself to a new day. Next, I do the plow and other poses, then 150 crunches, a headstand using a body lift so not to strain my neck, and then ten neck stretches. My ritual takes about an hour and really centers and calms me for the day.

I have been doing this for about five years. I know I need more if I ever find myself upset at someone in traffic. That is my barometer, my indicator that I need more yoga.

My mom and sister have been taking yoga classes for as long as I can remember. I like yoga because it is so calming, yet toning. I prefer to do my physical exercise alone. Men seem to enjoy sports and exercise that involve multi-participants, but I usually enjoy exercising in solitude.

Examples of serenity

One of the most impressive things to me about India, where Yoga originated, is the way many of the shopkeepers keep so calm, almost majestic, sitting in the lotus position in their three by three square feet of space. Amidst the terribly loud noises of horns blowing, people talking, bells ringing, the awful smells of cow dung, urine, diesel fuel, and the hundred and ten degree heat, there they sit, not moving, with completely celestial looks on their faces. Amazing.

Benefits of yoga

I personally have gained greatly from yoga. It really gets me calm and centered to start my day, but it was also the main force to get me to stop smoking. I knew it would be. I knew if I kept bringing these positive habits into my life, that my life would transform. Like most smokers, I had beaten myself up. I really wished I would stop, but cigarettes were like little friends I could always depend on to be there if I was hurt, angry, stressed, or bored. But when I started doing my yoga every day and began bringing so many other healthful things into my life, cigarettes just didn't fit anymore.

As I stated in the Quitting Smoking section of this book, I decided to forgive myself for smoking, but continued to add more and more positive things to my life. I was already doing my fresh carrot juice daily, drinking "pond scum" (juice, wheat grass, alfalfa, etc.), eating only fruit for most lunches, working out, walking daily, steaming, meditating, and so on. And one day, I got up just like any other day. I did my yoga. As I was sitting there in the lotus position doing my neck stretches, it came to me: I don't want to smoke anymore. Yes, that's it, I'm done. Finished. And I never smoked another cigarette. I am not saying that it wasn't difficult at times, but the choice had been made and I gave up immediate gratification for long-term health.

No matter who you are and what you want out of life, I highly recommend yoga. The benefits are too numerous to list here, but just to name a few: mental centering, physical toning and strengthening, stress relief, better posture, flatter stomach, tranquillity, and relaxation. It's easy, free, you can do it at home in almost any space, and it's simple.

Many of the poses enhance general health while nourishing all the vital organs, aiding them in their functions. Yoga is a great all-purpose energizer. It stretches muscles, stimulates circulation, strengthens the back, and supports the abdominal organs. It can eliminate constipation, refresh the mind, and it is a great weight regulator. No matter how perfect your skin is, no matter how many God-given gifts of good looks you were given, if your muscles are not toned and your vital organs aren't getting fresh blood, you are going to feel sluggish and look like jelly.

Yoga classes

Most of the yoga classes I have attended were through the Shambhava School of Yoga in Eldorado Springs, Colorado. One was a meditation and yoga combination class offered through Colorado Free University in Denver. In addition, I attended some classes at the Shambhava School's ashram. It has some spectacular teachers and rigorous classes, and I have to admit, after attending their classes I felt an extra bonus, in contrast to just doing my own little routine at home.

I highly suggest that you take a class to get you going and to make sure you are doing the poses correctly. Done improperly, the plow or shoulder stand can hurt your neck. There are many classes, retreats, videos, and books available on yoga. Look for them at your health food store. While there, check flyers and posters about nearby classes. You can also check out books and videos at your local library or locate them at your favorite bookstore.

Yoga camps and teachers' training

Serve, Love, Give, Purify, Meditate, Realize. Lead a simple life. Practice daily meditation and establish peace in your own heart. Then you will radiate peace to all who come in contact with you. Mysterious is this peace. If you enjoy this peace, you will be contributing peace to the whole world. Realize the peace that passeth all understanding and be free.

—Swami Sivananda

The Sivananda ashram has yoga teachers' training courses and retreats all over the world. In New York is the Yoga Ranch; in California, the Yoga Farm; and there is one I have mentioned on Paradise Island, Nassau, Bahamas. They promote "A Yoga Vacation Experience: Proper exercise, proper breathing, proper relaxation, proper diet, positive thinking and meditation."

Contacts

Sivananda Ashram Yoga Retreat
P.O. Box N7550
Paradise Island, Nassau, Bahamas
(242) 363-2902
Fax (242) 363-3783
(800) 783-9642 in US
(800) 263-9642 in Canada
email *syvcnas@batelnet.bs*

Sivananda Ashram Yoga Ranch
243 West 24th Street
New York City, NY 10011
(914) 434-9242

Ananda Yoga Ashram
International Centre for Yoga Education and Research
16-A/16-B, Mettu Street,
Chinnamudaliarchavady,
Kottakuppam 605 104, (via Pondicherry)
Tamil Nadu, India

According to the information that the International Centre for Yoga Education and Research (ICYER) sent me, it offers a six-month program. The Ananda Ashram and ICYER are located in a small fishing village on the coast of the Bay of Bengal, in Southern India, near Pondicherry. All meals are vegetarian. Meals and classes are held outside in the garden and meditation area. Most accommodations are single rooms with a shared bath.

This training offers a plus: taking pilgrimages to nearby temples and holy places, as well as participating in local religious and cultural festivals. Included are programs on Indian dance, music, and instruments. In addition, each student is expected to take up one facet of the Hindu culture or art and learn about it in depth to give him/her deeper insight.

According to one of the pamphlets, "The student learns that the real Yoga . . . Union with the Cosmos . . . can only occur when 'first works are done first.' The body, mind, emotions, must first be cleansed and purified. They must then be understood, explored, disciplined, controlled and made sensitive, so that the entire nature is capable of responding to and living in harmony with the Cosmic Rhythms.

"Most important of all, life in the Ashram Guru Kula is a constant study of one's own self—the student must come face-to-face with his or her own nature. There is no escape from self-knowledge in the Guru Kula. Change is possible only when one becomes aware in totality of one's faults and failings. This basic self-knowledge becomes the foundation on which to build a solid Yoga Life."

Other choices

For the more tame, there are many yoga training centers in the United States, the Caribbean, and Mexico. There are several in Boulder. The yoga training centers I know the most about are the Shoshoni Yoga Retreat Center and the Eldorado Mountain Yoga Ashram, which are both run by Shambhavananda Yogi.

The publication *Insight* states: "Shambhavananda Yogi's vision for Eldorado and Shoshoni is to create an environment conducive to inner growth nurturing practitioners toward the realization of their true Self or Buddha nature . . . the heart is the hub of all sacred places. Go there and roam in it."

The Shoshoni retreat center offers month-long "intensives" during the summer that are specifically set up for training, but when I stayed at the Shoshoni retreat center in the middle of the winter, there were a couple of resident guests in month-long yoga training. The center seemed to smoothly weave me into the ashram life of chanting, meditation, and yoga classes.

Shoshoni and the Eldorado Mountain Ashram are both beautiful, situated in or near the mountains. They have a quieting energy and the people are kind and friendly. I enjoyed being at each and highly recommend them.

The Eldorado Mountain Yoga Ashram offers a several-month non-resident program for working people. It is held on specific dates for six to eight months, two weekends a month and then one night a month.

This Ashram is approximately six miles from Boulder and is located in the foothills of the Rocky Mountains. Shoshoni is up the canyon about a half-hour, actually in the mountains. When you finish a class, you really feel the difference in your body. I have gone really uptight with all my muscles stiff and hurting and left after one hour feeling almost completely free of tension.

I like that their yoga classes are guided with imagery and positive words of wisdom. While the poses are not difficult, the teachers often have you hold them long enough to achieve ultimate stretching.

I have really enjoyed attending. Consider going yourself!

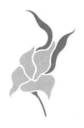

PART TWO

Ingredients for Beauty

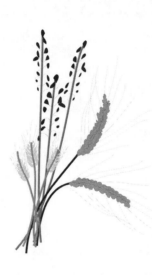

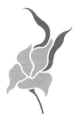

Concepts of Beauty

Everybody needs beauty as well as bread, places to play in and pray in, where Nature may heal and cheer and give strength to body and soul alike.

—John Muir

We fly to beauty as an asylum from the terrors of our finite natures.
—Ralph Waldo Emerson

Beauty, health, and happiness come from the same source—the harmony of daily life.

The concepts of looking good and feeling good are so intertwined you can barely tell the difference. Do you have to look good to feel good or do you have to feel good to look good? And if you have the recipe to look good and feel good and add a pinch of good attitude, then wouldn't you have the formula for happiness? That is the premise to this book.

As women, we want to be loved and admired. I think practicing a regular beauty routine reinforces loving ourselves, which is a magnet for attracting love and admiration.

Wisdom and beauty are inherent

Most of us do not look like Cindy Crawford, but all of us have inherent wisdom and beauty. I have seen many women who look beautiful because they take such good care of themselves that that effort, that expression of healthy self-love shines through. When you take the time to take care of yourself, it creates energy, a magnetic force. In other words, making friends with yourself helps you make friends with others. Loving yourself in a ritualistic way makes you more open to love from others. Expressing your appreciation for yourself makes it easier to express your appreciation for others.

Looking and feeling your best is beauty. Everything that you love is beautiful. So love yourself. Beauty is an attitude; love is beautiful; displays of kindness are beautiful.

If you take the time, even just two hours to prepare for a big evening through a homespa, steam or sauna, mask or facial, manicure, bath, washing and conditioning your hair, brushing your teeth, taking your vitamins, taking a healthy drink, applying body oils, taking your time getting dressed, you know you are going to feel more beautiful. Beauty is not only in the eyes of the beholder; it exudes from you. It emanates from every pore in your body. It is in your presence, your facial expressions. It comes from your laugh, your smile, your kind words. Beauty is held in your eyes especially when you are looking at something that you love. It comes deep from within you.

Caring for yourself

To start getting your health in order, start to eat properly, exercise, and take the needed supplements and herbs to enhance your health. Then practice healthful beauty treatments to enhance your good looks. Finally, practice the things that will bring happiness into your life. Polish your gifts from the Creator. Taking good care of yourself is an enjoyable expenditure of your time, not to mention a great investment that pays the best kind of dividends.

Beauty rituals bring together the art and expression of loving yourself, and can even be a spiritual experience, a type of meditation, as you deliberately, mindfully, take the time to appreciate yourself, your world, and your blessings.

The French have a saying: "Etre bien dans sa peau" (to feel good in one's skin). What could be more important? Both on the outside and the inside, God's creation is what we are talking about. It's an insult not to take care of this creation. Your body is the temple of the Holy Spirit. You are made of Divinity.

Creating harmony in our daily life is a great source of health. Balancing the aspects of our day between activities and rest, time spent inside with time spent outside, and mental activity with physical activity are life enhancing. Being near man-made objects and being near nature, being with people and being alone. If you live in the craziness of the city, be sure you get to the sea, mountains, or the forest enough. It is important to set a piece of each day aside to reflect on and reaffirm what is important.

How we see ourselves is imperative to how we look and who we are. Beauty's foundation is self-esteem. We all need to carve a peaceful place for ourselves in the world, a place on the planet where we feel as perfectly comfortable as is possible. We need to be mindful of any and all negativity, go to its source of pain and deal with it, and find a place to put it where it can't create havoc, but yet a place where we don't deny its existence.

We need to cultivate an attitude where we see our humanness complete with our flaws, where we can embrace those as well as our positive points, and cultivate acceptance for ourselves as integrated beings.

We need to see ourselves and others as beautiful, healthy, and happy and to live in harmony with ourselves first before we can live in harmony with others. It is important to allow yourself to visualize your beauty instead of focusing on your small imperfections.

Take control of what you can to be beautiful. First, you need to feel good.

Cosmetics: a universal idea

The word cosmetic is derived from the word "cosmos." The word cosmos was originally defined as "the order of the universe." Universal order can be expressed in every aspect of human existence. We seldom think of cosmetics in such esoteric terms. The relationship of appearance to one's own visual harmony was obvious, however, to the ancient Greeks and, before them, to the Chinese and Egyptians.

Although we modern people do not usually think of cosmetics in such deep and serious terms, that is, seeing the innate relationship of one's appearance to one's own inner harmony, this concept was clear to the ancients.

Throughout recorded history, a daily routine of beauty care has been an accepted ritual. The practice is considered by many to be a manifestation of civilized living. Men and women trying to enhance their natural beauty through the use of body care products and Mother Nature is nothing new under the sun.

The ancient Egyptians had a complex system that made it difficult to differentiate between religion, ritual, and cosmetics. Some historians say that the concept of using cosmetics just for adornment may have started in China nearly 4,000 years ago. According to Jessica B. Harris in *The*

World Beauty Book, "In Peking in the thirteenth century, upper-class women anointed their faces in the wintertime with a paste that was called 'Buddha adornment.' The paste remained on into the spring, when it was removed to reveal a complexion that was alleged to be as smooth and lustrous as jade."[*] We no longer have this formula. It has been lost in the mists of time.

Not all ancient wisdom is lost

Fortunately, there are places in the world where such ancient knowledge is still known and practiced. I experienced such a place during my visit to India. While I was in Goa, I tripped and hurt my foot. I could not walk. I was able only to hop on my other foot. A taxi took me to a small hospital. I was a little scared because it didn't resemble an American hospital in any way. It wasn't clean. No staff was visible, and it was out in the middle of nowhere. After waiting about a half-hour for someone to show up, a woman appeared and asked me what was wrong with my foot. I told her I didn't know, that I had tripped and now I could not put any weight on it without falling down.

She wrapped my foot in a bandage that she soaked in a yellow solution she said was from a local plant. It was Ayurvedic medicine, she added. Then she told me I should be able to walk within an hour. She didn't seem to appreciate Westerners. I asked her what plant the solution was made from and how it was formulated. She looked at me and said, "It's Ayurvedic." "Yes, I understand," I responded. "I am very interested in natural healing. Please tell me." The woman just shook her head and replied, "You Westerners wouldn't understand." I begged her to tell me about it, but she just said, "That will be 350 rupees," and stuck out her hand.

The solution felt wonderfully cool and diminished the pain. My foot felt better the moment she applied it. An hour later, just as she had said, I could walk. I couldn't believe it! All the pain and swelling were gone. I went back the next day to coax her again for more information and to thank her, but she was nowhere to be found.

---

[*] Jessica B. Harris, *The World Beauty Book*, San Francisco, CA: Harper Collins Publishers, 1995.

Rediscovery

We have just begun to rediscover our heritage of growing, learning, and using food and herbs for healing and enhancing, and getting back in touch with the subtleties of our most innate nature. It is in a true sense of appreciation and empowerment that we pursue a beautiful, healthy, and happy lifestyle.

We are just relearning the herbal healing that women traditionally passed down for generations since before recorded time. Perhaps with enough research, we could even approximate the ancient Chinese's "Buddha adornment." There is much the world has known and forgotten. With effort, we can rediscover the best of the old and blend it with the best of the new.

We are all interested in keeping and enhancing our health, beauty, and happiness, and we can. Many of the ways are included in this book.

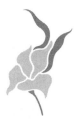

The Lily Method for Long-Lasting Beauty, Health, and Happiness

My method for long-lasting beauty, health, and happiness is for American women who want to have them but are already overwhelmed in their day-to-day life. It is for the women who want to drop their negative habits and bring new positive habits into their lives. The Lily Method is for the woman who wants to learn as much as possible about beauty, health, and happiness but just can't find the time to fit it all in. The Lily Method is for women of all ages who know they can be more beautiful, healthy, and happy, but haven't acquired their own techniques to implement these things in their daily lives.

Keep it fun

Note: The Lily Method is intended to be fun, mood-elevating, interesting, relaxing, mind-opening, exciting, beneficial, result-oriented, confidence-building, and to create long-lasting beauty, health, and happiness. Best of all, the Lily Method is simple.

My theory is that all of us have bad habits or addictions that we want to give up, but for so many reasons we have not been able to. Sometimes it's just the stress of even thinking about having to give anything up in a world where we seem to need so much and are getting so little. Or maybe it's an addiction such as coffee or nicotine. Maybe we are so busy we just can't seem to find the time to seriously think about how to go about breaking a bad habit. Maybe we see the habit as a friend. We all have our reasons.

In addition, I think we all want to bring positive things into our lives, but like the reasons we don't give up the bad things, we don't get around to bringing in the good ones. We know exercising is good for us, but we just never get around to it. We have heard some talk about herbal teas, but we don't have any handy when we think about trying some. We know smoking is detrimental to our health, but we're too stressed to quit and wonder what would take its place. It makes sense to us that eating a dead animal is not as good for us as eating fresh vegetables, but then what do we fix for dinner when we're in a hurry?

These thoughts and ideas spin in our heads creating more tension, more stress, and more anxiety.

Accept your bad habits!

The Lily Method emphasizes not beating yourself up for your bad habits. Accept your bad habits as part of your humanness. If you are going to buy that Snickers bar and if you are going to eat that Snickers bar, then enjoy that Snickers bar, savor every morsel, chew it slowly, thanking the good Lord for allowing you pleasure. The same goes with steaks, french fries, or coffee, and especially cigarettes. I have a good friend who is constantly puffing her cigarette while simultaneously talking about how bad it is for her and how she should quit. The smoking is one thing, but to beat yourself up like that is worse for your health. If you're going to smoke, smoke and enjoy it. The important thing is not to beat yourself up for it.

So many women never go to a restaurant without mentioning how many calories are in everything. If that stops you from eating something not good for you, okay, but if you are going to eat it anyway, don't think about all the negatives; just enjoy it.

Accept yourself

So the first step in the Lily Method is to totally accept yourself, complete with all your good and bad habits. Just let yourself relax about it, no matter what the bad habit. (The bad habits I am referring to do not include serious drug or alcohol problems. For those problems, seek medical attention and professional treatment.)

Okay, now that you have decided not to beat yourself up for what you are doing anyway, you need to start bringing easy, simple, healthful things into your life. Here is my list, but there are so many others that you can add. Go through the list and pick out *one* thing and try it for a week or a month, whichever makes more sense to you. See if making it a part of your daily or weekly life doesn't make you feel better, look better, or add confidence or happiness to your life. If it does, make a commitment to it, but only if you're benefiting and it suits you. After that positive thing becomes a ritual or you have deleted it, pick another healthful habit to try.

Choose what suits you

Slowly bring these positive things, practices, and habits into your life. Accept that many may not suit you. Vegetarianism may just not be for you at this point in your life, or maybe it is, but you're not ready to give up the Snicker bars, too; it's okay. One program doesn't fit all people.

What the Lily Method can do to improve your life:

❋ Help you let go of the negative thoughts you have about yourself because of your present bad habits

❋ Help you look and feel better because of the new positive habits you are incorporating

❋ Make your life more interesting by trying many new things

❋ Create self-confidence because you are taking control of your life

❋ Create self-discipline, which is the cornerstone to happiness

The Lily Method is just that you keep trying new things and keep a commitment to the things that are improving your life. Try my method. Just plan on being a *little* more beautiful, a *little* healthier, and a *little* happier. Consider:

❋ Wearing essential oils instead of synthetic perfumes

❋ Drinking a relaxing cup of chamomile tea one night a week

❋ Adding a fresh apple to your daily diet

❋ Taking a bath with essential oil of lavender to relax once a week

❋ Buying one pure body care product without any synthetic ingredients

❋ Giving up beef for one week

❋ Meeting your friends for a walk instead of a meal

❋ Buying organic produce for one week

❋ Buying and using an inexpensive water purifier

* Bringing carrots to work to snack on for one week

* Buying one fat-free healthy snack food to try

* Taking one good multivitamin every day for a month

* Using a shampoo without sodium laurel sulfate

* Saying one positive affirmation daily

* Buying a good book on herbal remedies and using one of them first instead of commercial products

* Planning your next vacation around a healthful activity (swimming, skiing, snorkeling, hot springs, hiking)

* Taking a sauna or steambath twice a week for a month

* Doing one yoga pose for 30 seconds every morning for a week

* Doing ten sit-ups every morning for a week

* Buying one more herb to cook with and using it

* Keeping a daily journal for one week

* Drinking more water each day for a week

* Drinking one less cup of coffee per day for two weeks

* Buying one herb of your choice in bulk and doing at least two different things with it

* Keeping an aloe plant in your kitchen for burns and pimples

* Doing a hot-oil treatment for your hair once a week

* Setting aside one or two hours to meander around a health food store, look at items, ask questions, and purchase a couple of things that you find interesting

* Buying one herbal book

Congratulate yourself on your achievements, no matter how small. Forgive yourself for any slip-ups. Enjoy the satisfaction of doing something good for your body. Enjoy taking more charge of your life.

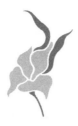

The Lily Theory

The Lily Theory and its application is this: Whatever you are using internally to treat your external skin problems, also use externally. So if you are taking brewer's yeast for acne or eczema, try using it externally by making a paste and applying it. If you're taking lecithin for psoriasis, also apply it externally on the affected area.

If you are taking vitamin E and PABA for hair growth, then also apply it externally. If you are taking vinegar to detoxify and cleanse internally, then also apply it externally as a toner or in your bath.

If you are drinking burdock tea for a skin ailment, try applying it topically. My theory states that whatever you are taking internally to treat an external skin problem will be much more effective if you also apply it externally at the same time. If you are eating more apples as a part of your nutritional therapy, apply them pureed as a paste to your skin. Whatever you are doing for the inside, you can do on the outside.

An additional benefit of this theory is that it may help keep you in check with not only the therapies you are treating yourself with internally, but also externally. For example, if you can't ingest it and it won't help detoxify you or build your system internally, then perhaps you shouldn't be applying it to your skin. In other words, you should be no less concerned with what you apply externally than with what you take internally. The Lily Theory uses both of these concepts. I believe using the same remedies externally and internally gives you much more benefit than if you only take the therapies or apply them. I have personally found this theory and application very advantageous, and I suggest you try it with all your skin care therapies.

I believe "if you can eat it, you can put it on your skin." Conversely, if you wouldn't eat it, don't put it on your skin. Please use your common sense with this theory, as there are some exceptions. There are few absolutes in life, but as a general rule I believe combining the internal and external has a beneficial synergistic effect and I think you will be delighted with the results.

Warning: Some herbs are beneficial externally but not internally, such as comfrey and arnica. Consult an herb encyclopedia or your physician if you have doubts or questions.

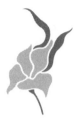

Ingredients Are Everything

One truism in the skin care field is this: A product cannot perform better than its ingredients. I'd like to repeat it: *A product cannot perform better than its ingredients.* If you get nothing else from this book, I'd like you to get this.

Checking ingredients

There are questions to ask yourself as you try to decide which skin care products you want to use. What is the ingredient that makes the product function? If it is an astringent, does it have herbs in it that are high in tannic acid? Does it contain witch hazel? Does it contain essential oil of lavender, which balances any skin type? What specifically is the astringent ingredient?

If it's a moisturizer, what are the moisturizing ingredients? Does it contain a humectant such as honey or vegetable glycerin that helps bring moisture from the air to your skin? How about high quality oils for lubrication? If you are using a moisturizer to help prevent wrinkles, does it have an ingredient that reputedly helps your skin regenerate itself such as horsetail, chestnut, comfrey, or rosehip seed oil? If you are using a lotion to soothe your skin, does it contain ingredients like calendula or chamomile that are anti-inflammatory and skin-conditioning?

Assuming that the product you have decided on has the desirable ingredients to perform its designated function, now you need to look at possible undesirable ingredients. These, in my opinion, can undo any good the desirable ingredients do.

So you have an astringent and it has witch hazel, calendula, chamomile, and essential oil of lavender, but towards the end of the ingredient list you see the entire paraben family. This includes ethylparaben, methylparaben, and butylparaben. Is the product still valuable? Do the synthetic ingredients take anything away from the herbs? I think you are the only one who can answer this question for yourself.

Like everything else in your life, it's a matter of acceptability. I do not think using synthetic ingredients is wrong. I do not like to put down synthetic, artificial, and petroleum ingredients. However, I do think the consumer should have a level of awareness high enough to understand the difference between these and natural ingredients. I think we each need to take responsibility for what we apply to our skin.

Many people do not care. Their interest lies in pretty packages or flamboyant promises. That is okay if that is what they want. These people probably aren't interested in using Lily of Colorado products. We make our products for that small but growing percentage of Americans who do not want parabens, urea, propylene glycol, and similar ingredients in the products they use.

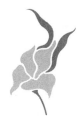

The Skin

As I and many of you know firsthand, our skin can profoundly affect our sense of well-being, who we are, and our confidence. Have you ever considered how important your skin is? Let's give the subject some thought.

A vital organ

Your skin, your body's largest organ, is what separates your internal organs from the hot sun, the cold, humid air, and harsh chemicals. The skin is our first introduction to the world. It protects us from outside influences including infection and pollution. It is a vital organ, involved in functions from temperature control to waste removal. It is our major sensory organ, relating to the environment with pleasure and pain.

Composition of our skin

The structure of the skin is composed of three layers: the epidermis at the top, the dermis in the middle, and the subcutaneous tissue below. (The skin and the layers of tissue below the surface can actually be separated into seven different layers.)

The epidermis. This is regularly being regenerated and consists of many dead skin cells being continually replaced.

The dermis. This layer contains the oil-producing and oil-secreting sebaceous glands. It is composed entirely of live skin cells. Here the skin maintains its strength level.

The subcutaneous tissue. This oil and water layer is composed of the sweat and sebaceous glands. It provides a pH balance and natural moisture to the skin and, because it consists of fat, provides a cushioning.

Vulnerability of the skin

The skin has tremendous powers of absorption. It takes in both healthful and harmful ingredients applied to it. Ingredients from skin care products have been found in the bloodstream. Essential oils applied to the skin can affect our central nervous system. (This underscores the importance of applying only pure products to your skin.) We must recognize that the skin is vulnerable and needs protection from harmful influences.

The outer layer of the skin, the epidermis, is renewed and replenished every eighteen days or so. The dermis, the second layer consists of the collagen and elastin.

Why is the skin important?

The skin fundamentally affects our health and sense of well-being, yet we continue to use mass-marketed, chemically filled skin care products without thought to their ingredients or the effects of those ingredients on our entire body and well-being. Many products cause allergic reactions and many more upset the skin's natural acid balance, the pH acid-base relationship, which protects us from the outside world.

The skin's pH balance

The skin's natural pH balance, which is the acid or acid mantle, is the measurement of acidity vs. alkalinity on a scale from 0 to 14. The skin's pH balance averages 5.5 and is usually between 4 and 6. Apple cider vinegar is a natural restorer of the acid balance. You can also help reintroduce acid to your skin with many acidic fruits and vegetables. This is very helpful for oily skin. Apply blended apples, strawberries, pineapple, papaya, horseradish, onion, and/or cucumbers to restore the natural acid balance.

Renewability

The body's skin is always renewing itself. The skin is a perfectly wonderful example of the ever-changing nature of human existence. To study and pay attention to our own skin helps us to be more aware of the ongoing process of change in our lives.

Energies from our emotions and from the environment, which are always entering the body through our pores in the skin, influence the flow of energy in the body. The quality of food we eat can change the quality of our blood that provides nourishment for new skin. Since the skin receives up to one-third of the body's blood supply, the quality of the skin can be greatly influenced by the quality of the food we eat. This is why it is so important to eat foods with a life force. The quality of food also influences the secretions of the sebaceous glands.

Cell transit time

Skin cells are formed in the deepest layer of the epidermis and are constantly moving outward and being discharged. The time this takes is often referred to as "cell transit time." If this doesn't happen fast enough, the dead skin accumulates on the surface. This can make the skin dry and scaly.

The cell transit time is approximately 22 days in people 18–28, while for people in their 70s, transit time could take an average of 37 days. Of course, age has a strong influence on this transit time. It is grossly influenced by the quality of energy flow through the body (e.g., diet, vitamins, overall health, and emotional status).

The same is true with body care products applied to the skin. The ingredients in these products affect the quality of energy that flows through the skin. These products are absorbed through the skin into the bloodstream through the cells.

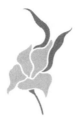

Labels, Claims, and Confusion— Now Clarity

"Cruelty-free"

We have to ask ourselves: Is animal testing a valid test for humans? There is a ton of information on the concept of cruelty-free and organizations to work with, so I am not going to say any more about it here. You can make sure the personal care products you buy are cruelty-free by simply shopping at health food stores. Almost all refuse to carry products tested on animals.

You can contact the following organization:

People for the Ethical Treatment of Animals (PETA)
P. O. Box 42516
Washington, DC 20015
(301) 770-PETA (7382)

"No animal products"

Did you know that a cosmetic product could contain animal ingredients like collagen and elastin and still be labeled "cruelty-free"? Cruelty-free refers only to whether or not the product was *tested* on animals. This is an entirely separate matter from the claim "no animal products," which means that the product does not contain any products from any animal. So a product can be cruelty-free (i.e., no animal testing) and still have animal products in it, or a product can have animal products in it and be technically cruelty-free. I think it is important that a product is both cruelty-free (no animal testing) and contain no animal parts, so you need to check out both.

Most people do not think of bee products as animal products. It is a debate, one I do not want to enter into; however, I will not be putting bee products in any new products we develop in the future.

Beauty products and the environment

The best reason to buy purely botanical™ body care products is because they work. They perform better than any other ingredients. Second, they are also less harmful. Third, by buying purely botanical™ products you are supporting sustainable agriculture. Making your own body care product from pure ingredients produces the least waste and provides you with the very best and freshest product.

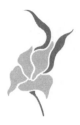

Preservatives

The first preservatives were cold temperatures, drying, and salt; the first cosmetic preservative was soap.

Preservatives are deadly by definition because they attempt to change and modify the life cycle, which we all know ends in decay and death. Preservatives can be dangerous, too, because they are a part of the synthetic belief system that says mankind can come up with something better than Mother Nature. I don't know about you, but I personally don't think all the men with all the degrees in all the labs in the world will ever be able to come up with anything better than Mother Nature.

Mother Nature has an inherent wisdom in every cell, plant, tree, and flower that will never be duplicated, never improved, and certainly never truly replicated by man. If you are of this mindset, read on; if not, you probably will not find this chapter interesting or helpful. It is not a matter of what is right or wrong; it is a matter of what you believe.

Decay and death are a natural part of life. Many synthetic preservatives simply mask the decaying process. Have you ever wondered how that bottle of lotion has stayed pearly and white in your bathroom closet for five years? I find that a little scary. I don't want a lotion to put on my face that looks the same as it did five years ago. Doesn't it age? Of course it does. It's five years old. You know that. Then why hasn't it changed at all? It is unnatural. Fresh fruit and vegetables age, decay, and spoil because they are natural.

Two questions

There are two issues here. One is a mindset, a philosophy. Do I think a company that makes a product knows better than Mother Nature? And do I want to pretend that neither I nor the cosmetic products I buy will never decay or die? The second issue is, do I think these petro-based and synthetic chemicals are going to benefit my skin?

More questions

There are sub-issues as well; for example, it is said these synthetic chemicals are necessary as preservatives because they are the best way to kill microorganisms. But are they more toxic than the bacteria they are supposed to kill? Plus, the testing is often done on animals. My question goes past the ethical question and into the validity issue: Does the fact that it was tested on animals prove that it is safe for humans?

Deciding what's acceptable

As I said in the beginning of the book, I am not a scientist, a doctor, a chemist, or anything like that. I am just an American woman struggling to find solutions to my own skin problems and trying to sort out what is right for me. I have more questions than answers, and a lot of the answers are not right or wrong. They are based on what I believe and what I think is acceptable for me. You can decide for yourself.

I think the first requirement of a preservative is that it must be free from toxins, irritants, or other harmful ingredients to the skin. Question: Are most toxic preservatives put in the product to protect you or the manufacturer? The mass marketers of cosmetic products make thousands of bottles a week. They then ship it to distributors where it may sit warehoused for months or years. The stores call in orders that are gradually shipped out. It is very efficient, making up large batches a couple of times a year. It lets companies focus on selling their products instead of *making* them.

I completely understand why they do it. It makes their lives easier, and their companies more profitable. What I don't understand is why people want to buy those products. By comparison, the way I and just a few other companies in the world make our products—in small batches, often, and with natural ingredients—is difficult, labor intensive, expensive, and problematic.

Difficulties in formulating all-natural products

Few recognize how difficult it is formulating an all-natural product. It requires patience, diligence, and discipline to take ten to fifteen years of trial and error to make these products work. I tried to get our first cream right for ten years, with literally thousands of different attempts. I am still trying to get it to naturally preserve longer, unsuccessfully. You have to try the same ingredients hundreds of different ways to get them right. Heat this, cool that, add this first, this second, this last. Sometimes it doesn't work right unless the three ingredients are the same temperature, and on and on.

Many companies don't even make their own products. They take the easy route. They simply call a private labeler, who makes many companies' products, onto which they slap their own labels.

We go through the formulating process weekly that many manufacturers go through only once or twice a year. It's just as much work to make a batch of fifty as it is 50,000. We ship them out directly and immediately to the store, bypassing distributors and warehouses. Our products may only be five days old when you buy them. Because we are so small, we also have to handcraft a lot of things. We are not automated and have no sophisticated filler machines.

Cost of ingredients

The labor is just one of many reasons it is so much more expensive to make a clean product. Most important, however, are the ingredients we use. They are expensive, but we prefer them because we believe in making synthetic-free, purely botanical™ products for our customers. We use rosehip seed oil, primrose oil, kukui oil, and essential oils. Many other body care products have a few cents' worth of these ingredients and are mostly composed of inexpensive ingredients. Also, as mentioned above, coming up with new products takes thousands of hours of manpower.

Natural ingredients

The preservatives we use are essential oils, vitamins, and citrus seed extracts that cost up to hundreds of dollars per gallon, while most synthetic preservatives are very cheap. Problem: Because our products do not last for years, we must make sure they sell fast. We guarantee them for one year, but they need to move quickly.

Using only agricultural ingredients also leaves my company vulnerable to Mother Nature. When you benefit so greatly from her, you must also pay the price. For example, a few years ago the almond crop was small due to poor weather, so the price of almond oil tripled overnight.

In many cases, the botanical ingredient varies in its chemical constituents depending on such variables as where it was grown, what kind of season the growers had, how much water and sun it was exposed to, and when it was harvested. Therefore, unlike synthetic ingredients where the chemical makeup is always consistent, purely botanical™ ingredients can vary. And so can the end products. Many people don't like that. Like McDonald's and their Big Mac customers, many consumers want everything to always be the same. Like Holiday Inn, they prefer no surprises. Working with Mother Nature's purely botanical™ gifts is challenging. But I prefer her natural products in the skin products I formulate.

Be aware that it is often the preservative that irritates the skin and makes people break out. Therefore, the preservative system is an important part of the product for the consumer to learn about and recognize. You need to decide for yourself what to believe and choose for your skin care.

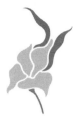

The Role of Herbs in Skin Care

In our daily lives we often take the fundamental role of plants almost completely for granted. Plants and plant products interact directly with our bodies, influencing the whole system with their powers and chemical components.

Unappreciated connections

As a society, we can be so removed from the natural world that most people don't know that aspirin was originally made from willow bark. How many of us realize that 12% of prescription medicines in the United States today come from plants, or that 75% of the world's medicines are botanical?

Furthermore, a lot of Americans don't see the daily importance and connection between plants and ourselves at all, much less on an almost constant basis. Do we think about how wheat in our toast is from the wheat plant, the corn flakes are from the corn plant, and the cotton we wear is derived from the cotton plant? When we go to work and sit at our hardwood desks, do we think of the strong oak tree from which our desks are made, or the gift of writing paper a tree gave us, not to mention the sheer beauty of trees, which filter and clean the air, give us shade, and convert the carbon dioxide we exhale into the oxygen we require to live?

Being biased toward apple trees, I don't think there is anything more beautiful than one in bloom. We are so fundamentally connected with the plants and the trees, yet when someone is hugging one, we laugh.

Time comparisons

Herbalism is based on over 10,000 years of trial and error. Western medicine is based on 200 years of trial and error.

Interestingly, different species of the same plants were used simultaneously for identical applications by Europeans and Native Americans before they ever crossed the ocean.

Herbs in skin care

Why use herbs in skin care? What makes them superior? Why not use the synthetic chemicals and petroleum-derived ingredients?

I came to use herbs from a process of elimination. In the beginning, I did not set out to find clean products free of harmful chemicals. I was a young girl who had serious acne and was desperate to clear it up. After ten or more years of trying everything else, I decided, what the heck, maybe a plant would work better than all these chemicals, because the chemicals were not working. To be quite honest, if the chemicals had worked, I probably never would have found my way to botanicals; my face would have cleared up and my search would have ended.

Even though my dad was a farmer and my sister a vegetarian, I didn't see the connection. Although my dad was a fruit grower and truly loved his farm, trees, and apples, he was not a "back-to-nature" kind of guy. He was a proponent of scientific agriculture, including, for example, the judicious use of insecticides. He really believed it made him a better farmer.

Even though my entire life my sister had not eaten meat, I still didn't understand the relationship between her vegetarianism and a Big Mac being part of a dead cow. Eating meat is just such a normal and established part of American life. We are not in touch with the connections between us and the animals, trees, or each other. I was probably in my late twenties before I really understood.

My search

So after I tried every other ingredient, I thought maybe herbs would be more effective. I knew the chemicals were not working for me, and they were expensive. I started to make homemade herbal cosmetics with things I already had lying around my kitchen.

I started trying a lot of toners and masks with fruit—apples and pineapple. I began reading and buying every book I could get my hands on, trying all of their recipes. I also started buying some products at the health food stores and trying to re-create and replicate them just to see if I could. Sometimes I could; sometimes I couldn't.

I read books on herbs, chemistry, and folk remedies and acquired an incubator, microscope, homogenizer, and sterilizers and started running tests. I felt a little like a mad scientist; it was exhilarating, rewarding, and fun. Making my own products, learning so much—it was empowering.

Why purely botanical™ skin care?

Why use purely botanical™ skin care products? Because it beats the alternative! Even if herbs didn't have the naturally occurring chemical constituents that promote health and heal us, I believe they would still be better than most mass-marketed cosmetic products.

Natural, synthetic, organic—what's in a word?

The modern medical profession rose with the synthetic era in the late 1900s. The cosmetic industry began to tap the synthetic chemical stocks for their products at the same time. In the early 1900s, 80% of all medicines and cosmetics were obtained from botanicals.

It would appear we live in a time and place that is completely supportive of synthetic chemicals with only recent faint knowledge of the possible damage they may create.

I am personally so much more at ease knowing most of the products I use come from Mother Nature. I think they are superior to any synthesized chemical.

The technical classification for substances is divided into things that are "organic" and things that are "inorganic." Organisms living or dead are called organic, and the rest are called inorganic. Chemists today refer to any substance that contains carbon atoms as organic, and they use inorganic to refer to any substance that does not contain carbon atoms.

So the technical definition of organic doesn't mean much to us as consumers. It is the same problem with the term "natural." Natural to me means produced from Mother Nature. Nothing from Mother Nature can really ever be successfully synthesized because it would no longer contain the essence of the earth.

Who knows better than Mother Nature?

Is any pharmaceutical company capable of coming up with any ingredient more perfect than a rose or a lily? As the overwhelming analytical discoveries of science continue, the simple basic conclusion will always be the same. The laboratory cannot successfully duplicate nature.

Versatility of herbs

Herbs and herbal products interact directly with our bodies, affecting the whole system with their active, naturally occurring chemical components.

Herbs influence the body internally and externally by changing the quality of the energy that flows through the body, just like food.

Synthetic chemicals are "use" specific only. This means that detergents are made to reduce surface soil and that is what they do. That is all they do. And they do it harshly. Sodium laurel sulfate is a detergent and that is what it does.

On the other hand, special herbs and oils have been selected for use in skin care throughout the ages. The mystical history of essential oils has its origin in ancient Egypt where herbs and essential oils were used in religious ceremonies. Three of the most widely used herbs in skin care are chamomile, comfrey, and calendula. All three of these herbs were used historically and are still popular today.

Nature always has provided us with the best ingredients for body care products. The basic chemistry of a healthy body care product is as old as mankind. The simple beauty applications of ancient cultures contained similar ingredients to any clean, natural product today.

How beneficial is Mother Nature?

American Indians believe the cure for every ailment is within twenty miles of where you live, that is, if you live in a natural environment where the native plants are allowed to grow.

One of the reasons why plant chemicals have such a dramatic effect on human physiology is because all living things are composed of families of related organic compounds. Proteins, enzymes, sugars, and vitamins from plants are bound to have some effect on similar substances in our own physiology. For example, antibiotic properties in plants perform the same effect on humans. They are present in the plants to provide an antibiotic function for the plant. In other words, the structure of botanicals corresponds identically to the structure of the human body. Bioflavonoids are in plants to protect them from the sun. Antibiotic properties in the plants perform the same effect on humans.

Botanicals' benefits

The benefit of using botanicals is valuable both on the aggregate and on the micro level. On the aggregate level, they help support the planet; on a micro level, you can derive the healing benefit of each individual plant.

In choosing a good natural cosmetic product, it is important to understand how beneficial the product is to the skin. A good product must have a healing ability as well as being absorptive, healthy, and not harmful.

Gentle herbal cleansers and body care products will cleanse the skin, tone it to restore the natural pH balance, and nourish it with plant oils and extracts.

What I want in products

As an American woman consumer, I want what I think all American women want in their body care products:

* a product to perform its duty (i.e., a cleanser to cleanse and a moisturizer to moisturize);

* a facial line product to have ingredients like essential oils, herbs, and vitamins that will benefit my skin;

* to support agricultural rather than chemical products.

I think that's what you want, too. That's why I've included recipes for you to make clean, healthy, and effective products in your own kitchen. (They are sprinkled throughout the book. Check the index.) And that's why I create clean, healthy, and effective products through Lily of Colorado.

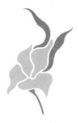

Preparation and Uses of Herbs

There are many ways to prepare medicinal herbs for consumption. Fresh herbs are best, but dried are good, too. Infusion or tea, decoction, tincture, powders, compresses, poultices, capsules, and ointments are various ways to take herbs.

Teas or infusions: This is the easiest and one of the most common methods of consuming an herbal remedy. Steep the herbs in boiling water for five to seven minutes to give the tea the taste and color of the herb. I use a teaspoon to a tablespoon of the herb, leaves, or flowers per cup of water. I often add honey for taste. Lemon can also add taste and vitamin C. I usually drink it warm to hot, especially to induce sweating or to break up a cough or cold. Otherwise you can take it lukewarm.

Decoctions: A decoction works best to extract bitter principles of the plant and is necessary for extractions of woody plants, barks, and resins. It is like a tea or infusion but stronger. I use one-half ounce of the herb soaked in cold water for two hours and then simmered in hot water for ten minutes. Cook until almost one-half of the water has evaporated, then use immediately.

Tinctures: Alcohol is probably the best extractor of herbal properties and is often used to preserve a tincture. I make mine by adding four ounces of cut or powdered plant to one pint of alcohol. I usually use high-grade vodka. *Warning:* Do not use rubbing alcohol. Many people from the Caribbean use rum, gin, or brandy. It is best to shake the tincture daily and allow two weeks for the extraction process. Then strain the herbs out. Vinegar can also be used with some herbs. Tinctures of edible herbs can be valuable for internal as well as external application.

Powders: Powders are made by mashing the plant until there are only very fine particles of the herb. Allow these to dry to a powder. You can make ointments and/or fill capsules with it (see below).

Compress or fomentation: This is a process by which the properties of the plant penetrate the skin topically. It is most often applied for flu, colds, pain, or swelling. It is similar to applying an ointment except it has the added benefit of heat. I boil two heaping tablespoons of the herb in one cup of water. Then I dip a cotton pad into the liquid and squeeze out the extra, placing it on the affected area immediately. Next I cover it with a piece of fabric (wool is best) to keep in the heat. When it cools, I do it again, over and over.

Poultices: I mash the herb and make a paste with water or oil, then heat it in a pan. When warm, I apply it directly to the affected area to relieve inflammation, draw out toxins, cleanse, or heal. Then I cover it with a heated towel to keep in the heat, and reheat and change when it cools.

Capsules: Empty capsules and a capsule filler can be easily purchased from any health food store, or you can purchase the capsules from the health food store already filled. To make your own, you just buy the powdered herb or powder and simply fill the empty capsules yourself.

Ointments or salves: To make an ointment, use three ounces of powdered herb to seven ounces of almond oil and one ounce of beeswax. Blend the ingredients together in a covered pot over low heat for one to two hours. When it cools, it is ready to apply. If it is not the consistency you desire, add more oil or beeswax.

Note: Never use aluminum pots in the preparation of herbs; use glass or enamel or porcelain.

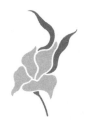

The Herbs

Aloe Vera

Aloe spp.

Liliaceae

There are many early references to aloe vera. The earliest recording of aloe vera appears to be 1500 B.C. in the *Papyrus Ebers*, the original copies of which are said to be at the University in Leipzig. These papers state the many beneficial uses of aloe vera.

Cleopatra and aloe vera

History records the all-time Queen of Beauty, Cleopatra, used aloe vera on a regular basis. Dioscorides, a Greek physician of the first century who compiled the first pharmacopoeia, made lengthy reports of aloe's many applications. The Greek philosopher and scientist Aristotle felt that aloe was priceless to treat wounds. Women of Asia used aloe to stimulate hair growth through external application.

Beneficial attributes

An aloe vera plant should be placed in every kitchen in the world. Not only is it one of the best cosmetic ingredients, it is the best first-aid kit for all kinds of kitchen and other burns. It is attractive and easy to grow, too. It is from the lily plant family like many important herbs, including garlic, onions, leeks, and tulips. Small enough to grow in a pot indoors, in places like Hawaii aloe vera plants grow as large as shrubs.

Scientific conclusions

Scientists have found that aloe has anesthetic, anti-bacterial, and tissue restorative properties, and they state conclusively that "aloe gel does indeed heal burns from flame, sun, and radiation. The gel soothes itching and burning, depending upon the severity of the burn, the tissue regenerates with no scar, and normal pigmentation of the skin returns,"[*] according to *Rodale's Illustrated Encyclopedia of Herbs. The Aloe Vera Handbook* states that "when applied to the skin, [aloe] is absorbed directly through the cells into the blood."[†]

Aloe is valuable in almost all skin care products—shampoos and conditioners, toners, astringents, skin stimulators—because of its reputation as a biogenic stimulator which activates and enlivens the cells in the skin, tightens tissue, and restores tone. It is perfect for moisturizers if it is used in conjunction with an emollient, oil, or vegetable glycerin. Used by itself, it is a wonderful cleanser. It is also an asset in mists and sprays, but it is especially wonderful for skin that is in dire need of soothing from burns, including sunburns, as well as insect bites.

Varied uses of aloe

In Mexico the women used to wet their hair at night with the juice directly from the aloe vera plant, allow it to dry, and the next morning rinse with water to make their hair rich and manageable.

According to *The Complete Book of Natural Cosmetics*, the U.S. Navy once kept aloe vera for radiation burns in case of an atomic attack.[‡]

Applying fresh aloe vera juice on scars daily for very long periods of time is said to diminish them. Try a mixture of aloe vera juice, vitamin E, and Madonna lily for six months. I have personally used aloe vera gel nightly for long periods of time to dry blemishes. I cleanse my face, apply a wonderful lavender and sage toner, let it dry completely, and then apply the gel directly from the plant or from a very high quality, organically grown product.

---

[*] Claire Kowalchik and William H. Hylton, eds., *Rodale's Illustrated Encyclopedia of Herbs*, Emmaus, PA: Rodale Press, 1987, p. 506.
[†] Max B. Skousen, *The Aloe Vera Handbook*, Cypress, CA: Aloe Vera Research Institute, 1982, p. 22.
[‡] Beatrice Travern, *The Complete Book of Natural Cosmetics*, New York, NY: Simon & Schuster, 1974, p. 128.

Many people have found that applying fresh aloe juice three times daily has reduced brown skin spots, also known as "age spots." For double effectiveness, try a half-and-half mixture with fresh lemon juice.

How good a deodorant is aloe vera? Native American hunters used the aloe vera juice to prevent animals from picking up their scent by rubbing aloe vera all over their bodies.

Many people say they are allergic to aloe vera. I always suggest that they try it directly from the plant before they assume it is the aloe plant they are allergic to. I think many times it is other less-than-desirable ingredients, usually preservatives, in the products that cause allergic reactions.

In an orchard there should be enough to eat, enough to lay up, enough to be stolen, and enough to rot upon the ground.
—James Boswell

Apples

Pyrus malus

Pomaceae

Apples are my favorite fruit, apple blossoms my favorite flower, and apple trees my favorite tree. Growing up with a beautiful apple orchard, plus my dad's affection for apple trees, could not but leave me deeply touched by their beauty and basic usefulness.

Preference for apples and apple blossoms

Apples have always held an unspoken meaning of "temptation." Thanks to the story of Adam and Eve, apples always remind us of this meaning. I believe apple blossoms should be preferred above all other flowers, including the rose, because when all the beauty of the rose is gone, it leaves a scent, but the apple blossom leads to the fruit.

Apples, cider, vinegar, and pectin are all extremely medicinal. (See section on Vinegar.) I think apples are one of Mother Nature's wonder health foods. The whole apple must be fresh and crispy; the cider is best when pressed without heat. The vinegar must be held up to the light before purchasing and have the "mother" floating visibly in it. The "mother" is what my dad and the other old-time farmers traditionally called the solid and quasi-solid stuff floating in high quality unfiltered and unrefined vinegar.

A good beginning

Apple products are an easy means to start making your own body care products. They are fun, familiar, available, and if you have some left over, you can just pop them in your mouth for a refreshing treat. Fresh raw apples make a wonderful mask mixed and mashed with honey or yogurt for irritated and sensitive skin.

When I first started making my own purely botanical™ skin care products, apples, of course, were my first choice for an ingredient. I made what I referred to as "apple mush" masks, cider astringents for the face and for the bath, and vinegar rinses for my hair.

Jeanne Rose recommends in her *Herbal Body Book* that "an excellent pomade for rough skin, elbows, heels, and knees is made by mixing apple pulp with equal amounts of solid fat and rosewater; the ingredients can be altered to suit your needs."*

A great apple mask can be made by blending one-half an apple, one tablespoon honey, one tablespoon cider vinegar, three tablespoons almond or olive oil, and one tablespoon cooked oatmeal. Apply while lying down or in the bathtub, and leave on for twenty minutes. This mask is very soothing, healing, and nutritious for the skin.

I find that apple tree bark makes a great facial skin tonic for dry and normal skin. Make a tea of approximately one-fourth cup apple tree bark in two and one-half cups water. Use within three days and keep refrigerated.

Components of apples

Apples contain amylase, which is an exfoliating enzyme beneficial in skin care products. Apples are an excellent source of malic acid, a protein digester, and contain vitamins A and C. Apple seeds contain toxins, so be sure to remove them.

Apples are a good source of boron, which boosts blood levels of estrogen and other compounds that prevent demineralization. Boron also increases brain alertness. Apples are mildly antibacterial, anti-inflammatory, and antiviral.

Other benefits

Eating "an apple a day" goes a long way to aid the digestive tract and to help eliminate toxins. According to Daniel B. Mowrey, in *The Scientific*

---

* Jeanne Rose, *The Herbal Body Book*, New York, NY: Perigee Books, 1982, p. 48.

Validation of Herbal Medicine,[*] apple pectin serves the natural purpose in plants of binding adjacent cell walls. It is believed that pectin operates by binding with bile acids, thereby decreasing cholesterol and fat absorption.

Especially beneficial to dry skin is an apple mush and brewer's yeast mask. Fresh apple juice made from the core and peel is a great source of pectin and an effective skin smoother. Just apply with a cotton ball or mix with honey as a mask.

Apples in my past

Since my dad was a sixth-generation apple grower and I grew up around an apple orchard, you can imagine the ways my parents prepared apples. Since they were "free" for us, and my parents had five kids to feed—and Mom and Dad were as frugal as you could be—we had apples every imaginable way. We had fried apples for breakfast, raw while working on the farm, applesauce for lunch, baked apples, apple crisp, and apple brown Betty for dessert, Dutch apple cake, stewed apples, and apples in tapioca. My parents tried a similar menu one year with corn, and after that year I did not eat corn again for ten solid years. But I never tired of apples.

Cherry and blueberry pies were not allowed in our house, and on the rare occasion we ate out it was not even wise to look at another fruit pie. Applesauce was made by the gallon, apple butter by the peck, apple cider by the barrel, and even love at our house was expressed in bushels.

Private enterprise began early at our house

My very first entrepreneurial job was selling apples door to door. My dad split up the neighboring housing areas between my brothers and me, and we each went door to door with wagons or a peck of apples with free samples for our potential customers to try. Teaching us the basics of business, my dad sold us each bushel for about $2 and then we sold our apples for up to $4 a bushel.

---

[*] Daniel B. Mowrey, *The Scientific Validation of Herbal Medicine*, N.P.: Cormorant Books, 1986.

Arnica

Arnica montana

Compositae

Arnica is one of the herbs most recognized for its external use. *Beware*: Taken internally it can be quite poisonous. The Greeks even used arnica for this purpose. It would be ground into a powder and used to poison enemies. Arnica wine was often made for this reason. The Greek naturalist Theophrastus wrote that when slaves became angry with their owners, they sometimes ingested tiny bits to make themselves ill and unable to work.

The external soothing qualities of arnica have been well-documented historically both in Europe and in North America. European herbalists concocted healing remedies with their arnica, while American Indians made healing ointments and tinctures with our native species.

A topical cream, lotion, or oil made from arnica helps relax stiff muscles, treat wounds, relieve pain, and reduce inflammation and bruises. A 1981 German study found two substances in this herb, helenalin and dihydrohelenalin, which produce anti-inflammatory effects.

To make your arnica oil, heat three ounces of the flowers in three ounces of almond oil, using a double boiler on low heat for four hours. Strain the oil and let it cool before applying.

Calendula

Calendula officinalis

Compositae

Calendula is from the plant family *asteraceae*. Many of calendula's historic uses are skin-related. Calendula is a native of the Mediterranean area. Today it grows in most temperate regions of the world.

The ancient Romans gave it the name calendula because the flowers bloomed on the first day of every month of the "calends," their calendar. The plant with the bright yellow and orange flowers was later given another name in honor of the mother of Jesus: Mary's gold. Later this was shortened to marigold.

Historical uses

One of its first uses was to treat scorpion bites. In the Middle Ages, it was widely used for warts, skin blemishes, and bedsores. It has long been a remedy to relieve pain and swelling of a bee or wasp sting. People used to just pick a calendula flower and rub it on the affected area.

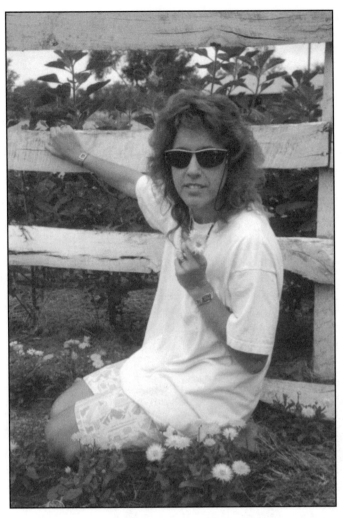

Calendula growing on my farm.

Current example

Years ago I was doing a demonstration of our products in Alfalfa's, a popular health food store in Boulder. A woman came hopping over to my table and said she had been stung by a bee just outside the store. She asked if I had anything to reduce swelling and help the pain. I gave her a sample of our herbal moisturizer, which contains a high content of calendula; she applied it immediately and went to do her shopping.

Less than five minutes later she came back and said, "What is in this stuff? It took away the pain and reduced the swelling already!" She was ecstatic; I should have had her write a testimonial then and there! I know it was a combination of all the healing herbs in our herbal moisturizer, but I'm sure the calendula was the foremost herb at work.

In 1987, a monograph on herbal medicinal substances presented by the West German Federal Health Authority confirmed that calendula flower petals have an inhibiting effect on inflammatory processes, and that an infusion of calendula has a healing effect on cracks, bruises, and burns.

Constituents of calendula

On a zero-moisture basis, the seed contains 30 to 37% proteins and 40 to 45% oils. The flowers contain the amorphous calendulin, analogous to bassorin, traces of an essential oil, and mucilage, along with other plant chemicals. The pigment consists of beta-carotene, lycopene, saponins, and phytosterols. The fresh plant material contains the analgesic salicylic acid, and the roots contain inulin.

Importance of carotenoids

Probably the most beneficial of the chemical constituents are the carotenoids, which are unsaturated pigments, mostly yellow, orange, or red. They occur widely in many plants. Carotenoids are recognized as substances of great importance for all bodily functions, particularly to help the skin regenerate itself. This would contribute to calendula's anti-inflammatory and wound-healing functions. Carotenoids are relatively stable compounds that are soluble in oil. This factor helps to determine what medium is selected for extraction when formulations are prepared.

Calendula can be used in the form of infusion, tincture, oil, and ointment. All are beneficial. Depending on the type of extraction used, however, different chemical constituents will go into the solution.

My experience is that both water and oil extractions are valuable for skin regenerative properties. The oil extraction is better for wound healing, moisturizers, and in products created for varicose veins. The water extracts are better for dermal inflammations and in products for astringency and blemishes.

In an oil-in-water emulsion, a formulator can, depending on his/her objective, do the extraction either in oil, water, or a tincture.

Benefits

Many baby products contain calendula due to its complete non-toxicity. It is perfect for astringent and acne products because of its ability to heal slow-healing wounds such as those from cyst acne, and because it is an anti-inflammatory and a bactericide. Since calendula can stimulate the supply of blood to the skin, it makes the skin not only more supple but also more resistant to mechanical and chemical irritants. This makes it great in a hand cream for people who have their hands in water and detergents a lot.

It is antiseptic and anti-bacterial. The sap from the stems has often been used for removing warts, corns, and calluses. It is probably most often found in creams and lotions for the face because of its regenerative properties that can possibly help reduce wrinkling. For the same reason, it's beneficial in after-sun products.

Calendula's benefits make it useful in almost all skin care products.

A magical reputation

In folklore, calendula was believed to have magical properties. A woman who could not choose between two suitors was advised to take dried calendula flowers, marjoram, and thyme, grind them to a powder, then simmer them in honey and white wine. Then she was instructed to rub the mixture over her body, lie down, and repeat three times: "St. Luke, St. Luke, St. Luke, St. Luke; be kind to me, and in dreams let me my true lover see." In her dreams she would see the man she was to marry. If he were going to be a loving husband, he would be kind to her in the dream, but if he were going to be disloyal, he would be unkind.

Calendula is an asset to any garden. It is an annual and blooms in Colorado from May to October.

Add some beauty to your yard by growing these hardy, brightly colored, showy, beneficial plants.

Coltsfoot

Tussilago farfara

Compositae

A.k.a.: coughwort, foals-foot, horse-hoof

Name derivation and uses

The ancient Romans called coltsfoot *tussilago* meaning "cough plant," which is what it has primarily been used for throughout history. Most herbalists recommended smoking coltsfoot for problems of the lungs and claimed that this use does not injure the lungs like regular tobacco. In Paris, apothecaries hung the coltsfoot flower on their doors as an emblem. In Scotland, they used the fuzz from the seeded flower as pillow stuffing.

Externally, it has been very popular to crush the leaves and roots and apply on areas where people are suffering from welts, hives, inflammations, burns, and itching.

Silica

The high content of silica is essential for connective tissue health and makes coltsfoot an excellent ingredient in skin and hair care products, particularly in products for dry and damaged skin and hair. (To read more on silica, see horsetail).

Calcium

The calcium content could also add to the reason it is so effective, as calcium with vitamin C is said to help form new collagen fibers as well as help keep wrinkles away by keeping the skin firm.

I personally have had great success using coltsfoot. I use it in my moisturizing cream for dry skin, my astringent, and my lotion for normal and combination skin. I have had many rave reviews for all of these products.

Chemical constituents: Silica, tannins, phytosterol, cystine, dihydride alcohol, faradial mucilage, alkaloid, saponins, zinc, potassium, calcium, and amorphous glucoside.

Caution: There is medical controversy regarding the safety of this herb.

Comfrey
Symphytum officinale
Boraginaceae

Comfrey's historical uses

Comfrey's reputation as a healing herb dates back to 400 B.C. The ancient Greeks used it to stop heavy bleeding. Greek physicians of the first century prescribed the plant to heal wounds and mend broken bones. Decoctions of the comfrey roots have been used topically in England since the mid-1600s to aid in wound healing.

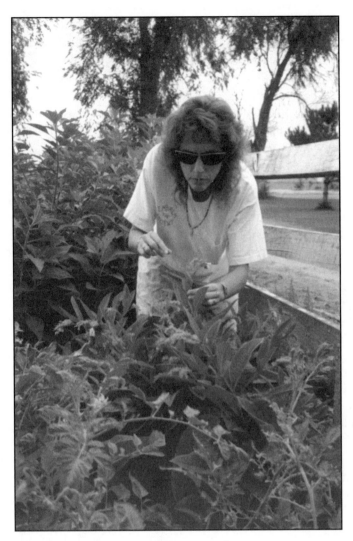

Comfrey on my farm.

Name derivation

Comfrey's botanical name comes from the Greek word that means "to unite." Comfrey, native to Europe and Asia, is also known as knitbone, bruisewort, and knitback, all names referring to its use as a wound-healing herb. It has a long history of use for fractures, bruises, and burns.

Nicholas Culpeper, a seventeenth-century herbalist, recommended comfrey poultices for gout, gangrene, and pained joints. He further stated that comfrey root put in a pot of boiling water with "severed flesh" will join it together again. Since 1887, similar uses were also reported in the United States.

Tannin

For cosmetic purposes, tannins in comfrey have important application. Comfrey's high tannin content is anti-inflammatory and astringent and thus aids in closing wounds and pores.

Allantoin

Comfrey's remarkable power to heal tissue and bone is due to allantoin, a cell proliferate that promotes the growth of connective tissue, bone, and cartilage and is easily absorbed through the skin. Comfrey's reputation goes beyond reweaving broken bones to healing skin lacerations and reweaving collagen. It appears allantoin in some way affects the multiplication of cells and tissue growth. Wounds and burns do heal faster when allantoin is applied. Besides its tissue-regenerative abilities, it seems to be effective in destroying harmful bacteria. Scientists have found allantoin in mother's milk.

The ethnomedical uses of comfrey root are also explained by the allantoin and mucilage content. Allantoin is a white crystalline powder that dissolves easily in hot water. It can be made synthetically or it can be extracted from a tincture. There is much data touting comfrey as a cell proliferate, which is why it has been used for so long for chronic burns, wounds, and ulcers. According to *Macalister's British Medical Journal*, January 6, 1912, allantoin in water solutions in strengths of 3% has a powerful action in strengthening skin formation and is a valuable remedy for external ulcerations.

Mucilage

The mucilage found in comfrey is also said to help new flesh grow and knit together. I suspect that the mucilage creates a gel or gum that pulls the flesh together and reconnects it. Certainly, the long reputation of comfrey as a curative has been considered due to its capacity to reduce the swollen area in the immediate neighborhood of fractures, causing union to take place with greater facility. John Gerard, a sixteenth-century British herbalist, affirmed that "a salve concocted from the fresh herb will certainly tend to promote the healing of bruised and broken parts."

Interestingly, comfrey also contains a small amount of necrotic properties that helps remove dead skin.

Is it possible comfrey works to heal in this way?

* The necrotic properties help remove the dead skin.

* The tannins reduce inflammation.

* The mucilage pulls the severed skin together.

* The allantoin increases the reproduction needed to make the mend.

If allantoin is a cell proliferate—meaning it increases and supports the healing process and cell reproduction—as folklore suggests, what could possibly be a better ingredient to include in anti-wrinkle products, lotions, creams, and astringents?

It is said that pouring a fluid extract of comfrey into a wound will often close the wound, avoiding stitches. Might that same extract help heal stretch marks, wrinkles, pimples, scars, and other blemishes?

We at Lily of Colorado use comfrey in many products very successfully. It is probably one of the most important herbs in cosmetic formulations because of its ability to re-knit collagen. It is valuable in any product that touches the skin. We put it in our herbal astringent, herbal moisturizer, botanical moisture mist, and botanical enzyme exfoliant mask.

Caution: Taking internally has been deemed potentially dangerous.

Elderberry

Sambucus

Caprifoliaceae (Honeysuckle)

Elderberry, it is said, is one of our earliest medicinal plants. It has been found in Stone Age sites.

Elderberry folklore

Like many herbs that have been around for a long time, powers of good and evil are associated with it. While physicians revered it, for a long time no carpenter would make baby cribs out of it for fear of bringing bad luck to the child. According to *Rodale's Illustrated Encyclopedia of Herbs*, the elderberry provided the wood for Christ's cross.[*]

---

[*] Kowalchik and Hylton, eds., *Rodale's Illustrated Encyclopedia of Herbs*, p. 178.

Elderberry music

There are many different kinds of elderberries, from short shrubs to trees as high as fifty feet. The American Indians used elderberries for many things. They even used the hollow stems, making them into flutes. From this use, the elderberry received its additional name, "Tree of Music." In fact, the Latin name for elderberry, *sambucus,* may have come from the Greek word "sambuke," a musical instrument said to be made of elderberry wood that has had the pith removed, leaving a hollow stem through which to pipe music. While the plant has had the reputation medicinally for healing the body, before that it may have been better known for making music to heal the soul.

Use of the berries

The wild variety of elderberries is one of the most potent sources of vitamin A, thiamin, calcium, and niacin. Tonics were often made from the berries to promote overall good health or to apply topically to reduce fevers and increase sweating. Eating the berries often was said to help relieve symptoms of arthritis and gout.

Use of the flowers

Elder flower water has been used widely in Europe as a mild astringent and skin softener for normal and dry skin. Try a handful of dried elderberry flowers thrown into your bath water to sooth your nerves.

A combination of the flowers and the fruit were used to make lotions, salves for burns, and to reduce swelling and joint pain. Some varieties were much more potent than others; these were used as antiseptic washes for hemorrhoids, broken blisters, sores, rashes, and to clear up pimples and acne.

One popular recipe was a concoction of elder flower tea mixed half-and-half with apple cider vinegar. This combination possessed both healing and cooling properties. Elderberry flower tea was often used topically for sunburn and as a helpful remedy to bleach freckles.

Native American uses

Native Americans made ointments from the flowers steeped in oils. After straining the cooked flowers, the mixture was poured into containers and used as a healing salve and skin cream. Other tribes used a similar mixture to treat rashes, inflammations, boils, contusions, scalds, and burns. It was used to treat ulcers, to relieve itching, and almost all other skin irritations. Another external remedy for healing the skin was to make a tea, cool the liquid in which the bark had been boiled, and use it as an overall skin wash.

Elderberries have long been used to dye hair black by simmering the berries in wine or vinegar.

Other tribes used an elderberry poultice for toothaches. Still others used elderberry poultices for headaches, while others for the pain of swollen joints.

Caution: Elderberry shrubs, leaves, and roots of some species can be unsafe, containing dangerous properties. Exercise caution.

Eucalyptus

Eucalyptus spp.

Myrtaceae

The name comes from the Greek *eucalyptos,* meaning well-covered, probably because the flower buds are covered with a membrane.

There are more than 500 species of eucalyptus plants ranging from shrubs to 480-foot giants, making eucalyptus some of the tallest trees in the world. Most are evergreen and all produce oils. Native to Australia, the eucalyptus constitutes much of the vegetation on that continent.

Aborigines play major role

The Australian aborigines deserve all the credit for the discovery of eucalyptus oil. Interestingly, the eucalyptus tree stores water in its roots. Many aborigines dig up a length of the root, blow into one end, and catch the water that comes out of the other end. The eucalyptus tree received one of its common names, "Australian fevertree," from its ability to help fight malaria. Aborigines planted the trees in mosquito-infested marshes. Soon the trees dried the marshes through their heavy feeding, thereby killing the mosquitoes by denying the insects the moisture they need to breed.

The oil, made from the leaves, is considered a germicide, antiseptic, and astringent. The leaves can be used widely, but never use the oil at full strength.

It is wonderful to throw a handful of the leaves in your bath or use it in a facial steam. One teaspoon of the oil in one cup of water rubbed on the skin makes a perfect insect repellent for animals and humans.

Respiratory aid

Eucalyptus is most notably used for the relief of the symptoms of bronchitis, asthma, and croup. Steeping the leaves in hot water for twenty minutes and then breathing the vapors is highly therapeutic. Commercially made cough drops often contain eucalyptus for this reason.

The leaves are useful in astringents, shampoos, and bath products, to relieve aching joints and muscles, as well as in soaps and massage oils. The scent helps open respiratory paths. Jeanne Rose, author of *Herbs & Things*, recommends the leaves be used in sleep pillows for asthma and bronchial problems.[*]

According to Mrs. M. Grieve, author of *A Modern Herbal*, "The medicinal Eucalyptus Oil is probably the most powerful antiseptic of its class, especially when it is old, as ozone is formed in it on exposure to the air. It has a decided disinfectant action, destroying the lower forms of life."[†] She further concludes that an ointment of eucalyptus is helpful for chapped hands, dandruff, and pains in the joints and muscles.

Chemical constituents include a terpene and a cymene. The oil also contains a crystallizable resin, derived from eucalyptol. One method for determining the eucalyptol depends on the conversion of the oil into a crystalline phosphate.

Fennel

Foeniculum vulgare

N.O. Umbelliferae

The wild perennial has yellow flowers and fragrant leaves. Oil is made from the fragrant seeds. The seeds have a licorice taste and flavor.

Appetite suppressing characteristic

The Greeks called the herb *marathron*, from *maraino*, which translates "to grow thin." Many people will be interested in this herb for this reason. The seeds act as an appetite suppressant.

Later, Nicholas Culpeper, a seventeenth-century herbalist, would write about fennel stating that it is "much used in drink or broth to

---

[*] Jeanne Rose, *Herbs & Things: Jeanne Rose's Herbal,* New York: Pergiee Books, 1972, pp. 59–60.
[†] Mrs. Maud Grieve, *A Modern Herbal: The Medicinal, Culinary, Cosmetic and Economic Properties, Cultivation and Folk-Lore of Herbs, Grasses, Fungi, Shrubs & Trees With All Their Modern Scientific Uses,* Vol. I, reprint, New York: Dover Publications, Inc., 1982, p. 289.

make people lean that are too fat."[*] Historically, the seeds were often eaten for the opposite reason, not for the well-fed to lose weight, but by the poor to diminish the pain of hunger. Fennel was often an asset in rituals for days of fasting.

Folklore

Like most herbs that have been around for a long time, there is an esoteric meaning for fennel. In medieval times, fennel was hung over doors to ward off evil spirits. There also are many references to fennel in poetry. In *Paradise Lost,* Milton speaks of the aroma of the plant: "A savoury odour blown, grateful to appetite, more pleased my sense than smell of sweetest fennel."

Fennel's many uses

The Italians love to use fennel in cooking. Throughout history, fennel was widely used with fish and meat, not only because of the culinary advantages, but because it aids in digestion. And it could make unsavory food edible. In fact, the tea was known to relieve vegetable poison caused by mushrooms and other plants. Perhaps this could be because fennel is anti-bacterial.

Fennel was even known to be good for serpent bites. A powder made from the plant is reputed to be effective in keeping fleas away from animals. Poultices of fennel were made to reduce swelling and inflammation of the breasts of nursing mothers. Fennel was taken internally to increase the flow of milk.

A poultice of fennel decoctions is wonderful for the eye area. I like honey masks with powdered fennel to help combat wrinkles.

It is said to stimulate estrogen production and is valuable for painful menstrual periods and cramps.

Historically, fennel has been used to scent soaps and perfumes. I have found fennel seed to be useful and anti-inflammatory in cleansers, shampoos, toners, and astringents. I find it works best in conjunction with other herbs having the same anti-inflammatory and anti-bacterial properties.

Chemical constituents: The seed contains volatile oil, partly comprised of anethole, fenchone, estragole, sulfur, organic sodium, limonene, camphene, and pinene, oleic acid, linoleic acid, and flavonoids, including rutin and vitamins, plus calcium and potassium.

---

[*] Nicholas Culpeper, *Culpeper's Complete Herbal & English Physician Enlarged,* Glenwood, IL: Meyerbooks, Publisher, 1990.

Feverfew

Chrysanthemum parthenium

Compositae

A.k.a.: pyrethrum parthenium, featherfew

Pyrethrum is derived from the Greek *pur* (fire) due to the hot taste of the root. There are many different varieties and species of feverfew. A member of the daisy family, the name comes from the Latin *febrifugia,* or "driver out of fevers." As its name suggests, it is best known for reducing fevers, prompting sweat, as well as its power to cure migraines.

A 1978 British medical journal report suggested that feverfew shares properties with aspirin. A later study reported that it does help stop the pain of migraines in possibly up to seven out of ten sufferers.

According to *Rodale's Illustrated Encyclopedia of Herbs*, "Researchers speculate that substances in the plant appear to make smooth muscle cells less responsive to body chemicals that trigger migraine muscle spasms." Further, Rodale's book quotes Varro Tyler, Ph.D., dean of the School of Pharmacy, Nursing, and Health Sciences at Purdue University: "If you take feverfew by eating the leaves, it should be in very small doses—from 50 to 60 milligrams, which is three or four of the little feverfew leaves each day."[*]

Feverfew makes medicinal claims by its very name.

Special benefits for women

Pedanius Dioscorides, a Greek physician and surgeon in the Roman army in the first century, who compiled the first pharmacopoeia, used the herb for its benefits to the uterus.

Nicholas Culpeper, the famous English astrologer and physician of the early seventeenth century, states in his *Complete Herbal and English Physician*, "Venus commands this herb, and has commended it to succour her sisters [women] and to be a general strengthener of their wombs, and remedy such infirmities as a careless midwife hath there caused; if they will be but pleased to make use of her herb boiled in white wine, and drink the decoction; it cleanses the womb, expels the afterbirth, and doth a woman all the good she can desire of an herb."[†]

---

[*] Kowalchik and Hylton, eds., *Rodale's Illustrated Encyclopedia of Herbs,* p. 192.
[†] *Culpeper's Complete Herbal and English Physician,* p. 73.

Variety of uses

Feverfew's uses are many and varied. John Parkinson used it to help people heal from overdoses of opium. It is a great insect repellent and can be applied externally to treat insect bites. It has also been used to ward off diseases, especially through the scent.

It has been used to diminish freckles, skin discoloration, and brown spots. I use it in our herbal moisturizer because it is anti-inflammatory, healing, skin softening, and a perfect ingredient for sensitive skin. It would also be a desirable ingredient for douches, in toners for dry or sensitive skin, for facial steams for sensitive skin, or as an added herb to a bath.

Chemical constituents: Sesquiterpene lactones, parthenolide and santamarine, volatile oil, and tannins.

German Chamomile

Matricaria recutita

Compositae

What is the world's most popular herb? Chamomile, of course! It is said more than one million cups of the tea are consumed daily. I believe it, because I am one of the many, almost daily chamomile tea drinkers. It is one of the best de-stressers known to the modern world.

Chamomile in ancient Egypt

The Egyptians had such great reverence for chamomile that they dedicated it to their gods and to the sun. They used it to cure ague, a malarial fever with chills and sweating that occurs at regular intervals. They also used it as a massage oil to reduce aching in muscles.

Name derivation

The fresh chamomile plant is strongly and agreeably aromatic, with a distinct scent of apples. This characteristic was noted by the Greeks and for this reason they named it "ground apple" (*kamai*—on the ground, and *melon*—an apple.) The Spaniards call it "manzanilla," which signifies "a little apple," and they gave the same name to one of their lightest sherries flavored with this plant.

When the chamomile plant is walked on, its strong fragrant scent will often reveal its presence before it is seen. For this reason, it was used as one of the aromatic stewing herbs in the Middle Ages and was often purposefully planted in green walks in gardens. Remarkably and unexplainably, walking over the plant seems especially good for it! In fact, the whole chamomile plant is very fragrant and of value, but the quality is chiefly centered in the flower heads or capitula, which is the part employed medicinally. The herb itself is used in the manufacture of herb beers.

Universality of use

The Germans have a saying for chamomile that translates to "capable of everything." America's nineteenth-century eclectic physicians recommended chamomile poultices to speed wound healing and prevent gangrene. The Greek physicians, the Roman naturalists, and India's ancient Ayurvedic physicians all employed chamomile for similar uses at the same time in different parts of the world.

Benefits of chamomile's flowers

Nicholas Culpeper gives a long list of complaints for which chamomile is "profitable": "The flowers boiled in lye are good to wash the head; the bathing with a decoction of chamomile takes away weariness, eases pains, to whatever part of the body it is employed."[*] It has been used in shampoos since the days of the Vikings, because it adds luster to blonde hair.

The flowers of the chamomile plant are recommended as a tonic for dropsy and for the abnormal accumulation of fluid in certain tissues and cavities of the body. Beneficial in their diuretic and tonic properties, they are combined with diaphoretics, which produce perspiration, and other stimulants with benefits.

Chamomile flowers are also extensively used alone or combined with an equal quantity of crushed poppy heads, as poultice and fomentation for external swelling and inflammatory pain. The extracted oil when diluted in vegetable oil eases the pain of rheumatism and gout.

Chamomile's essential oil

Chamomile's essential oil is very valuable in cosmetic preparations. The main component of chamomile's blue essential oil is a compound called azulene. Azulene is said to reduce inflammation and inhibit bacterial growth, which would coincide with why it was traditionally used to speed wound healing and prevent gangrene.

Up to 50% of the essential oil consists of bisabolol, which is highly regarded for its relaxing action on the skin. Bisabolol has numerous pharmacological effects that may account for many of its historic uses.

---

[*] *Culpeper's Complete Herbal & English Physician*, p. 39.

It is known to be effective for reducing inflammation, and its antimicrobial properties make it advantageous both on the skin and to aid in formulation preservation. A recent study shows that bisabolol taken internally speeds up the healing of ulcers and can prevent them from reoccurring.

Flavonoids

Other components of chamomile, principally the flavonoids, also contribute to the anti-inflammatory process. Flavonoids represent a widespread group of water-soluble compounds, many that are colored yellow to purple. The most active flavonoid, apagenine, a yellow-crystalline compound naturally occurring in many plants, is considered to have antispasmodic properties also contributing to its relaxing action on the skin.

Chamomile extracted in the water phase contains only about 10 to 15% of the oil present in the plant. However, the flavonoids, being water soluble, are better extracted by water or alcohol. The best method for extraction of the oil is through distillation, but some of the oil can be extracted by a hydroglycolic process.

Popularity of chamomile

Like calendula, chamomile is greatly loved and used often by cosmetic chemists because it is known to be virtually non-toxic, except to a few people allergic to ragweed. Chamomile penetrates the skin easily and seems to work well with all other herbs. In fact, my personal experience is that putting chamomile in a product aids in the penetration of all the herbal extractions and makes the product more effective. Many formulators also use it in products for marketing reasons—it is the world's best-known herb. Whatever the reason, chamomile is beneficial in all body care products, including, but not limited to, flower or massage oils, astringents, mists, bath products, steam facials, moisturizers, cleansers, lotions, creams, eye products to reduce puffiness, sensitive skin, and shampoos.

Ginseng

American: *Panax quinquefolius*
Siberian: *Eleutherococcus sentiocosus*

Araliaceae

Ginseng—Thomas Jefferson used it, and Daniel Boone sold it. It has probably been used in China since prehistoric times. It grows in Asia and America, and there are many different kinds. I prefer and use the Siberian ginseng, both as a tincture that I take internally and in cosmetic application. The Siberian is touted as one of the best immune system builders.

Medicinally, ginseng has been said to help every ailment under the sun. Lately, it has been recognized for being an "adaptogen" which helps the body in its resilience. After periods of serious stress on the system, adaptogens help the body and mind recuperate. Of course, it is most well-known for increasing longevity and prized as a perfect overall rejuvenator and tonic for inside or out.

Ginseng is a great rejuvenator, stimulant, and makes your skin glow when applied externally in a skin tonic. It is excellent in astringents, toners, creams, cleansers, or lotions.

Hops

Humulus lupulus

N.O. Urticaceae

Hops are native to Britain, although today they are grown in many countries. The English name hops is believed to be derived from the Anglo-Saxon *hoppan*, which means "to climb." This seems likely since hops is a tall-growing vine. Only the female plants are cultivated and used in brewing.

Culinary uses

Hops were mentioned by Pliny, the Roman scholar, as a cooking herb. The shoots were eaten. Hops have been used in brewing since the ninth century. Initially they were used widely as a preservative for beer, the brewers recognizing if they included hops the beer lasted longer. I have tried to use hops as a preservative with very limited success, even though they are said to have antiseptic properties.

Because of their widespread use, hops are globally a significant agricultural crop. The vine can grow up to 25 feet in a season, so hops growers build very tall trellises to support them. The blossoms are harvested for beer and other products.

Benefits of hops tea

Making a tea of the leaves, strobiles, and stalks is reputed to be beneficial for a sluggish liver and to promote hormonal balance, both of which could also have a positive effect on your skin. In addition, hops tea is said to be a stimulant for estrogen production and useful for intestinal cramps. In fact, Nicholas Culpeper states, "Half a dram of the seed in powder taken in drink kills worms in the body, brings down women's courses, and expels urine." He further states: "In cleansing the blood, they help to cure the French diseases, and all manner of scabs, itch, and other breakings-out of the body."* Hops can clearly be useful in a tea for a woman suffering from female troubles.

Hops and women

The effect of hops' estrogenic principles can be so strong that female hops pickers can experience disruption and even complete absence of their periods because of the absorption of the oil through the skin of their hands.

In minuscule amounts, hormonal effects can be beneficial. Thus hops can be very desirable as an ingredient for skin toners, lotions, and creams.

Because hops are known to depress the central nervous system, the tea can be great during times of PMS stress and irritability.

A sleep inducer

Hops are a sedative. Because of this quality, their most beneficial use may be in a sleep pillow. Historical figures as diverse as King George the III and Abraham Lincoln are said to have used this sleep-inducing aid. I have made many different herb pillows, but I think the best one is filled with a combination of hops for the sedative action, lavender for both the wonderful fragrance and its relaxant quality, and mugwort, because it is said to help you remember your dreams.

If you don't know how to sew and want to try this with minimal effort, just place one-quarter cup of each of these dried herbs in an empty pillow case, fold neatly until it is small enough to put in your pillow case with your pillow. Then tuck it in as flatly as possible on the underside of your pillow. I think you will be happy with the results.

Other cosmetic uses

Hops are very valuable in toners, creams, and lotions for dry or stressed skin, also because of its sedative properties. According to Culpeper, it is perfect for skin-lightening products. Hops poultices have been known to help skin discoloration.†

---

* *Culpeper's Complete Herbal & English Physician Enlarged*, p. 96.
† Ibid., p. 95.

Chemical constituents: Volatile oil, which includes humulene, myrcene, geraniol, linalool, citral, linionene, valeronic acid, lumulone, lupulone, tannins, flavonoid glycosides, oestrogenic, and asparagin.

Horse Chestnut

Aesculus hippocastanum

N.O. Sapindaceae

A.k.a.: European horse chestnut, Ohio buckeye, yellow buckeye

The native American horse chestnut trees are called buckeyes. American Indians prepared the starchy buckeye seeds for food by roasting and washing them thoroughly to remove the poison. They also made a powder of the raw seeds and threw it on the water to stupefy fish.

Derivation of name

Hippocastanum vulgare is the sweet chestnut and is not related to the horse chestnut. It is said that the prefix "horse" comes from the Welsh *gwres* meaning hot or bitter, to differentiate it from the "sweet" chestnut. The word *esculus* is derived from *esca,* meaning food.

Healing uses

The bark, fruit, and seeds of horse chestnut have all been used for healing. A tonic can be made from the bark and used for fevers. Historically, the bark has been used externally for ulcers. The fruits are widely used for rectal complaints and for hemorrhoids. It is an astringent and is believed to tone and strengthen the vein walls.

Horse chestnut has a positive effect on all skin it is applied to, so it is a perfect ingredient in astringents. It contracts the skin and is, therefore, especially valuable for people with enlarged pores.

Because it is very soothing and moisturizing to the skin, it is a benefit in any lotion or cream. It is also found in many anti-cellulite and cell-rejuvenation products. It is useful in lotions for sensitive skin and products that lighten the skin.

Chemical constituents: Escin, saponins, flavonoids, tannins, and coumarins.

Horsetail or Shavegrass

Equisetum spp.

Equisetaceae

Horsetail, it is said, has been around for 350 million years. To put that in perspective, cockroaches have only been around for 300 million years.

In prehistoric times, horsetail grew as high as trees. Native Americans used bundles of horsetail stems to scour their cooking pots. Later, cabinetmakers used horsetail for polishing wood finishes. This is how it received its nickname: "shavegrass."

Silica

A large quantity of silica is deposited in the stems of horsetail, especially in the epidermis or outer skin of the plant. Silica in the human body is said to benefit the hair, the skin, and is in the skin's connective tissue. Horsetail has long been used to increase connective tissue tone and resistance in skin treatments.

Nature provides silica in high amounts in horsetail, coltsfoot, and rosehip seeds. These herbs are said to make a vegetable collagen. Collagen is the dermal protein that holds your skin together. Young collagen is flexible and its molecules are displaced in relation to each other. This means it can absorb water and swell slightly. In the aging process, collagen becomes cross-linked, inflexible, and insoluble, like tanned leather. The cells in the dermis lose water and the skin becomes dry and then inelastic.

Plant-derived silica is believed to encourage the formation of new fibers. Experiments have shown that a deficiency in vitamin C suppresses the formation of collagen in the fiber growth called fibroblast. It is believed that vegetable silica has regenerative powers, contributing biologically catalyzing elements to start up the fibroblast again, permitting tissues to regain their tone and elasticity.

Distilled water infused with horsetail is used on the face to clear up pimply breakouts. Horsetail tea is good for broken nails and lifeless hair. It is also useful for white spotting on the nails, a symptom said to indicate a calcium imbalance in the body. Silica encourages the absorption and use of calcium by the body and also helps guard against fatty deposits in the arteries. Horsetail's astringent action makes it perfect for reducing pores.

In Russia, horsetail has been used experimentally to cleanse the system of lead poisoning. Studies have shown fractured bones heal much faster when horsetail is taken. Applied externally it will help stop bleeding and speed healing. It has been found to be very beneficial in reducing the swelling of the eyelids. It has also been used as a diuretic and astringent for bleeding and wounds.

According to *Silica, the Forgotten Nutrient* by Klaus Kaufman, silica is the "ultimate remedy that has the power to transform our aging years into golden years."[*]

For many reasons, horsetail is a beneficial ingredient in any moisturizing or astringent product for your skin or hair. Distilled water infused with horsetail can be used on the face to clear up acne. Just apply a tea or tincture of horsetail to the skin and leave it there for several minutes.

I use horsetail in many of my products. It is beneficial in most cosmetic products: astringents, toners, creams, lotions, steam herbs, masks, shampoos, and conditioners.

Importance of ingredients

What makes horsetail so wonderful is that it can be used instead of animal collagen, which is an ingredient in many commercial skin care products. Personally, there is no way I am going to put any part of a dead animal on my skin. I cannot buy into the idea that this is a good thing. It is not only the moral issue; I just don't think it could be good for me or for my skin.

Worse, there is a multi-level skin care company that uses human placenta as an ingredient. I find that disgusting and most unhealthy. I do not want to apply that to my skin under any circumstances, or to even think for a moment of how it is obtained, preserved, stored, and processed. I do not want to even discuss it further, but this is a good time to make my case on how important it is for you to carefully look at your cosmetics' ingredients. You just might be horrified to what extent some companies go to come up with some new, trendy, hyped ingredient.

Cosmetic astrology

Herbalists interested in astrology place horsetail under the influence of Saturn, and Saturn rules over all aging and chronic processes: bone structure, teeth, spine, minerals in the blood, and the bladder.

Beware: Excessive use of horsetail may cause irritation to kidneys and to intestines; it is recommended a person not take horsetail for more than two and a half weeks at a time. Do not take it if you are pregnant or nursing.

---

[*] Klaus Kaufman, *Silica, The Forgotten Nutrient*, Burnaby, B. C.: Alive Books, 1990.

Irish Moss

Chondrus crispus

Rhodophyceae (Red Algae)

A.k.a.: Carrageenans, Lichen

Scientists with the U.S. Department of Agriculture state that 100 grams of edible sea moss is very nutritious and contains very high amounts of potassium, calcium, phosphorus, sodium, and iron. It also has magnesium, chlorine, sulfur, copper, iodine, and other trace minerals.[*]

Irish moss is extremely soothing whether taken internally or externally. Historically, it has been used for respiratory disorders and as a nutritious food for the elderly and invalids. It is also used to ease the pain of gastric problems.

Drying and reconstituting qualities

Irish moss can be stored for years when it is dried. It maintains its nutritious value and swells up to its original size again when remoistened. This is one of its attributes that make it such a valuable ingredient in cosmetic preparations. I love working with it; it seems almost magical the way it can be stored dry for years and then grow back to its original size.

A natural thickener

Irish moss partially dissolves in water and forms a viscous gel. It reacts with mild protein to form a thick gel. Instead of synthetically derived emollients in thickeners, Irish moss can be used effectively.

It is an emollient and enhances any skin care product. I use it in a seaweed cleanser, and it works well to help the product feel soothing and wonderful on the skin. It nourishes the skin with all of its precious botanical constituents.

Irish moss is a seaweed that is harvested in shallow water. When my mother was a teenager, she and her brothers and sisters packed it into large burlap sacks. She remembers that they got paid two cents a pound by a company that sold it to a milk processor. The Irish moss kept the chocolate milk in suspension.

Chemical constituents: Five polysaccharide complexes known as carageenans, sulphur, iodine, bromine, and iron.

---

[*] Bradford Angier, *Field Guide to Medicinal Wild Plants*, Harrisburg, Pa.: Stackpole Books, 1978.

Ivy

Hedera helix

N.O. Araliaceae

Ivy is best known today as the cover for unsightly buildings and is highly ornamental.

Ivy was formerly held in high esteem. Poets' crowns were made of ivy leaves. Because ivy is a symbol of marital fidelity, Greek priests used to make wreaths of it for newlyweds. It is said that drinking the wine in which ivy leaves were boiled will take away intoxication.

Ivy has held meanings of friendship and matrimony because ivy clings forever to a tree once entangled. This is the major point of its symbolism. Even though ivy maintains its own root system and life force, nothing can separate it from a tree it has once embraced.

Throughout history, the flowers were used to aid in healing burns. Culpepper in *The Complete Herbal and English Physician* writes: "It also quickly heals green wounds, and is effectual to heal all burnings and scaldings." He also states: "The fresh leaves of Ivy, boiled in vinegar, and applied warm to the sides of those that are troubled with the spleen, ache, or stitch in the sides, do give much ease. The same applied with some Rosewater, and oil of Roses, to the temples and forehead, eases the head-ache, though it be of long continuance."[*]

Ivy is often found in bath products, lotions, creams, and anti-cellulite products. I use it primarily in my herbal moisturizer because of its healing effect on burned, scalded, or stressed skin, and it works synergistically very well with other herbs, such as chamomile, hops, and bladderwrack.

Chemical constituents: The leaves and berries contain saponins, ederin, chloroginic caffeic acids, and flavonoids.

Kelp or Bladderwrack

Fucus vesiculosus

The seaweed kelp has several common names: Bladderwrack, Black wrack, Sea wrack, and Black tang.

There are many different types of species. All are good to eat, even though they can vary dramatically in chemical makeup. There is the giant kelp from the Pacific Ocean, often reaching eighty feet in length, which whales and sea lions enjoy snacking on. Some grow to 150 feet

---

[*] *Culpeper's Complete Herbal & English Physician*, p. 100.

and can form underwater forests. Then there is the less impressive looking kelp that is often green or brownish but is also valuable.

Many and varied uses

Kelp is the original source of iodine, a discovery made in 1812 by Cour-
tois. It is high in potash salts, potassium chloride, sodium, calcium, and
many trace elements, and a superb food supplement benefiting the skin,
fingernails, and hair. Kelp is also a skin smoother. One of its main uses is
to re-mineralize the body. All of the seaweeds are advantageous for
poultices for cuts and bruises, and to treat chronic psoriasis and reduce
inflammation and pain from arthritis. Many Native Americans used
kelp to relieve pain and to heal scalds and burns. It has also been used as
a blood purifier and, in general, to bring good health.

My view

Anything as nutritious and containing so many essential properties for
your body must be beneficial to your skin. Seaweeds in the bath leave
trace elements on your skin and, if you take a hot bath, those minerals
enter your body through your heat-opened pores. I love seaweeds. The
mucilage they produce is very healing, cleansing, moisturizing, and
feels good. Kelp is high in silica so it is extremely beneficial to the skin
and hair.

There's more: Kelp is renowned for being a weight-loss herb because
of its effects on the thyroid gland. Twenty-five grams taken before each
meal is often recommended.

Chemical constituents: Mucilage, mannitol, potassium, iodine, volatile oil, sodium, calcium, potassium chloride, potash salts, and many
trace elements.

Lavender

Lavandula angustifolia

Labiatae

Many old books on lavender say that its smell has the power to conjure
memories of other times and places. I have seen this statement proven
time after time. I use lavender in many of my products, and when people
smell the product full of the essential oil, they say, "This reminds me of
the first girl I ever loved" or "This reminds me of my grandmother's
house" or "My mother used to wear this scent." I love lavender and I

think it is one of the most wonderful flowers, fragrances, and cosmetic ingredients known to womankind.

Lavender has a very clean, spare, and classic fragrance. Its very name derives from the Latin verb "to wash," and both the Romans and the Greeks scented their soaps and bathwater with the flower.

Lavender is balancing

Both historically and today, lavender has so many uses it would almost be confusing, except for the fact that it is so balancing. This is one word you must remember whenever you hear anything about lavender. For example, in the Middle Ages, lavender was thought to be an herb of love, and it was often used as an aphrodisiac. However, it seemed to work both ways because it is also said that lavender sprinkled on one's head is helpful in keeping one's chastity. For more about this versatile plant, see the section on Lavender under Herbs and Essential Oils.

Lavender is used in just about every kind of skin care product, and all correctly, because lavender is so balancing. It is perfect for dry skin, normal skin, and oily skin. One of lavender's most important uses is to normalize the oil flow of the glands. Lavender stimulates the skin, but it is also the universal calming and soothing oil. Lavender in any form is valuable in all body care products, including, but not limited to, facial steams, masks, cleansers, astringents, toners, lotions, creams, oils, bath products, and sleep aids. It is applied as an antiseptic for swabbing pimples, wounds, acne, or sores.

I personally love lavender oil, and I put the essential oil in my bath. I make my own perfume using lavender as one of the key ingredients. I put it in all my oils for my bath and my hair.

Lavender is one of the best remedies for burns and bee stings. Before World War I, lavender was used as a disinfectant for wounds because of its strong anti-bacterial action. Traditionally, it has been used to freshen sickrooms, to soothe troubled minds and bodies, and as a medicine for hysteria, nervous palpitations, and headaches. Lavender has even been used for embalming corpses, curing animals of lice, repelling mosquitoes, and taming lions and tigers.

Sleep pillows

Probably my favorite use for lavender is in the sleep pillows I make. I take one-half cup of lavender, one-half cup of hops, and two tablespoons of mugwort herb, and for simplicity's sake, I fold them up in an old pillowcase and then put it inside my regular pillowcase. More ambitious people can choose delightfully appropriate fabrics featuring moons, stars, and angels—whatever appeals to them—and make small pillows, say 6 to 8 inches square, or round, triangular, or even free form. Choose whatever pleases you.

Lavender has the most wonderful scent; the hops scent is a sedative and helps you relax and prepare for a wonderful sleep. The mugwort helps you have better dreams and remember them.

Many stores sell these dream pillows; however, I think it is probably best to make them yourself, because it is said that negative vibrations can be passed from the person making them to the herbs. Why take the chance? You can lovingly make these for yourself and those around you.

Lily

Lilium

Liliaceae

Lilies are one of the most underestimated herbs. From the time of man's earliest recording, the lily was noted as the flower of purest beauty. Special virtues were once thought to be possessed by water distilled from the flowers, known as *aqua area* or golden water, and it was deemed worthy to be preserved in vessels of gold and silver.

A distilled water of lilies was historically employed as a cosmetic, and oil of lilies was supposed to possess nervine powers. The odorous matter of lilies of the valley, though very powerful, is totally dissipated in drying and entirely lost in distillation, so no essential oil can be obtained from them through this process. However, the petals can communicate their fragrance to almond oil. The only effective method to collect this scent is to take a container of almond oil and fresh lily of the valley flowers and soak the flowers in the oil for two weeks. After that time, strain and squeeze the oil from the flowers, and repeat the process using fresh flowers each time, as many times as it takes to impart the scent to the oil.

Native American uses for the lily

Native Americans found many special uses for lilies. Lilies of particular value to the Rocky Mountain region Indians included the yellow pond lily. The Indians would eat the entire plant. They dried lilies, roasted them like popcorn, or ground them into meal for bread and porridge. They also used the leopard, or tiger lily, which Western Indians and the Eskimos still eat like corn.

One of the best remedies known for healing burns and scalds without leaving a scar is an ointment made from Madonna lily root. Many of the lily bulbs, in ointment form, are excellent to remove the pain and inflammation from burns and scalds leaving no scar. The ointment is also used to remove corns.

Ointments of lily have had the reputation of being excellent as an application for contracted tendons. John Gerard, a sixteenth-century British herbalist and author of one of the most famous of all herbal books, said that "the root of the garden lily stamped with honey gleweth together sinewes that be cut asunder. It bringeth the hairs again upon places which have been burned or scalded, if it be mingled with oil or grease."*

Pond lilies

White pond lily root is used for inflamed skin. The European yellow pond lily contains nuphar-tannic acid and the flowers contain a fragrant, volatile oil with tannins, sugar, gum, and chlorophyll. If the flowers are too old, they may produce symptoms of narcotic intoxication.

Country people sometimes steeped the fresh lily blooms in spirits and used the liquid as a lotion for bruises in the same manner as arnica or calendula.

The French call lily of the valley *muguet*. According to *Perfume Album*, although the scent is not passed through the distillation process, "The chemist knows almost nothing about the composition of lily of the valley oil," and "Jasmine and rose oils mixed with ylang ylang and orange blossoms can give a lily of the valley scent."†

The lily was always known as a symbol of majesty, and as a formal flower almost needing other flowers in contrast to make its majestic impression. The lily of the valley is regarded as a "return of happiness."

"The light of its tremulous bells is seen/ Through their pavilions of tender green," Shelley writes of the exquisite lily of the valley.

Legend says that the fragrance of the lily of the valley draws the nightingale from hedge and bush and leads him to choose his mate in the recesses of the glade.

---

* John Gerard, *The Herball or Generall Historie of Plantes*, London, 1597; fac. ed., London: John Norton.
† Jill Eva Jessee, *Perfume Album*, Huntington, NY: Robert E. Krieger Publishing Co., Inc., 1951, p. 52.

Artistic and religious use of the lily or lotus

In Greek mythology, the lotus plant represented distaste for active life and was known to induce luxurious dreaminess. In India, there is a large temple made of concrete built in the shape of the lotus lily that holds hundreds of people. Many Buddhist and Hindu deities are pictured and sculpted sitting on lotus flowers. The goddess of the lotus is Prajna-Paramita, the highest female personification in Buddhism, the most spiritual feminine symbol. "The lotus of the world supports the symbol of the enlightenment that dispels the darkness of the naïve ignorance inherent in all beings."[*]

The lotus symbolizes how we should live life: Although it has its roots in the mire, it pushes upward through the water and raises its blossom head above the earth.

The lily has historically been the flower chosen to represent the Easter season, commemorating the resurrection of Jesus Christ, perhaps because it blooms at that time of year.

Lilies are mentioned numerous times in the Bible. It is believed that the Madonna lily was around in biblical times. Many believe that the flower's revered place partly stems from its beauty being constantly painted by medieval artists who always showed it as the symbol of purity, most referring to the Virgin Mary.

It seems to me that if roses represent romantic love, then lilies represent pure unconditional love.

Mint

Mentha piperita

N.O. Labiatae

I grow wild mint at my house. I simply put the clean, fresh leaves in boiling water and steep a few minutes. It makes a very refreshing beverage. I also cut the stalks of the plant and place them on me or around me when I am trying to enjoy my porch in the summer, because the mint keeps away the flies that the nearby horses attract.

External uses

There are several varieties of peppermint. According to Mrs. Maud Grieve, author of *A Modern Herbal*, "Among essential oils, peppermint

---

[*] T.C. Majupuria and D.P. Joshi, *Religious and Useful Plants of Nepal and India*, Lalitpur Colony, Lashkar, India: M. Gupta, 1989.

ranks first in importance."[*] Peppermint essential oil is used widely both commercially and medicinally. Due to its anti-spasmodic action, it relieves pain and is often applied externally for this purpose, for toothaches, colic, rheumatism, sudden pains, and cramps in the abdomen. It acts as a local anesthetic and vascular stimulant, and it is anti-bacterial.

Internal uses

Internally, the tea is a stimulant and is a wonderful carminative, aiding greatly in reducing flatulence and the pain therefrom. It is said that drinking mint tea on the onset of a cold or mild flu will expel it within a day and a half.

When you are suffering from any sort of stomach problem, whether it be female cramps or too much food or disagreeable food, peppermint tea is helpful. It is inexpensive and delightful to drink. I like the tea mixed with a little honey.

There are many branches in the mint family. Two are peppermint, a perennial that is primarily used for cosmetic purposes, and spearmint, used for culinary purposes. The fragrant oil from the peppermint plant's smooth, sharply pointed leaves is extracted from the plant by steam distillation. (Commercial mint growers have mint distilleries.)

Menthol, useful in giving a sensation of coolness in the mouth, is made from peppermint oil.

Peppermint is highly stimulating on the skin and at low doses, mixed with other appropriate ingredients, accelerates the sloughing process. Thus, it is a favored ingredient in botanical enzyme exfoliant masks, facial steams, cleansers, and toners.

Chemical constituents: Menthol, menthyl acetate, isovalerate, menthone, and cineol.

Myrrh

Commiphora myrrha

Burseraceae

So precious was myrrh that it was one of the gifts the Wise Men brought to Bethlehem. Tradition holds that myrrh was used 2000 years before Christ. Its uses are varied. The ancient Egyptians often used myrrh as an ingredient in embalming corpses. It also has been used in incense and in perfume.

---

[*] Grieve, *A Modern Herbal*, Vol. II, p. 541.

"A Syrian legend, later adopted by the Greeks, associates myrrh with the goddess Myrrha, daughter of Thesis, the king of Syria; she was forced by Aphrodite to commit incest with her father and then escaped being murdered by him when the gods transformed her into a myrrh tree. The drops of gum resin that come from cuts on the tree are said to be Myrrha's tears."[*]

Myrrh is often used as an ingredient in gargles and mouthwashes, because it is anti-fungal, antiseptic, and astringent. This is the same reason I use it in skin care products. It is infection fighting, anti-inflammatory, and is able to reduce oiliness and cool the skin, making it a desirable ingredient for creams, lotions, and any skin tonics. Myrrh is only partially soluble in water.

Chemical constituents: Volatile oil that contains heerabolene, limonene, dipentene, pinene, eugenol, cinamaldehyde, cuminaldehyde, commiphoric acids, ash, salts, sulphates, benzoates, malates, and acetates of potassa.

Rosemary

Rosmarinus officinalis

Labitatae

A.k.a.: Compass weed

Symbolism of rosemary

The ancient Greeks, it is said, wore sprigs of rosemary in their hair to promote good memory. Because of its reputation for strengthening the memory, it was also the emblem for fidelity in marriages and represented friendship. Rosemary is a symbol of love and loyalty. It has been used in incantations particularly to ward off evil spirits. It was worn by brides at weddings. Together with an orange and cloves it was given as a New Year's Eve gift.

Benefits

Roger Hacket stated in a sermon, "A Marriage Present," published in 1607: "Speaking of the powers of rosemary, it overtoppeth all the flowers in the garden, boasting man's rule. It helpeth the brain, strengtheneth the memorie, and is very medicinable for the head."

The Treasury of Botany states that "rosemary will not grow well unless where the mistress is master; and so touched are some of the lords

---

[*] Kowalchik and Hylton, eds., *Rodale's Illustrated Encyclopedia of Herbs,* p. 396.

of creation upon this point, that we have more than once had reason to suspect them of privately injuring a growing rosemary in order to destroy this evidence of their want of authority."[*]

A formula dated 1235, made of rosemary and called "Hungary water," is said to be in Vienna in the handwriting of Elizabeth, the queen of Hungary. According to Mrs. M. Grieve, author of *A Modern Herbal*, "Hungary water, for outward application to renovate the vitality of paralyzed limbs, was first invented for a Queen of Hungary, who was said to have been completely cured by its continued use. It was prepared by putting 1.5 lbs. of fresh Rosemary tops in full flower into one gallon of spirits of wine, this was allowed to stand for four days and then distilled."[†]

Jeanne Rose recommends in her *Herbal Body Book*, "Rosemary with lavender is an excellent herbal stimulant tea if you are allergic to caffeine."[‡]

Culpeper states in his book, "Take what quantity you will of the flowers, and put them into a strong glass close stopped, tie a fine linen cloth over the mouth, and turn the mouth down into another strong glass, which being set in the sun, and oil will distill down into the lower glass, to be preserved as precious for diverse uses both inward and outward, as a sovereign balm to heal the diseases before mentioned, to clear dim sights, and take away spots, marks, and scars in the skin."[**]

Uses

Rosemary is known as a great purifier, an antioxidant, and is antimicrobial. It soothes sprains and bruises and helps wounds in the healing process. It is found in acne products, aching-muscles toners, cleansers, facial steams, creams, lotions, and astringents. A couple of drops in the bath are very relaxing.

Rosemary should be included in high quality hair products of any kind as it is an effective remedy for dandruff and is recommended in shampoos, conditioners, and rinses. It is touted for its effectiveness in footbaths and facial steams to stimulate the skin.

---

[*] John Lindley, *The Treasury of Botany*, rev. ed., London: Longmans, Green and Co., 1889.
[†] Grieve, *A Modern Herbal*, p. 683.
[‡] Rose, *Herbal Body Book*, p. 120.
[**] *Culpeper's Complete Herbal & English Physician*, p. 156.

It is said to stimulate the hair bulbs to renewed activity and therefore to aid in preventing baldness. Essential oil of rosemary mixed with almond oil and slowly heated to use as a hot-oil hair treatment is wonderful also mixed with a little lavender. A small amount of rosemary and lavender is nice to put on your hairbrush to stimulate the scalp daily.

Chemical constituents: volatile oil; the primary constituents of the oil are borneol, bornyl acetate and other esters, rosmarinic acid, carnosic acid, tannins, and oleanolic acid.

St. John's Wort
Hypericum perforatum

Hypericaceae

Many old-time superstitions relate to this plant. The name *hypericum* is derived from the Greek and means "over an apparition," referring to a belief that the herb was so obnoxious that one whiff and it would send the demons straight back to hell. I've been told of the legend that if you stepped on the plant at dusk, you may be carted off on a magic fairy horse and not be back until the next day.

Connection to St. John the Baptist

For hundreds of years this plant has been used to fend off evil spirits and the devil. The plant is named after St. John the Baptist. It was said to bloom first on his birthday, June 24th, and to bleed red oil from its leaf glands on the day he was beheaded in August. It is believed that the plant is most potent medicinally if it is harvested on June 24th.

Benefits

Preparations are derived from the leaves and flowers. St. John's wort contains compounds with potential immune boosting, wound-healing, and antibiotic properties. It is astringent, and the tea is helpful for children to drink at night to stop bedwetting.

The oil of St. John's wort is made from the flowers infused in a high quality vegetable oil. It is widely used to soothe the skin. It has also been used as a sedative and painkiller and to take the sting and pain out of sunburn. It is being investigated as a bactericide. The blossoms soaked in a high quality vegetable oil make a soothing dressing for cuts. St. John's wort is also used to increase and induce a sense of well-being and is gathering wide acceptance today as an antidepressant.

It is used to reduce blotches and varicose veins. Cosmetic manufacturers use it to texturize, as an astringent, and add it as a soothing agent. It is useful for wrinkles, dry skin, or as a general healing agent. And a dye of yellow and red can be obtained from the flowering tops and stems.

St. John's wort contains terpenes and sesquiterpenes, tannins, flavonoids, rutin, hypericin.

Caution: There are reports of animals being photosensitive after digesting the plant.

Witch Hazel

Hamamelis virginiana

Hamamelidaceae

Witch hazel is an herbal product that individuals have used and probably do not even know it is botanical. It is great for astringents because it is very high in tannins, which are highly astringent. It is good for acne-skin, blemished skin, or just to tighten pores. However, you can have normal or dry skin and still use witch hazel.

What can tend to be drying with the witch hazel is the alcohol many companies use to make it. If you make a product on your own, you can either boil the witch hazel in water or do an alcohol tincture and then use a slow heat process to evaporate out most of the alcohol. Or simply add other more moisturizing ingredients, for example, an herb high in polysaccharides such as Irish moss or comfrey, or add a humectant, which draws moisture to the skin, such as vegetable glycerin or honey.

In the dictionary, astringent is defined as "tending to contract or draw together organic tissues; binding." I try to always make this important point. Many people think astringent means drying. Not so if you minimize the alcohol.

Yarrow

Achillea millefolium

Compositae

Yarrow has many names, including Nosebleed, Milfoil, Thousand-leaf, Soldier's Woundwort, Devil's Nettle, Devil's Plaything, Bad Man's Plaything, and Yarroway. The name *yarrow* is Anglo-Saxon.

From Trojan War to American Civil War

The sixteenth-century British herbalist John Gerard states that Achilles stopped the bleeding wounds of his soldiers with yarrow in the Trojan

War some 3,000 years ago.* Thus, historically it was called *herba militaris*, or the military herb. In fact, the herb was found on the battlefields right up to the American Civil War.

Yarrow's broad use

Yarrow enjoyed widespread use. The Native American Utes applied yarrow to injuries and sores. At least 46 American Indian tribes used yarrow. The first century Greek physician Pedanius Dioscorides used yarrow on ulcers to prevent inflammation. John Gerard recommended yarrow to relieve "swelling of those secret parts." An English shopkeeper used yarrow with brandy and gunpowder, plus comfrey, for back pain. Yarrow appears in the U.S. pharmacopoeia from 1836 to 1882. In 1982, it still appeared in most European pharmacopoeias.

Long history of healing

For centuries, yarrow has been used for healing wounds. And in the 1950s, an alkaloid from the plant was found to help make the blood clot faster. Its anti-inflammatory and anti-spasmodic property is azulene, the same volatile oil found in chamomile.

Probably because of its close association with bleeding, the early seventeenth-century herbalist Culpeper recommends yarrow for women's complaints, including menstrual cramps. Interestingly, like many herbs, yarrow has the power to both stop and start nosebleeds. Its popular name "nosebleed" comes from its ability to stop nosebleeds; contrariwise, if you roll up the leaf and apply it inside the nostrils it will cause a nosebleed. According to folklore, it could be a positive sign if your nose bleeds.

It was used historically in witchcraft, hence its nicknames, Devil's Nettle, Devil's Plaything, and Bad Man's Plaything. There was a spell where the leaf was inserted in the nose while the following lines were recited:

Yarroway, yarroway, bear a white blow/
If my love loves me, my nose will bleed now.

Yarrow is very astringent, a tonic, a stimulant, and mildly aromatic. It is reputedly a wonderful preventative of baldness and should be in any shampoo that makes that boast. Oily hair also benefits from it in rinses. I include it in facial steams for normal to oily skin. It is fine in

---

* Gerard's *Herball*.

herb baths. It is a perfect ingredient for a cleanser, especially for oily skin or toner. Yarrow's anti-inflammatory properties make it great for skin care. It is often used in cosmetics as a soothing agent. Yarrow has also been historically known as one of the best remedies for a fever.

Yarrow in Scandanavia

In Sweden, yarrow is called "Field Hop" and has been used to make beer. It is considered much more intoxicating than when hops are used. It is used in Norway for the cure of rheumatism, and the fresh leaves are chewed to cure a toothache.

Planting yarrow next to other herbs increases the essential oils of the surrounding plants.

Chemical constituents: flavonoids and salicylic acid; yarrow contains a volatile oil that contains achilleine, which is said to be identical with acontitic acid; acontitic acid is a white to yellowish crystalline solid that is soluble in water and alcohol; it can also be obtained from sugar cane; it is used as a wetting agent and as an antioxidant; yarrow also contains resin, tannin, gum, and earthy ash.

Caution: Taking yarrow internally can cause sensitivity to the sun.

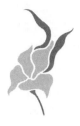

Essential Oils

The sense of smell is the most powerful of senses. It is capable of bringing up long-forgotten memories, feelings of delight and sorrow, as well as stimulating sexual responses. Our noses are said to be able to identify over 10,000 scents.

Aromatherapy

Aromatherapy developed because of the far-reaching effects of our sense of smell. Aromatherapy is simply the science of using oils distilled from plants, including trees, flowers, and herbs, to heal the spirit, mind, and body. A plant's life force is stored in the oil. When penetrated into the skin or inhaled, these oils have the power to alter moods, heal cells, stimulate circulation, and enter the bloodstream to heal the body.

Aromatherapy has been used for eons to heal and enhance our sense of well-being. It has been used in skin care since the Egyptian culture, some 5,000 years ago. For thousands of years, man has used the sense of smell ritualistically through incense, perfumes, lotions, and in healing.

Distilling essential oils

Essential oils are the essence of the plant. Plants usually contain 1 to 10% essential oil. The oils are usually extracted by a distillation process.

Extracting essential oils

Extraction is sometimes done with alcohol. Sometimes it is done mechanically, like for citrus fruits. For example, the citrus peel is squeezed and the essential oil oozes out.

Robert B. Tisserand, author of *The Art of Aromatherapy*, suggests that the essence of a plant "is like its personality. All animals, including humans, have their own characteristic smell."[*]

There is little doubt of the importance scents play in our lives. Scents affect our sexuality and arousal, relaxation, memory, moods, emotions, and help the body by promoting healing. It is estimated there may be up to 500,000 different scents on this planet.

The function of essential oils

One theory is that the function of essential oils is to regulate the rate of transpiration in plants. Moisture from essential oils has different heat conductivity than of just moisture alone, so the essential oil and its scent is a protection to retain moisture and to maintain temperature.

Many things can affect the essential oil within the plant. In some plants, the essential oil can be found in different parts of the plant during different times of the day or year. During the fecundation process, flowering, the essential oil can change drastically; also many external conditions such as fertilization, light, heat, moisture, altitude, even parasites can change the anatomical structure of the plant, hence the essential oil.

Most essential oils are formed at an early part of the plant's life, and it is best to extract it before the fecundation process.

Definition

The Condensed Chemical Dictionary defines essential oils as "volatile oils derived from plants, and usually carrying essential odor or flavor of the plant used. Chemically, essential oils are often principally terpenes (hydrocarbons), but many other classes of compounds are also found. They are to be distinguished from fixed oils such as linseed oil or coconut oil in that the latter are glycerides of fatty acids and hence saponifiable, meaning capable of being converted into soap by reaction with an alkali. Essential oils (except for those containing esters) are unsaponifiable. Some essential oils are nearly pure single compounds, as oil of wintergreen, which is methyl salicylate. Others are mixtures as spirits of turpentine (pinene, dipentene), and oil of bitter almond (benzaldehyde, hydrocyanic acid). Some contain resins in solutions and are then called oleoresins or balsams."[†]

---

[*] Robert B. Tisserand, *The Art of Aromatherapy, The Healing and Beautifying Properties of the Essential Oils of Flowers and Herbs,* Rochester, VT: Destiny Books, 1977, p. 15.

[†] *The Condensed Chemical Dictionary, Fifth Edition.* Revised and enlarged by Arthur and Elizabeth Rose, New York: Reinhold Publishing Corp., 1956, p. 440.

Derivation

Essential oils are derived from the flowers and plants to which they supply the characteristic odors commonly identified with those plants.

Methods of extraction

❋ by steam distillation

❋ by pressing (fruit rinds)

❋ by solvent extraction

❋ by enfleurage (employed for those very delicate oils whose odors are destroyed by even moderate heat; i.e., exposing odorless fats to the exhalations of flowers until they become strongly charged with the perfume)

The Chemistry of Essential Oils and Artificial Perfumes defines essential oils as "odoriferous bodies of an oily nature obtained almost exclusively from vegetable sources, generally liquid (sometimes semisolid or solid) at ordinary temperatures, and volatile without decomposition." It also states that "an absolute scientific definition of the term essential or volatile oils is hardly possible."[*]

Sometimes the essential oils come from the entire plant, sometimes from the tree gum, or the bark, leaves, or root, or as in the orange family, the peel of the fruit. Many theories state that the majority of essential oils are by-products of the "metabolic processes of cell life, such as are many of the alkaloids, colouring matters, and tannins."[†] The essential oil can be part of the excretionary functions, pathological or fibrovascular functions, or the fundamental tissue.

Odors and chemical constitution: Substances of high molecular weight are usually odorless. In order for a substance to be odorous it also must be somewhat soluble in both water and the lipoid fats of the nose cells.

Twenty-two essential oils

Caution: Essential oils can cause irritation when used full strength. Consult a professional herbalist for more information.

---

[*] Ernest J. Parry, *The Chemistry of Essential Oils and Artificial Perfumes*, Vol. II, 4th rev. ed., London, England: Scott, Greenwood and Son, 1922, p. 1.

[†] Ibid.

Essential oil of benzoin gum

Styrax benzoin

A.k.a.: Benzoin tree gum and gum benjamin

The extraction of benzoin oil is usually done tincture-style with high quality grain alcohol. It is often used as a fixative in making perfume and has a nice pleasant scent. The benzoin trees are usually from Thailand or Sumatra. When the trunk of the tree is cut, the gum or resin exudes, which technically makes it a resin. Historically, benzoin tree gum has been used for incense to drive away evil spirits.

It is an antiseptic, deodorant, sedative, and skin tonic for irritations, wounds, dry and cracked skin, and used as a preservative. Although I enjoy using benzoin tree gum in my products for its warming, toning, and healing skin effects, I have never found it to be an adequate preservative although I have run many tests with it.

A very old recipe recommends benzoin tree gum and cinnamon for tiredness, physical and psychological. It is warming, drying, and energizing. It is often used in aromatherapy to help overcome misery, fear, anger, and self-doubt.

Essential oil of bergamot

Citrus bergamia

The essence of bergamot is captured by pressing part of the peel of the fruit. Citric acid is sometimes made from the pulp. Having a wonderful citrus, yet warm and floral scent, it is widely used in the perfume industry.

Bergamot is used as an anti-depressant; it is refreshing and helps people realize the joy in life, to deal with burnout, grief, and loneliness.

It is antiseptic, anti-spasmodic, and relaxing; it is a deodorant, a healing agent, and beneficial for eczema and psoriasis.

Bergamot oil can cause photosensitization and should never be used "neat," that is, full strength, or applied before sun exposure. A mixture of almond oil with 1% bergamot can be used. It should not be used by individuals with sensitive skin.

Used in low doses with kukui nut oil, it can be applied directly on acne. You can put it in your favorite mist and make a spritzer with which to spray your pimples. I make a wonderful acne mist with bergamot, rose geranium, lavender, and tea tree oil. I spray it on my face many times during the day, and it really helps keep my skin clear. While I enjoy the scent of bergamot alone, many people prefer it blended.

Bergamot oil was one of the essential ingredients in Queen of Hungary water, which was said to keep the skin youthful. It may also be beneficial for varicose veins. Also, it is often used to defer appetite and to flavor tobacco and Earl Grey tea.

Chemical constituents: linalyl acetate, limonene, and linalol.

Essential oil of bois de rose

Aniba rosaeodora

A.k.a.: Rosewood oil (can refer to other species as well)

Bois de rose oil is from the rain forest and so is considered by some to be endangered and not recommended. The oil is high in linalol, which is a sedative; it is also highly antiseptic.

Essential oil of camphor

Cinnamomum camphora

Camphor is anti-inflammatory, helps stimulate the skin, reduces pain, and acts as a sedative. A gum, it is a very soothing ingredient at low levels in skin care products. It makes a nice addition to many perfumes and calms the mind. It is used to reduce tired and sore muscles. It is excellent in cleansers for its clean and classic scent.

Essential oil of cedarwood

Juniperus virginiana

Juniperus virginiana is the only cedarwood oil I have worked with, but there are many varieties from all over the world. It is very useful in drying acne but should not be used by people who have sensitive skin. It is a great fixative in a blend. It is often used in aromatherapy to gain self-esteem and improve self-image and confidence. It helps me to face mood swings and even death. Cedarleaf oil, also known as Thuja, although an irritant to the skin, can be applied carefully to remove warts.

Essential oil of cypress

Cupressus sempervirens

Cypress oil is steam distilled. Traditionally, it was inhaled for respiratory problems. It is uplifting, anti-spasmodic, and astringent, reduces fluid retention, is beneficial for cellulite, especially in baths and massage oils, helps with varicose veins, and acts as a sedative.

Jeanne Rose states in her *Aromatherapy Book* that inhaling cypress oil helps heal diseased lungs, and that a drop in a glass of water can be gargled for sore throat or laryngitis.

Cypress oil is wonderful for oily skin, acne, and hair, and helps balance oil glands. It aids healing hemorrhoids and is said to act strongly on the female reproductive system.

It is deemed to help people emotionally who are frustrated, unstable, and full of turmoil and is used in aromatherapy for confusion, mood swings, regrets, and rejection.

Essential oil of fennel

Foeniculum vulgare

Fennel is known for being antiseptic, toning, weight-reducing, diuretic, and anti-bacterial. It contains potassium and sodium. Fennel has been used to scent soaps and perfumes for centuries. It is a stimulant and great in a cleanser or astringent. I find it is one of the best essential oils to inhale during menstrual cramping. It is also reputedly beneficial in building confidence and dependability. (See fennel herb.)

Essential oil of frankincense

Boswellia carteri

A.k.a.: Oil of olibanum

Distilled from frankincense gum resin, frankincense oil is used in many religious ceremonies. I recently attended a traditional Mexican funeral, complete with mariachi band and the burning of frankincense. It was a double funeral that left two orphans, sad in any case, but when they burned the frankincense, it seemed as though everyone went into deep prayer and meditation.

In Roman times, oil of frankincense was used with cremation, either to appeal to the gods or to disguise the odor of burning flesh. When I was in Varanasi, India, which is the holiest of Hindu cities, people brought dead bodies from all over the country to be burned at the ghats (the steps) of the Ganges River; they burn the bodies there almost 24 hours a day and pour the ashes into the river. This practice leaves a very unpleasant odor and causes terrible air pollution. It might be wise for them to burn frankincense with the bodies, drastically improving the smell and air quality. It definitely (it seems to me) would be more pleasing to the gods as well.

Tisserand states that "the Egyptians did not use it for embalming purposes, but it was used in many of their rejuvenating face masks."[*] Frankincense is a valuable skin care ingredient and has been for thousands of years, especially for wrinkled and dry skin in soaps, skin oils, cleansers, and astringents.

And who can forget that frankincense was brought by the Three Wise Men as a fitting gift for the infant Jesus?

Essential oil of German chamomile
Matricaria chamomilla

Chamomile oil is anti-depressant, anti-spasmodic, and antiseptic. It is widely used in shampoos for light or blond hair and in skin care products for dry skin. It soothes chapped and dry skin and lips, and is used in toners and hair care products. Aubrey Organics has a wonderful Blue Chamomile shampoo. (See Chamomile under Herbs for more about this versatile herb and oil.)

Essential oil of immortelle
Helichrysum italicum

A.k.a.: Everlast

Jeanne Rose states in her *Aromatherapy Book:* "According to Dr. Penoel, [essential oil of immortelle] is outstandingly effective in stimulating production and protection of new cells, even in the case of deep, bleeding wounds. This regenerative effect is also apparent in minimizing and smoothing scar tissue when mixed with Rosa rubiginosa (wild rosehip seed oil)."[†]

Immortelle works wonders used diluted on acne, but I have had success applying it directly to the pimple. It is resinous and sticky and is best used at night because it has a brown color to it and needs to be left on. It is said to help combat negative emotional crises, blockages, and tension.

---

[*] Tisserand, *The Art of Aromatherapy,* p. 226.
[†] Jeanne Rose, *The Aromatherapy Book,* San Francisco, CA: Herbal Studies Course/ Jeanne Rose, 1992, p. 98.

Essential oil of jasmine

Jasminum officinale, J. grandiflorum, J. sambac

Jasmine oil is often used as an anti-depressant, antiseptic, anti-spasmodic, aphrodisiac, sedative, and to reduce anxiety. It is both uplifting and soothing.

Jasmine oil is one of the most expensive essential oils and is extracted through enfleurage, a method of extracting the scent of flowers without heat. The scent is warming, sensual, sweet, and exotic. It reputedly works well on an emotional level to create optimism and openness, as well as to combat guilt, low self-esteem, and jealousy; therefore, it is used heavily for psychosomatic purposes.

It is very useful for menstrual cramps or other pain. It is used as an aphrodisiac and often applied to the male sex organ for strength.

It is the most welcomed ingredient in any skin care product, but is particularly beneficial for dry and very sensitive skin. I have some jasmine oil, but it costs so much that I mostly just inhale its lovely scent before I go to bed.

Essential oil of juniper

Juniperus communis

I love adding fifteen drops of juniper oil to my morning bath. It is both stimulating and detoxifying, and helps reduce cellulite. My cellulite has been reduced noticeably over the last couple of years due to bathing in juniper, plus getting lots of fresh air, exercising, and eating right.

Juniper berry oil has a great positive effect on the circulatory system and is known as a blood purifier. It is a diuretic and detoxifying. It is valued in bath products, cleanser soaps, massage oils, products for acne and oily skin, and is perfect as an ingredient in toners and astringents.

Since it also has a great effect on the kidneys, juniper oil is very useful in products to reduce puffiness. Make juniper tea to apply externally to reduce puffiness around the eyes and to use as a compress on other swollen areas.

When you can't sleep because of worry and tension, try putting a drop of juniper berry oil on your pillow to bring slumber. I have a wonderful juniper shrub in my yard, which I love to smell on a warm summer night. Interestingly, gin is made from juniper berries.

Essential oil of lavender

Lavandula vera
Lavandula officinalis

The lavender plant is a small, low-growing evergreen that belongs to the mint family. It originally grew in the high altitudes of Spain and North Africa, but it now grows in England, Norway, France, and even the United States. Most lavender for commercial purposes is grown in southern France, but some claim that the lavender grown in England has a finer fragrance because of the moist climate there. It didn't grow very well on my farm in central Colorado. The climate was too arid and the flowers looked dried out and scanty, hardly imparting a scent. However, I have seen them proliferate under controlled conditions such as at the Denver Botanical Gardens.

It is said that lavender oil was first originated by Hildegard of Bingen, a German Benedictine nun and mystic who lived from 1098 to 1179 in the Rhine Valley. While she was making her herbal remedies, she discovered that the lavender flowers could be distilled and employed for additional healing powers. I always thought a nice and appropriate name for a product would be "Hildegard's Water" or "Hildegard's Cream."

Not just for the ladies, lavender was among the roses, lilies, violets, and sage in kings' gardens, and it is said they scented their linens with lavender and rose essential oils.

Essential oil of lavender is distilled. Lavender water was often prepared by crushing the fresh flowers in alcohol and then distilling the mixture.

Lavender's great versatility

To me, lavender means balancing, neutralizing, and normalizing. Historically, many people used lavender to fight fatigue. Contrariwise, others prescribed it in a pillow to induce sleep. Lavender in a bath can be stimulating in the morning but relaxing at night. It balances the skin, recommended for both dry and oily skin. Lavender essential oil is widely used as an anti-depressant, antiseptic, anti-spasmodic, anti-toxin, deodorant, diuretic, and sedative, for acne, depression, eczema, and to relieve headaches.

It has the ability to aid in nervous tension and irritability. After spending so many days in a row visiting my mother in the hospital following her car accident, I always thought it should be used extensively in hospitals, in the heating and air-conditioning ducts so it permeates everywhere to disinfect as well as uplift not only the spirits of the patients, but the staff and visitors.

I use my mist with ylang ylang and lavender essential oils while in traffic, the office, or whenever I feel moodiness or anger arise in myself. I find the combination of the two essential oils very calming.

All essential oils are antiseptic. This is very valuable in any skin care ingredient because we always want to be fighting unwanted bacteria, keeping our products and bodies clean and free from parasites. Anti-spasmodic and anti-inflammatory, lavender is wonderful for skin care ingredients because it is calming and relaxing to the skin, especially skin that has been damaged, stressed, and irritated.

Lavender is anti-toxic and is used as a deodorant; the very derivative of the word means " to wash." It is one of the least toxic of all essential oils, so it is excellent in any cleansing product. Its anti-bacterial action makes it effective for acne and acne products. Lavender is cytophylactic, or skin regenerative. It helps the body produce new skin cells. This is probably why it is known to be so effective on burns.

I think lavender is the most versatile essential oil, naturally providing you with what you need in essential oils. If you want to get started with essential oils by starting with just one, I would say use lavender. You can use it for so many therapies. Use in your bath, as a perfume, as an insect repellent, or put a few drops on your pillow. I use lavender oil extensively in my product line because it is full of properties that make it one of the most desirable skin care ingredients on earth. (See also Lavender under Herbs.)

Lavandin, a hybrid

Lavandin is a hybrid of lavender. I tried it once by mistake when an essential oil company sent me samples of about twenty essential oils. I thought it was lavender at a glance, until I poured it in my hot bath and swished around the water to smell the scent. Personally, I thought it was awful. It seemed artificial to me, but others may like it.

Essential oil of lemon

Citrus limon

Toning, astringent, cleansing, and antiseptic, essential oil of lemon is a disinfectant and a very effective ingredient used in cleansers and to treat acne. We use it in our cleanser for all skin types. It is used for emotional purposes to help combat fear, forgetfulness, and moodiness and to fight fatigue.

Essential oil of lemongrass
Cymbopogon citratus
Antiseptic and anti-bacterial, lemongrass oil is used widely in Asian cooking. It has a high amount of citral, which is a terpene, a chemical composed of ten atoms of carbon and sixteen atoms of hydrogen. Citral is an oxygenated terpene. Lemongrass is usually from India or Guatemala. It is one of the best ingredients for oily skin and hair.

Essential oil of lemon verbena
Lippia citriodora
This oil is distilled from the leaves of the verbena plant. It is perfect for cleansers and soaps because it leaves you with that squeaky clean feeling and scent. It is astringent and adds a sharp note to perfumes.

Verbena oil is calming, cleansing, and helps to relax and produce sleep. It is used in cleansers, toners, shampoos for oily hair, facial steams, and for acne. The leaves are used for oily and blemished skin.

Essential oil of mandarin
Citrus reticulata
Mandarin oil smells just like the mandarin orange. It is very pleasant and is used widely for massage, being very soothing and calming. Mandarin oil is expressed from the peel of the fruit. Many find it wonderful in helping to reduce stretch marks.

Essential oil of melissa
Melissa officinalis
A.k.a.: Lemon balm
Melissa is a vibrant oil that is an anti-depressant antiseptic, and anti-spasmodic. It helps reduce the pain of menstruation, and relieves anxiety, especially when people are supersensitive.

According to Tisserand, "It is one of our earliest medicinal herbs, and was highly esteemed by Paracelsus, who called it the elixir of life, and combined it with carbonate of potash in a mixture known as 'primum ens melissae.'"*

---

* Tisserand, *The Art of Aromatherapy*, p. 253.

Essential oil of myrrh

Commiphora myrrha
Balsamodendron myrrha

Myrrh is stimulating, antiseptic, somewhat anti-fungal, and an anti-wrinkle agent. I like to blend it with almond oil, primrose, rosehip seed, wheat germ, frankincense, palmarosa, rose geranium, and sandalwood. I apply the mixture lightly on the dry places on my face around my eyes and mouth, and then I spray an acne mist over it to help it penetrate. A few minutes later, I put on my makeup.

Essential oil of myrrh is captured from the myrrh tree, whose trunk exudes the oil. It is usually obtained by distilling the oleogum resin.

Myrrh has a long history. "Gold, frankincense, and myrrh!" All Christians remember myrrh as part of the three kings' gifts to the infant Jesus. Widely varied in its uses, myrrh was used as an offering to the gods, in incense, for embalming Egyptian mummies, for fumigation, and in perfumes.

Myrrh is also a good incense to use during meditation. (See Myrrh herb.)

Essential oil of neroli

Citrus vulgaris

A.k.a.: Orange blossom oil

Neroli comes from the bitter orange's white blossoms. It is said that the Chinese have been using neroli oil for centuries in cosmetics and that the orange tree is originally from there. Some believe that the beautiful, famous, and popular "blue onion" pattern on Chinese porcelain does not depict onions at all, but oranges!

Neroli oil is an anti-depressant and is known to calm people down who worry themselves and spin around in their dramas. It is also used in aromatherapy for people who are fearful.

Neroli is a prized skin care ingredient known as a cell regenerative, and it helps your skin exfoliate itself. It is a stimulant, yet relaxing, and acts as a sedative on the skin. It is a valuable ingredient in any cosmetic product, including creams and lotions (especially for dry skin), toners, mists, and is luxurious in the bath. Try a couple drops on your pillow to induce sleep.

Essential oil of niaouli
Melaleuca viridiflora

Niaouli is used a lot like tea tree oil. As a daily acne prevention treatment, I like to put it on my face after my bath, while my skin is still moist in the morning, and let it soak in a while before I put on my moisturizers. It is both a stimulant and an antiseptic.

Essential oil of palmarosa
Cymbopogon martini

Palmarosa oil is an excellent skin care oil, reputedly a rejuvenation oil and an aid in cell reproduction. It works spectacularly on wrinkles and seems to keep your skin pliable. Palmarosa oil is often used in cosmetics and soap, adding a rose-like scent to products.

This has recently become one of my most used essential oils. I mix it with primrose oil or rosehip seed oil and apply it nightly around my eyes, mouth, and on my forehead. I also like to put this blend below my eyes before and after I have applied makeup to make sure my skin is moisturized.

Often from the East Indies or India, palmarosa oil is distilled from a grass. It contains geraniol.

Essential oil of patchouli
Pogostemon patchouli

Patchouli, also from the East Indies or India, has an oriental, sweet, and earthy scent. It has many uses: a good deodorant; an aphrodisiac; and a fixative in floral perfumes, soaps, candles, and potpourris. It is an antidepressant, antiseptic, astringent, and sedative. It is very grounding, soothing, and stimulating, and appears to aid people in seeing problems more clearly. It also helps with meditation. Patchouli oil is reported to promote the healing of scars. Patchouli oil itself seems to improve with age.

Essential oil of peppermint
Mentha piperita

Peppermint oil is probably the most popular essential oil in the world. Its high content of menthol makes it both very soothing and cooling. It is an anti-depressant, stimulates the mind, and yet helps calm an overactive mind. Tisserand says, "If you think too much, or have a hot head, it will cool you down."[*] Peppermint is antiseptic, anti-inflammatory, anti-toxic, a cleanser, and is used for varicose veins and aching muscles. I like it in aftershaves, cleansing products, shampoos, and for an invigorating bath. Go easy. A drop or two will do. I have irritated my skin putting too much in a bath. I like to use it when I fly to keep me refreshed. I find that using the peppermint oil "aromatherapeutically" and drinking lots of water help prevent the negative effects of traveling.

Dilute peppermint oil; do not use "neat" or full strength; 2% is often enough.

Essential oil of rose
Rosa alba

> A rose is a rose is a rose.
>
> —Gertrude Stein

No other plant has had as much praise from literature and art as the rose, the queen of the flowers. The first-century Roman, Pliny, listed 32 remedies that were derived from the petals or leaves of the rose. The Greeks best loved roses for their religious and social rituals. The Persians and the Romans also used rose oil lavishly in bathing, burials, and ceremonies. To the perfumer, rose oil adds smoothness, depth, and warmth. It is used in exquisite perfumes.

The finest roses come from Bulgaria. The rose growers pray for a wet season because rain helps intensify the scent of the oil in the flowers. Harvest takes place during May and June. Like most flowers, roses should be picked while still covered with the morning dew, or during the night.

Roses are very feminine and are often prescribed for female problems. They are used widely to help regulate the menstrual cycle. Roses are anti-depressant, aphrodisiac, and astringent. Many say that Native Americans used roses to treat gonorrhea.

The rose is perfect for all skin types: supersensitive, mature, and dry. Because it is astringent and cleansing, oily and younger skins also seem to benefit from its use. As one of the most antiseptic oils, it has a soothing, cleansing, and toning effect on the skin.

---

[*] Tisserand, *The Art of Aromatherapy*, p. 272.

Essential oil of rose geranium
Pelargonium graveolens

Rose geranium oil is antiseptic, astringent, anti-depressant, a cell regenerator, and a help to aging skin. It is perfect for therapeutic facial oils, lotions, creams, and shampoos. Like lavender and sandalwood, it is useful for both dry and blemished skin because it is balancing. I like it best blended with a very light or healing oil such as kukui or wheat germ to put around my eyes, forehead, and mouth before I go to bed. It stimulates the skin and gives you a rosy, healthy glow. I also often put it in the bath with juniper and sage in the morning.

Essential oil of rose geranium is used widely in perfumes to add an oriental note and blends well with rose. It is high in geraniol and rhodinol.

Essential oil of rosemary
Rosmarinus officinalis

Rosemary, grown in Spain, Morocco, Tunisia, and Turkey, is the symbol of eternity. Thus it was often planted near tombs. Rosemary is frequently associated with enhancing memories, as in Shakespeare's *Hamlet* when Ophelia says, "There is rosemary, that's for remembrance." The name of rosemary derives from the Latin *ros marinus*, meaning sea dew.

Antiseptic, anti-spasmodic, and an aid for baldness, rosemary is widely used in skin and hair care products. Rosemary oil is camphoraceous (i.e., contains camphor) and blends well with peppermint and lavender. It is eye opening and invigorating as a bath oil.

I prefer it best in cleansers, especially with seaweeds because the combination leaves your skin feeling squeaky clean. Also, after the cleanser is rinsed off, there is a reminiscence of the rosemary that feels divine. Rosemary is also great for aching muscles and pimples. It is also perfect for a hair rinse, especially for brunettes. You can just put several drops in with your rinse water. It stimulates the scalp, helps with dandruff, and removes any product buildup in your hair.

I often put rosemary in my bath in the morning because it is stimulating and refreshing. I also like adding it to my kukui, lily, and lavender oils, and applying it to my hair often as a hot-oil treatment or just a few drops to freshly shampooed hair for shine and manageability.

The oil is obtained by distillation and is often used in the scenting of soaps and colognes. Rosemary is thought to be an excellent nerve stimulant, the one word I would use for rosemary.

Essential oil of sage

To capture their oils, the clary sage (*salvia sclarea*) and dalmatian sage (*salvia officinalis*) are both distilled. I prefer clary sage, and I love oil of sage mixed with lavender for a classic cleansing effect. It is often recommended with lavender and rosemary as a hair conditioner. It is a stimulant to the skin and helps heal breakouts because of its cooling effect. It is effective on normal, blemished, or over-hydrated skin. Sage is great in the bath and is an effective deodorant.

It is wonderful in toners and astringents and has a clean scent. I also like it in the bath with lavender and juniper for a relaxing, pleasant, detoxifying experience.

Sage is antiseptic, healing, disinfectant, astringent, so is used in sick rooms, directly on insect bites, and as a mouthwash. Clary sage is used to regulate hot flashes for women during menopause. The essential oil is used as an anti-depressant. Because it is euphoria-producing, it is also known to be an aphrodisiac.

Clary sage oil has a high content of linalol. Pure essential oil of clary sage is very expensive, often used in skin care products for older women to maintain youthful appearing skin.

Essential oil of sandalwood

Santalum album

Sandalwood is used as an antidepressant, an aphrodisiac, and an anti-spasmodic as well as for all skin disorders including wrinkles and acne. It is calming and sedative and is said to help expel bad spirits. It is prized for its use in very expensive perfumes and is nice in a bath mixed with lavender.

Sandalwood was used by the ancients of Egypt and India in incense, cosmetics, and for embalming. In India, many carvings of Buddha and other crafts and statues are made of sandalwood; they are sold not only to tourists but are also valued by many Indians. In Mysore, India, the entire town smells of sandalwood; there are many sandalwood soaps from Mysore.

Oil of sandalwood is perfect oil for the skin. Although it is very well known for dry and dehydrated skin, it is also perfect for adult acne, hydrating where the skin is dry and antiseptic where the skin has breakouts. I like to apply it all over my face with primrose oil or rosehip seed oil, mixed with palmarosa essential oil. Due to its mildness, it can be used in high strengths.

My interest is always piqued by the essential oils that have been used in embalming. If these oils can preserve a corpse, what could they do for an active, healthy, well-taken-care-of body? Is this not a testament to their effectiveness?

Essential oil of tea tree
Melaleuca alternifolia

I apply tea tree oil full strength on my acne and find it works better than the chemical products the dermatologists used to prescribe me. I just put it directly on the pimple and then rub it around my whole face to prevent acne. I do this at least once a day to keep the acne away. It has necrotic properties that help eat dead skin, making it a great exfoliant. Since skin types vary, test tea tree oil on a very small area of your skin before using it.

Valerie Ann Worwood states in her book, *The Complete Book of Essential Oils and Aromatherapy*, that "the antiseptic action of tea tree oil is thought to be one hundred times more powerful than carbolic acid—and yet is nonpoisonous to humans!"[*] I find this extremely interesting because in the *Chemical Dictionary* under carbolic acid it says "See phenol." Under phenol, under derivation, it states: "treating the coal-tar oil fraction boiling between 170 and 230 degrees C, with caustic soda to form phenolate."[†] This is a pretty serious disinfectant. The dictionary further defines "phenol coefficient [as a] method used to determine the effectiveness of a disinfectant using phenol as a standard of comparison. The phenol coefficient is obtained by dividing the highest dilution of the test disinfectant by the highest dilution of phenol which sterilizes a given culture of bacteria under standard conditions of time and temperature."[‡] Suffice it to say that tea tree oil is a powerful disinfectant!

---

[*] Valerie Ann Worwood, *The Complete Book of Essential Oils & Aromatherapy*, Novato, CA: New World Library, 1991.
[†] *Condensed Chemical Dictionary*, p. 847.
[‡] *Condensed Chemical Dictionary*, p. 848.

It is amazing that it can be so powerful and yet completely non-caustic. When I first began my company, I had some tea tree oil on my hands when I picked up a silk-screened bottle. A few minutes later when I looked at the label, the silk-screened letters on the bottle were jumbled and rearranged. Interestingly, they were not smudged or messy, just completely rearranged. The tea tree oil somehow removed the adhesive without ruining the letters!

Tea tree oil kills bacteria, disinfects, and is beneficial to any kind of skin affliction such as bites, itching, infections, burns, cuts, and even open wounds. For very sensitive skin, it may have to be diluted, and not everyone appreciates the scent. Tea tree oil is perfect for creams, cleansers, astringents, facial tonics, and most important, acne products.

Essential oil of thyme

Thymus vulgaris

Thyme has many varieties. It is an antiseptic, antibiotic, disinfectant, and a mild sedative. It is used in hair growth products, lotions, cleansers, in massage oils for cellulite, and to bring stimulation to an area of the skin where applied. It is an air freshener and helpful to the respiratory system. Use only diluted, however.

Essential oil of vetiver

Vetiveria zizanoides

Vetiver oil is produced from distilling the plant's roots. Vetiver oil is a wonderful skin oil. It is stimulating to the skin and a humectant that brings moisture to your skin from the air. It is especially beneficial in a skin oil for people over 35. Years ago, almost all perfumes had vetiver.

Essential oil of ylang ylang

Unona odorantissimum

The name ylang ylang means "flower of flowers." The trees grow as high as 60 feet in Sumatra, Java, Madagascar, and the Philippines.[*] The finest ylang ylang comes from the Philippines because of the heavy rainfall and fertile ground. In the 1950s, Madagascar produced around 66 tons of ylang ylang oil each year.

---

[*] Jill Eva Jessee, *Perfume Album*, Huntington, NY: Robert E. Krieger Publishing Co., Inc., 1965.

Ylang ylang is personally one of my favorite essential oils, one I have used extensively. Because of its anti-frustration, anti-depressant, and aphrodisiac scent, I have put it in my original cream for dry skin, original facial lotion, and mist mixed with essential oil of lavender. I like to put a drop on my pillow or use it by itself as a perfume. The scent is heavy, sweet, and sensual.

Men love the scent of ylang ylang. Everywhere I go, every time I place my cream with the fragrance of ylang ylang under a man's nose, he enjoys the scent, almost without exception. When I tell them, "It is used as an aphrodisiac," they smile.

Ylang ylang is widely used by perfumers for its lovely fragrance. It is also used as a fixative and a modifier. It blends well with lily, violet, and jasmine. It can often round out harsh notes in perfume compositions.

Ylang ylang also blends well with lavender, rosemary, and sandalwood. It has a soothing effect on emotions, especially frustration, and on the skin. It is said to affect the nervous system as a sedative and is used for anxiety and tension.

Caution: Do not use ylang ylang in high concentrations as it can cause headaches.

Classifications of essential oils

Essential oils capture the essence of plants, or specific parts of plants.

Flowers from which essential oils are made include rose, jasmine, orange flower, ylang ylang, violet, narcissus, jonquil, hyacinth, tuberose, acacia, cassia, and mimosa.

Grasses from which essential oils are drawn are lemongrass, gingergrass, vetiver, and palmarosa.

Spices and herbs also are used to make essential oils. Clove, ginger root, nutmeg fruit/nut, thyme, vanilla bean, costus, clary sage, lavender, and rosemary are among those favored.

Citrus chosen for their essential oils are orange, bergamot, lemon, lime, and petitgrain.

Woods used for their essential oils are sandalwood, cedarwood, and rosewood.

Gums and balsams in demand for their essential oils include labdanum, myrrh, galbanum, olibanum, benzoin, opopanax, storax, balsam peru, and balsam tolu.

Emotional healing with essential oils

Essential oils have a history of use in enhancing relaxation as well as diminishing negative emotions.

Essential oils used to *combat fears* include sandalwood, cypress, lemon, chamomile, lavender, cedarwood, vetiver, and neroli.

Essential oils that *bring calm relaxation* include lavender, neroli, sandalwood, chamomile, clary sage, and ylang ylang.

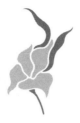

Other Ingredients

Bee Propolis

The word *propolis,* meaning "defenses before a town," comes from the Greek. It is one of the bee's building materials. The bees use this sticky substance in making and repairing their hives. The raw material is a resinous substance exuded by the leaf buds of trees such as the horse chestnut and poplar, and is found in cracks in the bark of trees such as spruce, larch, and other conifers. The bees collect it, take it back to the hive, and use it as a cement. In addition, whenever a foreign insect is in the hive, the bees encase it in propolis; because of its antibacterial qualities, the propolis disinfects the foreign object, thus protecting the hive and its occupants.

According to *Propolis, the Natural Antibiotic*[*] by Ray Hill, propolis is a sticky substance which protects leaf buds and prevents them from drying out. Its biologically active components may vary according to its plant source. A test of propolis collected in fifteen different districts of the USSR showed uniform constituents, the approximate breakdown of which was 50 to 55% resin and balsam, up to 30% wax, about 8 to 10% fragrant essential oils, and about 5% solid matter. It is said to be rich in fats, amino acids, organic acids, composite ethers of univalents alcohols, and trace elements such as iron, copper, tannic acid, phytocides, and antibiotics.

---

[*] Ray Hill, *Propolis, the Natural Antibiotic,* Wellingborough, Northhamptonshire, England:Thorsons Publishers Limited, 1981.

Antibiotic properties

The antibiotic properties of propolis are believed to come from the flavonoids it contains, particularly galangin. The name comes from galingale, an aromatic plant root from the East, which is related to ginger and has always been used medicinally. Plants containing flavonoids have been used as healing agents for centuries before these active substances were ever scientifically identified.

According to Ray Hill, it was quite accidental that Dr. Lavie, while studying the natural biochemical defense of insects, learned that bees killed recently and put into a liquid medium without any preservative developed no bacteria. Dr. Lavie proved that the bees and their surroundings provided over seven antibiotics.

Interestingly, Dr. Lavie found that extracts he made from the buds of poplar tree resin were identical in chemical consistency and potency to the propolis.

Propolis can be valuable for anything involving bacteria or germs. It is said that any propolis treatment should work within three weeks or it is not going to work. The best way I have found to extract the properties from propolis is through an alcohol/water extraction. You can apply it with the alcohol, or you can slowly heat it, after straining, to evaporate the alcohol. Be careful never to get it too hot; many chemical constituents are heat sensitive.

Because of its anti-bacterial properties, propolis has received rave reviews for blemishes. Bee propolis in a product helps keep the skin clean and free from germs. For serious blemishes or acne, it can be applied topically as well as taken internally.

Propolis is often recommended for dry eczema with wonderful results; however, it has been known to aggravate wet eczema. It is also an age-old remedy for corns. Apply a propolis cream with a small gauze pad.

In the first century A.D., Pliny mentioned the uses of bee propolis. His recommendations included to reduce swelling, to soothe pain, and to heal sores when they seemed hopeless to mend. In Russia during World War II, propolis was applied to wounds.

Other uses

Propolis ointment was often recommended for second-degree burns, and healing took place without scarring. Propolis has a stimulating effect and works with the skin's natural regenerative process.

I use bee propolis in many of my products; I find it most advantageous in astringents, creams, and products for blemishes.

Caution: About 0.05% of the population is allergic to propolis.

Honey

The Romans believed honey endowed those who ate it with grace and elegance. The term "honeymoon" is said to come from an old European custom in which a newly married couple drank honey wine daily for 30 days following their wedding. I have read that honey has been associated with the concept of truth. Honey is mentioned in the Bible and has been a prized item since before recorded history.

Honey is the first and one of the best humectants and, therefore, moisturizers. A humectant attracts moisture from the air and brings it to your skin. Honey is sweet and very viscous, made from the nectars of flowers and then partially digested by honeybees. It is said that honeybees tap two million flowers and travel 55,000 miles to bring us one pound of honey.

A popular ingredient for any formulator of at-home products, honey consists of protein, calcium, phosphorus, iron, niacin, and vitamin C. Honey is a great wound healer; it protects against infections and may be superior to many dressings. Honey is highly antibiotic as well as an energy-producing food. It has been said that bee pollen is the world's richest food.

A natural hydrator

Honey is a natural rejuvenator and leaves your face feeling refreshed and invigorated. Skin does not age because it loses its ability to hold oil, but because it loses its ability to retain moisture. Honey is also a natural hydrator. It has the ability to maintain or restore the normal proportion of water in the skin. Honey applied to your skin feels smooth and leaves the skin tight and firm, feeling light and clean. Because honey is acidic, it also helps rid the face of blemishes and blackheads.

As a skin rejuvenator, honey is perfect for all skin types. It is wonderful for sensitive skin that breaks out from any synthetic ingredient. It is predigested natural sugars, easily assimilated, full of vitamins and minerals. Honey is a great carrier for powders or ground herbs in masks.

Benefits of honey

Honey aids in:

* Repairing skin that is clogged

* Restoring moisture

* Restoring a youthful look to complexions because of its moisturizing and humectant qualities

* Bringing color to skin

* Reducing coarseness in skin

* Refining pores

Homemade recipes

To soften, cleanse, and refresh skin, make a mixture of two tablespoons honey with one-half teaspoon organic vinegar and one-half teaspoon lemon juice. Mix well and apply to the face. Leave on for one-half hour. Do this daily to restore a youthful appearance. It aids in cleansing, protecting, and drawing moisture to your skin.

Honey is a perfect base for masks. You can use honey alone or you could make thousands of different kinds of masks. Try grinding to a powder the following herbs and mixing them with honey to make a paste to apply to your face: lily, lavender, rose, chamomile, and calendula. Or come up with your own herbal blend.

Try any of the following or apply honey to your face alone:

* Use two tablespoons honey and add a few drops of one of the following essential oils: rose, blue chamomile, lavender, or ylang ylang.

* Use equal parts of honey, yogurt, and your favorite powdered herb and apply to your face.

* Try equal parts of honey, milk, and powdered lavender.

* Try equal parts of honey and oatmeal.

* Try equal parts of honey and freshly peeled papaya.

Seven Exotic Oils

Here in the Rocky Mountain state of Colorado, we love our oils, almost every kind of oil applied everywhere on our bodies. We like them in our hair, especially kukui, almond, rosehip seed, and primrose oil. We like them on our faces, alone or blended; we like them around our eyes, mouths, and necks. We use them as makeup removers, cleansers, and in our baths. We like them scented, unscented, and with herbs. My Seven Exotic Oils, which includes the seven listed below, is my personal favorite blend of oils. You can use these oils alone or together in any way that suits you. Don't let my limited suggestions stop you from trying them every way.

Kukui Oil

Aleurites moluccana

The kukui nut trees flourish on Hawaii's hills and gulches and are commonly found around the Islands. In 1959, the kukui nut tree became the official state tree of Hawaii.

The kukui tree produces a cluster of small white flowers as well as kukui fruit. The fruit has a hard green covering about one-fourth inch thick when it is immature. As it matures, it turns a dark grayish-black and softens. Within the fruit is a large nut with a hard shell and an inner core or kernel. The shell is dark brown to black and looks like a small chestnut. The inner core is white and characteristically oily. A mature tree can produce 75 to 100 pounds of fruit a year.

In native Hawaiian medicine, kukui had many uses. The nuts were lightly baked so that the hard shells cracked open. To obtain the oil, the shells were removed and the kernels lightly roasted; a clear oil could be pressed out. For hundreds of years, the Hawaiians have found this to be an excellent, penetrating oil for their skin care needs.

Kukui nut oil has been tested and rates among the best of the polyunsaturated oils. It is high in linoleic and linolenic acids, which are essential fatty acids beneficial for healthy skin. Kukui oil helps smooth, soften, and relax irritated skin. It has a reputation for being excellent for the treatment of superficial burns and chapped skin.

Many people who don't like the more traditional heavier oils do enjoy kukui oil because it is so light and highly absorbent. It is wonderful to use after sun exposure as an all-over body oil, and it is highly desired for hot-oil hair treatments.

Kukui nut oil is minimally refined and highly unsaturated, has a wonderful emolliency, and is non-greasy.

Almond Oil

Prunus dulcis

The almond is a medium-sized tree of the rose family. The bushy, round-crowned almond tree normally reaches heights of 20 to 30 feet. There are numerous biblical references to the almond. In Genesis 43:11, the patriarch Israel commanded his sons to carry into Egypt gifts from Palestine, which included almonds.

Almonds were mentioned in Greek mythology and the Muhammedans associated almond flowers with hope, since the beautifully scented blossoms appear on bare branches.

In Elizabethan England, "An almond for a parrot" was a popular proverb in which the almond was considered to be a mouthwatering temptation: thus, in Shakespeare's *Troilus and Cressida*, Act V, Scene 2, Thersites says, "The parrot will not do more for an almond."

Symbolism

Almonds have symbolized good luck for many centuries in southern Europe. Traditionally, candied almond nuts are given away at weddings in Greece as tokens of long life and happiness. When two good friends of mine were married a few years ago in a Greek Orthodox church, they had candy-coated almonds at their reception for this purpose.

John Gerard (1597) observed that "fove or sic [almonds] being taken fasting do keepe a man from being drunke." My mom is among those who eat "five almonds a day to keep cancer away."

In the seventeenth century, Ninon de Lenclos, a French woman of fashion, recommended an almond-based cold cream, which was said to have preserved her beauty and kept her face free of wrinkles until she was 70.

Ripe almonds can be ground up in a blender into almond meal that is wonderful as a skin conditioner, pore cleanser, and refiner. You can use this alone or mix the almond meal with honey or yogurt and apply as a mask.

You will find almond oil as a top ingredient in most quality skin care products. It is perfect to use alone as well. It has been used for centuries as an all-purpose, soothing oil, as an emollient, in face lotions, shampoos for dry hair, massage oils, bath oils, and is a key ingredient for making your own herbal oils. Extracted from the almond nutmeats, almond oil has been used for centuries for the entire body.

Almond oil is a wonderful remedy for dry skin. It can also be used as a gentle non-soap makeup remover. It is healing and soothing to the skin and is included for those reasons in many face creams and emulsions.

Vitamin E Oil

Tocopherol

Vitamin E oil is often made by diluting natural vitamin E with soya oil, usually light-colored and odorless. Wheat germ oil is the best source of vitamin E; however, it can also be made from alfalfa or almond oils.

Vitamin E is an important nutrient for humans and must come from an outside source; the body does not produce its own. Natural vitamin E protects the skin from ultraviolet light, aids in increasing moisture levels, and helps slow down the natural process of decay.

Vitamin E prevents oxidation of unsaturated fatty acids. It keeps the skin healthy and youthful by slowing down the aging of cells resulting from the interaction of oxygen with other chemicals in the body. It works to protect against cell deterioration.

Vitamin E is a superb beauty aid; it is great in facials and day and night creams. It may be applied fresh from the capsule to any part of your skin alone or mixed with wheat germ or other oils.

Vitamin E is absorbed through the skin, and because of its beneficial effects, it is an excellent addition to any blend of oils, creams, or lotions. You may add the contents of a pierced capsule to your favorite cream. It is said it can eliminate scarring and speed healing when applied to an open wound. It is a great skin-care product ingredient that softens and lubricates the skin.

Alfalfa, dandelion, sesame, watercress, and wheat germ are all very high in vitamin E. It is an antioxidant, skin smoother, and hair shiner.

It is said that vitamin E can work favorably at slowing down overactivity of the sebaceous glands. It is a well-known anti-inflammatory agent. It assists in healing by aiding the formation of smoother skin and promoting softer scar tissue, which can diminish the scarring.

Wheat Germ Oil

Wheat germ oil is a valuable source of vitamin E, coming from the heart of the wheat kernel. Wheat germ oil makes tired skin look fresher, more resilient. It is a skin nourishing and softening oil. It is perfect blended with other fine oils and in creams, masks for dry or dull skin, and as an ingredient in fine bath oils. Wheat germ contains fatty acids and is high in protein. It can be used as a massage oil or as a complexion oil to massage the face, particularly effective in wrinkle-prone areas. Soaking your cuticles in wheat germ oil so you may gently push them back is an effective practice for prettier fingernails.

Rosehip Seed Oil
Rosa aff. Rubiginosa
A.k.a.: Rosa mosqueta

The rosa mosqueta, from which rosehip seed oil is commercially derived, is grown in South America. This is one of the finest oils and one of the most expensive oils you will find in a skin care product. From the rosehip fruit come the tiny amber seeds to make the oil. The oil is high in essential fatty acids and is used for severe burns, sunburns, and damaged hair, and for reducing wrinkles, scars, and marks on the body. Skin-smoothing and reportedly regenerative, rosehip seed oil is great for UV sun-damaged skin and deep lines. It is said this oil is excellent as a treatment for prematurely aging skin and acne scars. Because it is so high in essential fatty acids, it is often used not only in healing but in preventing continued wrinkling.

Rosehip seed oil is useful for grooming normal to oily hair; after washing, dry your hair with a very small amount of oil massaged through it for luster and normalization. Rosehip seed oil can be used as a hot-oil hair treatment for dry hair. It is particularly beneficial to hair that has been damaged by chemical treatments, sun, or cold weather.

Evening Primrose Oil
Oenothera biennis

Evening primrose flowers are nocturnal, the yellow flowers opening only at night. Evening primrose oil is high in essential fatty acids, including gamma-linolenic acid (GLA). It is said that the high GLA content in the oil is what makes it so beneficial. GLA also occurs in mother's milk and black currant oil.

Evening primrose oil has been used for moisturizing the skin, to treat eczema and psoriasis, inflammation, redness, itching, and diaper rash. The oil is useful used alone or blended with other oils and applied topically to the face, neck, or all over the body in or after a bath. I think it is one of the most desirable oils in creams and lotions and hair care products.

In hair care products, evening primrose oil helps reduce the oil secretion without causing dryness, and it moisturizes dry hair. It is wonderful in shampoos, conditioners, rinses, and can also be applied lightly and directly to clean, dry hair for luster.

Evening primrose oil has reportedly been used successfully for the following:

- Hair loss
- Wrinkles
- Dry scalp and hair
- Overweight
- PMS
- Brittle nails
- Acne, when taken with zinc
- Eczema

Lavender Essential Oil

Lavandula officinalis
Lavandula vera

Lavender essential oil is oil distilled from the lavender flower. Today, the largest percentage of the blooms goes into perfume products. One acre of lavender yields 15 to 20 pounds of oil. It is very popular and enjoyable to put a few drops in a bath or to simply enjoy as a perfume. For more about this versatile plant, see the section on Lavender under both Herbs and Essential Oil.

Vinegar

The word *vinegar* is from the French vin aigre, meaning sour or acid wine. It is a dilute acetic obtained from the fermentation process. When fresh apples are pressed into cider and are fermented organically, they make vinegar that contains natural sediment with enzymes, pectin, and good bacteria.

Please note: When I say vinegar, I mean only pure, natural, unrefined, unfiltered, raw, organic apple cider vinegar. You can tell it is the genuine article if when you hold it up to the light, it has the "mother" floating in it, a sediment and web-like substance. I always thought it looked like a jellyfish in the bottom of the jug. It is best purchased at a health food store or a farm market where the grower makes his own naturally.

My personal connection with vinegar

As mentioned previously, I have a personal affinity with apples, both as part of my history as well as that of my family. Not only did I grow up working on the family apple orchard, but my family has been composed of apple growers for 200 years.

My dad used to make his own vinegar, which he used heavily in cooking. He put it in coleslaw. He pickled eggs and beets together with it, turning the eggs purple as well as preserving them. All were delicious.

I remember Dad speaking of the "mother," the cloudy substance in the vinegar, as the giver of its life. He used to speak of the energetic old farmer who drank a shot of vinegar daily just like people do shots of tequila or whiskey. He said that the vinegar gave the farmer the substance and power to keep up with his hard work.

Vinegar elixirs

I make several different, perfectly wonderful vinegar elixirs, which I drink daily. In one of them, I soak garlic, horseradish, and onion in vinegar for a month and then I add about 20% of a tincture of elethro ginseng, dong quai, and vitex. This is a consummate health drink for women. I have not been sick in the last two years since I began taking it daily, not even with a cold. It gives me the strength and energy to keep up and stay on target with my ever-so-many activities. I highly recommend this formula for everyone. Men can just do the vinegar mixture without the herbs.

Versatile vinegar

Vinegar must be one of the most useful things on earth for humankind. Just to name a few things, vinegar is used to clean windows, disinfect, in the laundry to brighten colors, on the carpet to absorb odors and remove stains, polish furniture, remove ink stains, absorb cat box odors, dissolve chewing gum, remove perspiration stains, make an air freshener, and clean the entire household for "pennies on the dollar" without any harm to the environment.

As a medicine, it kills infection, soothes coughs, eases the pain of a sore throat, and calms nausea. Taken with honey before bed, it instills sleep.

A few of the skin remedies vinegar has been used for are to treat burns, soothe sunburn, help aching feet, and relieve the itch of welts, hives, and bee stings. It also fades age spots. Vinegar helps control appetite and aids in digestion, and therefore can aid in weight reduction.

Vinegar's history and importance

Vinegar has a long history. It is literally a key player in the overall destiny of mankind. Vinegar may have been a major ingredient in getting rid of the black plague in Europe in the Middle Ages.

Vinegar is so important in folk medicine because it associates minerals with potassium. Vinegar contains phosphorus, chlorine, sodium, magnesium, calcium, sulfur, iron, fluorine, silica, and many trace minerals. Folk medicine holds potassium to be the most important mineral, in fact, the key mineral in the constellation of minerals. Potassium is found with acids. P. C. Bragg, in the book *Apple Cider Vinegar Health System*, refers to it as the "mineral of youthfulness."[*]

Vinegar's role in skin care

Apple cider vinegar is helpful to both dry and oily skin. It acts to refine the skin pores, and reestablishes a natural acid balance while softening the skin. When the skin is acidic, it seems to attract blood. The presence of the needed amount of blood in the skin gives it a wonderful glow. Soap is often needed to remove dirt and makeup, but following the cleansing process with a rinse of an herbal astringent or apple cider vinegar is beneficial to restore acid balance.

If your skin has a reaction to soap, such as itching, you may want to stop using soap and use apple cider vinegar instead, particularly in the bath. Vinegar is a natural deodorizer and acid balance restorer. Just add one cup of vinegar to your bath water and let it soak into the pores for at least twenty minutes.

If you have an itchy scalp, try dipping your hairbrush in a glass of water with one-teaspoon vinegar enough times to get your hair wet. This will not only help reduce itching but it will make your hair soft and easy to manage. *One caution*: Vinegar may straighten perms.

For skin blemishes

Vinegar helps soften skin and restore the skin's natural acid mantle. It is a great rinse for blemished skin. Steam the face with lavender to cleanse the skin. Bring a pan of water to a boil, put a small handful of lavender

---

[*] Paul C. Bragg and Patricia Bragg, *Apple Cider Vinegar Health System*, Santa Barbara, CA: Health Science, 1987.

flowers in the water, and remove from the heat. Hold your head over the pan and drape a towel over your head to allow the lavender-enhanced steam to loosen the grease and dirt. Then, take a cotton ball drenched in vinegar and lightly pat on the skin. Repeat this twice. Then pat on vinegar that has been chilled in the refrigerator, to close the pores and tone the skin.

For tired muscles and joints, take a vinegar bath. Soak in warm water to which one and a half cups of vinegar have been added.

Making a cosmetic vinegar

Add one tablespoon of apple cider vinegar to one cup of rose water. This can be used to tone oily skin, as well as after shampooing to restore the hair's acid balance.

Rose Vinegar:

1 cup vinegar

1 tablespoon fresh or dried rose flowers

1 cup purified water

Heat the rose flowers with the vinegar and water. Bring to a boil and steep for 30 minutes. After cooling, place mixture in a jar with a tight-fitting lid and let sit for two weeks. Strain the rose flowers from the vinegar and use the liquid for bath, hair rinse, or facial soak.

For a vinegar facial soak, heat the rose vinegar slowly until it is a comfortable temperature to apply to the skin. Soak a clean, warm washcloth in the vinegar and lay over the face for five minutes, each time redipping the washcloth to reapply. For best results, keep the washcloth on the skin for a total of 20 minutes. This is an excellent exfoliant and skin stimulant.

Water

Water is the source of life, health, and prosperity. It makes it possible for life to exist on Earth.

Water, H_2O, is the liquid that descends from the clouds as rain, forming streams, lakes, and seas, which turn to vapor and become clouds again in a never-ending cycle. Water is a major constituent of all living matter. Your body is 80% water. The surface of the earth is 66% water.

Held sacred

Water is purifying, life-sustaining, and calming. There is still much sacredness associated with water. Consider its use in baptisms, and the burning of the bodies at the ghats, or steps of the Ganges River in India. The ashes are lowered into this holy river.

Historically, many of the Eastern cultures held water in the highest esteem for cleansing and cooling and thought it healed both the body and soul.

We in industrialized, well-fed nations each use an average of 150 gallons of water per day directly; but indirectly we use about 1990 gallons per day. About 1660 gallons are used to grow the crops and meat we eat, and 180 gallons are used in industry to provide us with the products we use.

Purifying water

It is wise these days to purchase a water purifier for your kitchen. There are many on the market in all price ranges. Go check them out at your health food store and get one that best suits your needs. Remember, one of water's most important functions is to cleanse the system, to flush out toxins. Use the purest water possible to accomplish this. Water is the secret to growing anything, even bacteria and molds.

Uses of water

According to the Colorado Farm Bureau, to produce our food it takes:

- 150 gallons for one loaf of bread
- 120 gallons for one pound of tomatoes
- 22 gallons for one pound of potatoes
- 37 gallons for one bushel of corn
- 120 gallons to produce one egg
- 223 gallons per quart of milk

Households use:

- 30 to 40 gallons per bath
- 7 to 9 gallons per minute of shower (up to 90 gallons per ten-minute shower)
- 3 to 4 gallons per toilet flush
- One or more gallons to brush teeth

* 24 gallons to wash dishes by machine

* 30 gallons to wash one load of clothes

* In-house use averages 40 to 60 gallons per person, per day

We are each deeply connected to one another, in fact, to the entire planet, by this colorless liquid, water. We all need water to live.

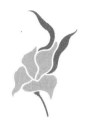

PART THREE

Treatments for Beauty by Skin Types and Conditions

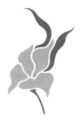

Treatments for Skin Types

No one can shed light on vices he does not have or afflictions he never experienced.

—Antonio Machado

Dry Skin

Good news/bad news

The good news is that people with dry skin seldom have to suffer from acne when they are young. The bad news is they may pay a price as they get older.

Dry skin can be especially difficult to deal with in cold and dry climates such as Colorado's. Most people here have dry skin. The situation is even more extreme in New Mexico. A good moisturizer is worth its weight in gold under these conditions.

Low moisture is one major reason for dry skin. This can occur as the result of age, climate, race, general disposition, excessive cleansing, or physiologic factors. Constant lubrication of the skin is absolutely necessary if you don't want a dried-out, wrinkled prune face.

Dry skin responds well to oils and heavy creams. You need to apply enough moisturizer to give your face and body the elasticity they need to function without straining the skin. You need to make sure that when you smile, your face doesn't feel like it's going to crack.

Traditional tried-and-true remedies to help combat dryness of the skin include taking herbal teas with reputations for improving the blood, such as sarsaparilla, burdock, yellow dock, and nettle. Also:

* Eat lots of nuts and high-quality vegetable oils.

* Cleanse the skin with a non-drying cleanser ensuring that all debris of dead skin is removed.

* Use a moisturizer, such as a cream or lotion.

* After the cream soaks in, apply a nut or vegetable oil with a tissue and pat off the excess; allow the rest to soak in.

* Rub the inside of an avocado skin all over a clean face and let sit for twenty minutes to moisturize and nourish dry skin.

* Take vitamin E internally and apply externally.

* Take evening primrose oil and apply topically.

* Drink aloe juice and apply topically.

* Add a cup or two of cider vinegar to your bath.

* Use a bag of oatmeal as a wash cloth.

* Give your skin a break; only wear natural fabrics: cotton, linen, and wool.

* Make a fresh apple juice and brewer's yeast mask by blending together into a paste.

* Add one tablespoon of brewer's yeast to eight ounces fresh apple juice for a daily drink.

* Put a humidifier in your bedroom to provide moisture while you sleep.

* Take unsaturated fatty acid oils or GLA; taking zinc supplements also is helpful.

Remember, dry skin loves:

* Olive oil
* Primrose oil
* Rosehip seed oil (topically only)
* Almond oil
* Wheat germ oil

* Kukui oil (topically only)
* Avocado oil
* Flaxseed
* Apples
* Brewer's yeast
* Honey

Further suggestions for improving your skin:

* Exercise; get lots of fresh air and sunshine; walk, skip, hike, take deep breaths of air; get your circulation going.

* Use botanical enzyme masks or just apply fresh pineapple and papaya to the skin.

* Do yoga; especially postures that reverse the body: headstand, plow, and shoulder stand; a milder way is to lie on a slant board.

* Frequently moisturize; carry moisturizer with you at all times.

* Frequently hydrate with moisture mists.

* Do seasonal internal cleansings.

* Think kind thoughts; among its many benefits, it gives you a softer look.

* Take spirulina.

* Use products that contain horsetail, coltsfoot, rosehip seed, and primrose oil.

* Use a skin brush or a loofah sponge to remove dead skin from your limbs and stimulate circulation.

Avoid synthetic chemicals as much as possible because those of you with dry skin don't have as much sebum on your face. It is less acidic and, therefore, doesn't have as much of a protective barrier as oily skin. This is one reason you are so much more sensitive to products than your more oily-skinned sisters.

Make a dry skin therapy oil containing frankincense, myrrh, patchouli, and sandalwood, diluted in almond oil. Apply to areas of dry skin.

Mix any of these essential oils with pure sweet almond oil for dry skin during cold weather:

* Frankincense
* Myrrh
* Patchouli
* Sandalwood
* Clary sage
* Geranium
* Jasmine

* Rosewood
* Rosemary
* Rose
* Palmarosa
* Neroli
* Lavender

Dry Skin Regime

Cleanse

Cleanse your skin twice daily with a mild soap or cleanser and then use a good astringent or toner. This removes any residue, all makeup, and leaves the skin squeaky clean.

Be sure that whatever cleansing method you use does not leave your skin feeling tight and dry afterwards. If everything does leave your skin feeling dry, try cleansing your skin with an herbal oil: a blend of almond oil with lavender or calendula. Just apply to a warm, wet washcloth and wipe your face.

You will want to use oil and water emulsion soap with ingredients of almond oil, lily, seaweeds, sage, or lavender. I would also recommend an astringent or toner with ingredients such as lily, lavender, seaweeds, elderberries, or chamomile.

Masks/Exfoliate

Dry skin needs a mask that is going to help bring in and seal in moisture. Honey, glycerin, and yogurt are all beneficial for dry skin.

Use ingredients that have a life force. A couple times a week you may want to use a botanical enzyme mask with pineapple or papaya. You can make your own by blending fresh pineapple with honey and applying to your skin for twenty minutes.

I would avoid alpha hydroxy and those sorts of products as they can be very harsh; I have seen many women in health food stores looking for the antidote to their burned skin. Apply fresh pineapple or papaya instead, which have necrotic properties that eat the dead skin while not adversely affecting the live skin.

Toner/Astringent

Use a great toner to help close the pores after cleansing or doing a mask. Look for ingredients like lily, coltsfoot, calendula, horsetail, and essential oils of sage and lavender. A good toner/astringent should never be drying. It should smell wonderful with pure plant essential oils, and it should feel good the moment it touches your skin. Then as you apply it and let it penetrate your skin, it should give you a slight, almost tingling sensation. The toner should remove all residue and dirt without drying your skin. It should make for a delightful experience every time.

Moisture

This is the most important factor for dry skin. You really must moisturize as much as necessary to keep your skin pliable and flexible. You will instinctively know how your skin should feel. When smiling, for example, you never want to feel your skin resist.

In climates like Colorado's, you may have to moisturize almost constantly, as many as five to ten times a day. This is where an herbal oil-free moisturizer is a good item to carry, so you can apply it throughout the day over your makeup. I carry a trial size of my herbal moisturizer with me wherever I go in the winter, to keep the skin around my eyes moistened. Lots of people here use heavy oils like my Seven Exotic Oils after cleansing their skin and before applying their makeup. Many women tell me that for a real added boost they apply the Seven Exotic Oils with the herbal moisturizer. My moisturizing cream for dry skin is my most loved product among dry-skinned women in dry climates.

This is not just because our products are fantastic, but because these women really need good moisturizers. Dry skin not only causes long-lasting lines and loss of elasticity; it makes women look older. So never let your skin look or feel dry. Moisturize, moisturize, moisturize! A mist and moisturizer should be your constant companions.

Moisturize when you get up in the morning with something heavy-duty and rich. Try a really rich cream made with lily, comfrey, shea butter, or rosehip seed oil. Or make your own blend of any of the following: almond, olive, sunflower, kukui, wheat germ, vitamin E, primrose, lavender, or rosehip seed oil. Then blend in your own favorite essential oils. Many of these cosmetic-making processes need not be difficult.

I have seen many people look as old and dry as dead cacti, mostly men, because they do not moisturize. It's a rare woman in Colorado who doesn't have to moisturize just to be able to smile. I recommend women cleanse their skin and then apply astringent, my herbal moisturizer, and as a sealant for super-protection, my Seven Exotic Oils. Top off with our Lily Mist and you will look years younger just because you have removed the obvious layer of dead skin and debris and applied lubrication and hydration.

Mist

Mist is valuable for people with really dry skin. You can easily mist your skin throughout the day even after you have applied your moisturizer and makeup. It is also a refreshing pick-me-up. Look for essential oils that are balancing and refreshing like lavender, and uplifting and anti-depressant like ylang ylang.

Oil your skin

If you have really dry skin, I'd recommend you have quarts of quality oil around like almond or olive oils, or purchase a face and body oil with lily, calendula, and chamomile, or make your own. Constantly put oil on your skin when at home and not concerned about how you look.

Make your own herbal oils by simply placing your favorite herb in your favorite fixed oil. For example, buy eight ounces of almond oil at your local health food store and one ounce each of your favorite herbs. A wonderful blend for dry skin is lily, lavender, rose, chamomile, calendula, and arnica. Blend in a little vitamin E and essential oil of lavender. Of course, you can make any blend of herbs and add any blend of essential oils. Experiment! Discover what most pleases you.

Normal and Combination Skin

If you have normal skin, you just need a good all-around nutritional plan and a simple skin-care regimen. If you have combination skin, follow the same advice as for normal skin, using the ideas in the sections on dry skin or acne where applicable.

Cleanse

Cleanse with a good cleanser or soap, whichever suits your skin. Just make sure it does not leave your skin feeling stripped of oil and dry. If you have combination skin, you may want to use products with lavender because it is so balancing.

Steam or Mask

For combination skin, steam with lavender, eucalyptus, nettle, and/or shavegrass. Both skin types can benefit from a gentle botanical exfoliating mask with ingredients of honey, papaya, pineapple, and lily. Once or twice a week should be adequate.

Toner/Astringent

Use a toner or an astringent both delightful to use and with therapeutic essential oils that make your skin and senses rejoice. Again, if you have combination skin, look for products that contain lavender to balance.

Moisturize or mist

All skin types need moisture after 25 years of age. Maybe you only need to moisturize around your eyes and/or mouth, or maybe your forehead gets dry. Just moisturize where you are dry. You do not necessarily need to apply moisture all over your face. If you are a combination skin type, you may want to use a light lotion that contains tea tree oil, rosemary, seaweeds, and lily, or maybe an oil-free herbal moisturizer that contains lilies, seaweeds, and calendula.

Oily Skin

You know you have oily skin if you have had pimples, acne, blackheads, or if at 5:00 P.M., your skin has oil oozing out of it. Fortunately, oily skin looks better as you age because it maintains its natural oils later in life.

Recommendations

Eliminating animal fats and fried foods can help many with oily skin. After every cleansing, use a toner with lavender, sage, or vinegar, or make your own. Oily skin can benefit greatly by applying a grated raw potato as a mask or just rubbing the potato on the skin and leaving the juices on for one-half hour, rinsing off with water and vinegar. Apply an oil-free herbal moisturizer. Buy almond butter at the health food store and use it as a cleanser to give the face a light scrubbing.

You might find taking the B vitamins (especially B6), whole grains, beets, oranges, and lemons helpful. I take one tablespoon a day of brewer's yeast, preferably in my spirulina, wheat grass, alfalfa, and apple juice blend.

Rose geranium, lavender, and lemon make a nice blend for oily skin. Grape-seed oil is one of the lightest oils. Kukui oil is light and highly absorbent and can be used on oily skin. These are good to blend with the essential oils for oily skin. Mix several drops of rose geranium, lavender, and lemon to grape-seed oil or kukui oil as a nighttime application. You could also mix these essential oils in with your present unscented lotions, oils, or creams.

Do-it-yourself treatments

For blemishes, you can apply tea tree oil, lemongrass, peppermint, or myrrh directly on the eruption. Be careful, because peppermint and lemongrass should not usually be applied directly on the skin at full strength. You can also use these essential oils to make yourself a refreshing mist. Just add several drops to a cup of purified water and mist your face several times throughout the day. Mist will not disturb your makeup. (See section on Acne.)

More skin care recipes to make at home

Another great toner you can make for yourself is one cup of purified water with several drops essential oil of lavender and one tablespoon of organic vinegar. A cleansing rinse of equal parts of water and organic apple vinegar helps to fight infections, tone, and reduce enlarged pores. A couple of drops of coriander oil in a cup of water is great for oily skin to help remove impurities.

In one cup of purified water, add one tablespoon each of lemon juice, lime juice, pineapple juice, and apple cider vinegar. Use every day the first thing in the morning and after cleansing at night. You can drink this, too!

Try two tablespoons Fuller's earth clay and mix with water so you have enough to cover the entire face. For seven days in a row, apply a thin layer and let dry for twenty minutes, then wash off with warm water. This is a one-week detox program; some may break out before their skin clears up.

Papaya is best for oily skin. Make a mask by blending the entire fruit, minus the peel and seeds, which you can use to rub all over your cleansed face to promote circulation before applying your mask. You can use it alone or mix it with honey.

For a brewer's yeast mask, mix brewer's yeast with water until a paste of desired consistency is achieved, apply, allow to dry for twenty minutes, and then rinse it off. You may also add a couple drops of your favorite essential oil and some honey to this mask. While doing this three times a week, you may also take brewer's yeast internally to get a noticeable result.

Making a strong infusion or tea of yarrow and drinking it daily is said to cut down the amount of sebum production.

Inhale and apply any of the following essential oils diluted in almond oil: bergamot, tea tree oil, camphor, cedarwood, cypress, eucalyptus, juniper, lavender, lemon, lemongrass, peppermint, or rosemary.

Homemade masks for oily skin

The following kitchen and garden cosmetics are helpful to oily skin and can be made at home in a blender. To make your own mask, use any of the following alone or blend any of the following with honey or yogurt:

- Buttermilk
- Cucumber
- Brewer's yeast
- Brandy
- Lemon
- Tomato
- Cornmeal

- Vinegar
- Peppermint
- Parsley
- Sour cream
- Fuller's earth
- Onions

Remedies for blackheads and pimples

✳ Steam your face with peppermint, sage, and fennel seeds in two quarts of water and a total of half a cup of herbs for eight minutes. When all the pores are open, go very quickly to a mirror and with very clean hands, gently dislodge the blackhead. You may need to steam a few days in a row before you can loosen the lodged material. Use a cold astringent, preferably refrigerated, immediately after treatment.

✳ Mix two tablespoons buttermilk with two tablespoons of fresh, mashed strawberries and a little Fuller's earth to make into a paste. Apply and leave on for twenty minutes before rinsing.

✳ Lemons are degreasers. Apply fresh lemon directly to the blemish or dilute with water, or put in a spray bottle. Keep in the refrigerator and apply throughout the day.

✳ Apply raw onions directly to the blemish. Or soak a peeled and chopped onion in water for one day and apply the resulting onion toner to your skin after cleansing.

✳ Juice or take the liquid from one squeezed cucumber and add one tablespoon of vinegar, and use this for a perfect after-cleansing skin tonic. Apply with cotton ball or spray bottle.

✳ Make a tea of parsley and peppermint and apply as a toner.

* Using sour cream as a base for an herbal mask reputedly helps close large pores. Use two tablespoons sour cream with powdered parsley and peppermint, or any of the appropriate herbs for oily skin. Sour cream, like yogurt, is high in lactic acid, which is beneficial and has astringent properties that will help with blackheads.

* Mix two tablespoons oatmeal in a little water to make a paste and apply as a mask.

* If you like the feel of a scrub, take your regular cleanser and while you are washing your face just add a little corn meal or salt to get the grainy feel. That way you can have a scrub handy any time. Don't add it to the entire container; just add it to your hand at the time of each individual cleansing.

* Use a good astringent after each cleansing; either use one of the simple recipes above or you can buy a few high-quality astringents. (See section on Astringents.)

My daily program

For optimal results, oily skin needs daily care. Develop your own regimen. As an example, here's mine:

Cleanse

Twice a day, I cleanse with a quality cleanser, making sure it does not have any harsh chemicals. Look for cleansers that contain ingredients such as homemade soaps with almond oil, vegetable glycerin, lemon juice or essential oil, seaweeds, witch hazel, lily, lavender, camphor, grapefruit seed extract, tea tree oil, sage, comfrey, aloe, eucalyptus, and calendula.

Steam

Once a week after cleansing, I steam a variety of herbs, perhaps lavender, lily, chamomile, rose, calendula, comfrey, or seaweeds. Sometimes, I will just do chamomile. Pour a cup of the infusion for tea, and then to the rest, put a couple drops of any of the essential oils recommended for oily skin. I particularly like lavender, juniper, or sage. Be ready to put the towel over your head because the essential oils will evaporate very quickly, and you want their benefit to go directly to your skin. Be careful not to use too much of these essential oils in the water, as they are very strong and concentrated. I learned the hard way. I actually put so much in the first time that I couldn't breathe.

Mask/Exfoliate

For maximum results, you can do this daily for a week to see if your skin is benefiting. Again you can try so many things. I like to use my botanical enzyme exfoliant mask with honey, pineapple, papaya, mint, lily, and comfrey. Sometimes I apply yogurt with one of the above-mentioned herbs with brewer's yeast blended into a paste. Be creative and come up with your own mask.

Vinegar peel

You can do this right after the steam, after the mask, or alone anytime. Warm organic apple cider vinegar, about one cup, so it is hot but not too hot to apply to your skin. I dip a clean washcloth in the vinegar and then put it on my entire face. You may want to cut a hole in the cloth so you can breathe easier. Let it sit for a while and keep re-applying until the vinegar is gone. (You may want to dilute the vinegar in water.)

Astringent/Toner

I like to do this at least twice a day and after cleansing. If you do not wear makeup, you could apply astringent up to three to five times a day to keep your skin impeccably clean. Your astringent should be free of any synthetic chemicals and full of herbs and essential oils instead. Look for ones that tone, cleanse, and help close and tighten pores, like sage and lavender essential oils, and herbs like lily, eucalyptus, elderberries, horsetail, coltsfoot, calendula, and chamomile. I keep a bottle of my astringent by my computer to apply several times a day. (You do not need to use an astringent if you just did a vinegar peel.)

Moisture

Even people with oily skin usually need to moisturize facial areas around the eyes and mouth. I like using a lightweight lotion with almond oil, lily, primrose oil, rosehip seed oil, myrrh, and aloe, and essential oil of tea tree. I just simply apply it to wherever I feel dry.

If you prefer oil-free products, look for an oil-free moisturizer made with aloe and vegetable glycerin, with herbs like comfrey, hops, lilies, seaweeds, horsetail, calendula, chestnut, and ivy. If you don't want to apply anything, at least mist your skin with moisturizing mist made of pure water and herbs like lily, comfrey, seaweeds, chamomile, calendula, and with essential oils like lavender and ylang ylang. Or simply make your own. Focus on what makes you and keeps you looking beautiful.

Sensitive and Allergic Skin

While everybody talks about the sun, aging, or ingesting poor foods as the skin's enemies, another real culprit may be many beauty products themselves. The very products that we are buying to protect us may just be accelerating the process of aging due to the irritation they may cause.

It is estimated that nearly 20% of all women suffer from serious, continuous problems when they apply almost anything to their skin. I think these estimates are accurate because about half of the women I talk to in health food stores say they are ultra-sensitive. It makes sense to me that the incidence of sensitive-skinned people shopping in health food stores would be at least twice as high, because this is one of the main reasons that people end up shopping there instead of at mainstream stores.

Sensitive skin

Sensitive skin is described as being unable to tolerate over-stimulation. The face is often the most sensitive, and light-complexioned women seem to have the most trouble. People with sensitive skin seem to be much more sensitive to the sun and wind, as well as more prone to allergies. Itching, blisters, scaling, or redness indicate allergies. The words "allergy tested," "hypoallergenic," and the like don't seem to have much influence on the undesirable ingredients some manufacturers use.

Constant irritation to the skin is potentially damaging. If you suffer from asthma, allergies, and hay fever, you are more likely to have irritation with many cosmetic products. The condition of not being able to apply anything to your skin is termed *status cosmeticus*. Many times, however, if you patch test women with this condition, they do not come up allergic. I think a lot of the problems stem from the harsh ingredients in many products on the market today. Between the strength of many of the chemicals, the preservatives, and now the alpha hydroxys, people are much more likely to disrupt the skin's natural barrier function.

The dead layer of skin, the outermost layer, has as its primary function to provide protection against the outside world. If you use harsh chemicals on this outermost layer of skin, it may cause irritation. The skin can become degraded. It may be that both elastin and collagen can be destroyed by the constant inflammation, which could ultimately cause premature aging of your skin.

Moisturize

Moisturizer is needed to slow down the evaporation of water from the layers of skin. Dryness is often the beginning of skin sensitivity, *so keep your skin moisturized all the time.* My recommendation is: Do not use any product that contains any ingredients that are not purely botanical.

A good suggestion for those with sensitive skin is to begin by using only products from your kitchen. Oils for moisture, teas for toners, and fresh vegetables and fruits, honey, and yogurt as masks. Keep it simple. Use plain oils, almond or kukui, for example. Then after a few months free of irritation, make your own pure products, or move up to an impeccably clean body-care line from your health food store. Check to see if they are "clean." *Read the labels..*

I personally heard so many complaints from so many women for so long saying they couldn't use any products (e.g., they couldn't tolerate vitamin E, aloe vera, essential oils, etc.), that I made an ultra-sensitive skin cream with only the gentlest ingredients. So far I have not had one woman tell me she broke out from it. It contains only purified water, almond oil, shea butter, vegetable glycerin, lily, xanthan gum, lecithin, soy protein, and grapefruit seed extract.

Kukui oil is another great ingredient for people with extremely sensitive skin. People who are allergic to everything else can usually use it. (See more in the section on oils.)

Sunscreens are extremely harsh. Even the only natural SPF-sunscreen PABA, which I prefer, causes breakouts in about 20% of the population.

Depending on your skin and body's tolerance I would follow a regimen like the following:

First, you are going to have no choice but to become completely educated in all phases of reading ingredients. Usually, health food stores will be the only places you will be able to buy products at all, and even then you are going to have to become the pickiest. You will probably not be able to use any products with any synthetic, animal, or petro products. Those with sensitive skin will probably break out from urea, propylene glycol, and all of the parabens.

Many companies put "derived from" after chemical ingredients to let you know that at one time this ingredient was botanical. However, I don't think it matters if the molecular makeup of the ingredient has been altered. It is not the same as natural. You may not be able to use any ingredients that have been chemically reacted to other substances. You will also not do well with products that are preserved with alcohol. This leaves you with very few choices. The only preservative you will probably be able to tolerate is grapefruit seed extract.

Ultra-sensitive

The very best thing to do if you are ultra-sensitive and everything makes you break out is to make your own body care products. We have many recipes in this book; in addition, there are many more great books. (See bibliography.) If you are very sensitive, it will be worth the trouble. You can also ask at your health food store for the cleanest products they carry without any synthetic or petro chemicals.

Regimen for sensitive skin

Cleanse

Cleansers are by nature going to be a little harsh because their job is to reduce surface tension. If you do not have any blemish problems, you may want just to cleanse with almond oil on a clean, warm, wet washcloth. If you can use a cleanser from the health food store, try the sample sizes first and do patch tests, first on your arm and then on your face. Seaweed cleansers can often be tolerated. If all soaps bother you, you may want to try using only a toner/astringent on a cotton ball to cleanse.

Toner/Astringent

You can try sample sizes of many of the toners at the health food store or you may be better off making your own. I would simply make a tea of calendula, place it in a glass jar and keep it in the refrigerator. Apply it with a cotton ball after cleansing.

Moisturize

Depending on how dry your skin is, you may need to try many different moisturizers before finding one that really suits you. I make an unscented cream for ultra-sensitive complexions. It has very few ingredients and works beautifully for most people who can use nothing else. But you need to patch test everything all the time. My herbal moisturizer is another gift from nature you may want to try. I also make a face and body flower oil, but it is scented with essential oil of lavender. Or try unscented kukui oil. Another choice: make your own herbal oils. Make your own blend of any of the following essential oils diluted with almond oil, alone or together: jasmine, neroli, chamomile, and rose.

Mask

A good mask for sensitive and dry skin is the following:

Take two tablespoons cooked oatmeal and mix with honey or milk to make a paste. Apply the mask all over your face, then lie down and relax. Leave on for twenty minutes and rinse off with cool water, pat dry, and apply a quality astringent/toner and moisturizer.

Final note on sensitive skin

If you are ultra-sensitive, you probably want to do as little to your face as possible. Leave it alone and let it breathe and heal. You may also want to see an herbalist, nutritionist, or naturopath to see what you specifically need to be doing internally. There is also a myriad of great books at libraries and health food stores on the topics of allergies, skin sensitivities, and homemade skin care remedies.

Wrinkled Skin

Facial lines are caused by the collagen fibers in the skin's dermis, or lower layer, losing their tone. Collagen moves, changes, and must retain its flexibility in its unique arrangement of fibers. These fibers bend and move so we can chew, smile, yawn, and talk. These movements pull the skin into different shapes.

The skin has a great tolerance for returning to its original state, but as the years pass, the collagen fibers begin to wear and lose their exact arrangement. There is a breakdown of the collagen, which begins to harden, becomes less elastic, and loses its flexibility. The stretching and sagging first appear as fine lines around the eyes and mouth where there is the most movement.

Some believe that the underlying fatty tissue of the skin begins to shrink more rapidly after 45. There is therefore an excess of skin, giving the appearance of aging skin. The English and Irish as well as all people with fair complexions usually have thinner skin, which ages more quickly. Frequent weight gain and loss (the yo-yo effect) can accelerate the stretching of the skin. It's a fact that smokers have more wrinkles than non-smokers, because smoking slows the circulation of the blood to the skin.

So, what can you do to minimize wrinkling?

✤ Follow a good, clean skin-care regimen. Moisturizers lubricate the skin and reduce the stress of the skin when facial expressions are made. Moisturizers also have the ability to puff up the skin somewhat, making the skin look less lined.

* Take good care of yourself. That includes exercise, good nutrition, and being happy.

* Sleeping face up really helps, so that the skin doesn't get so distorted. Spending eight hours a day with your face pressed hard against the pillow may accelerate aging.

* Watch your facial mannerisms. While smile lines are attractive, frown lines are not. I get a lot of questions about lines on the forehead. We all have them, but the serious worrying type have much deeper lines on their foreheads; if you don't know what facial expressions you engage in, put a mirror on your desk at work and watch yourself in the mirror when you talk on the phone.

* Use a blend of any of the following essential oils diluted in almond oil: lavender, neroli, rose, frankincense, patchouli, rosemary, sandalwood, cypress, fennel, or myrrh.

* Focus on getting your body in shape. There is nothing more beautiful than a woman who looks like she takes impeccable care of herself.

* Notice your beautiful attributes whether they be your smile, your laugh, etc.

* Accept and love yourself and the fact that God has allowed you to continue life on the planet.

* Celebrate your continued existence. Remember, life is a gift.

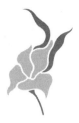

Treatments for Skin Conditions

Acne

Two glaring realizations came to me regarding acne: the first is how little anyone understands or knows about its cures, and the second is how all-encompassing painful acne can be.

Sometimes I lose patience with people who have never even experienced a blemish giving advice on acne. Incredibly, many of the 50-plus books I have read on natural skin care have dedicated less than two sentences to acne. When you have it, acne is a major thing in your life, worthy of more than one sentence.

Obviously, these authors have never had a blemish and certainly never felt completely insecure about their appearance because of skin problems. Is it possible acne might be a little more complicated to cure than simply giving up chocolate?

If during the entire four years of high school you hardly had a date or you didn't get invited to the prom, if you had to develop a glowing personality, your brains, or your sense of humor because your good looks were not going to open any doors for you, then you know what I am talking about. It reminds me of a joke a friend of mine told me about when his niece was born. She was kind of an unattractive baby and the baby's grandfather said, "Don't worry; we'll get her a good education." It's the truth: being attractive in America is a lot better than not being attractive. It's also a fact that attractive people are more successful in business, and we all know how much easier they have it socially.

Some doctors are worse than authors. Many times blessed with clear skin they simply (and inadequately) tell patients just to avoid chocolate and mustard and take an antibiotic. If it were that easy, I don't think you'd be reading this. It's like the commercial for a health gym that states: "Come on, if great bodies came in a video or a can, everybody would have one."

I make no claim to being any kind of health care practitioner. I hold no degree in medicine or nutrition or anything else even close; however, I offer something few others can—personal, firsthand experience and decades of concentrated effort and research on the subject of acne and other skin-related subjects.

Acne is primarily hereditary and hormonal

My humble, non-medical theory is: Acne is hereditary and 90% of acne in adult women is hormonal.

The fact that you haven't had acne is not an indicator you have done anything right! It only shows you picked the right parents and you were born lucky. So beware of giving your advice; please, spare those who are suffering from acne. Instead, be supportive. Show empathy. Focus on the positive aspects of your acne-suffering friends. Tell them what is great about them. Remember: A friend is one who reminds you of your good points when you may be forgetting them.

Many books say that "no one should have to suffer from acne." All you have to do is eat right and avoid chocolate. Or "your skin is the window to your general health." If those books are right, why is it that people dying of liver disease, cancer, or kidney failure don't all have acne? How come many drug addicts and alcoholics don't have acne? Why don't all smokers have acne?

I am not saying that poor nutrition has not been the culprit in many cases of acne. Good nutrition is certainly an important part of good general health, as well as trying to clear up your skin, but only *one* part. You can eat impeccably and still suffer cyst acne.

Food and lifestyle

The greatest relationship between food and acne is that your body does need proper nutrients to perform its functions correctly. In that sense, food and lifestyle become very significant. Hormones are manufactured best when your body is functioning optimally. An excess of saturated fats can increase the sebaceous glands and create more oil. Poor elimination through the bowels, liver, and kidneys can put excess work on the pores of the skin.

What is acne?

There are up to 5,000 oil glands found on the face. Acne is inflammation of these sebaceous glands. The sebaceous glands are most plentiful and active on the face, neck, back, and chest. The excess oil or sebum blocks the hair follicles and pores, and the bacteria builds up and inflammation occurs. Acne happens when the amount and/or quality of the oil secreted by the glands become abnormal.

Acne is ongoing inflammation of the sebaceous glands. Cyst acne is the most damaging physically and emotionally. Cysts are infections below the skin. Corynebacterium acne is usually responsible for the secondary infection, which often times causes deep tissue scarring. The cysts are very painful to the touch.

Less painful and less harmful kinds of skin eruptions include blackheads, whiteheads, and papules, which are red hard areas of inflammation caused by a blockage of the sebaceous duct. These conditions are often found in adolescents and often do not stop there, as is usually believed. Acne, closely related to hormone activity, can stay with afflicted women until their early forties or until after menopause.

Different theories offer different remedies

Nutrition

If acne could be cured simply by eliminating sugar, chocolate, white flour, dairy, wheat, meat, etc., I don't think you would see too many women with breakouts. I know you wouldn't see me ever again with a blemish, because I would consider that a very small price to pay for clear skin.

Lack of sufficient essential fatty acids can cause all kinds of skin problems, including acne and eczema in addition to thin hair and flaky scalp. It is said that taking supplemental EFAs may not always be effective if the EFAs are inhibited by insufficient vitamins B6 and C or magnesium or zinc. Taking all with primrose oil with zinc has helped some sufferers with the problem.

Toxins

Many, many, many people say acne is caused by toxins being released from the body. This could be the case for some people. I just doubt it in the hundreds of women I talk to who work out and steam daily, shop wisely, and are vegans.

The liver's contribution

Liver-cleansing herbs can often be helpful in clearing up hormonal-related acne because the liver metabolizes estrogen and testosterone. It is believed that if the liver cannot metabolize the estrogen, it can cause pre-menstrual syndrome (PMS), acne, and irritation. If the liver cannot process testosterone, it can also cause acne, increased sexual energy, and aggressive mood swings. Follow the instructions under the detox section, if this may be the case.

The sebaceous glands process the nutrients from the bloodstream. They take substances from the blood, which come from the diet, and utilize the fatty acids as secretion that is sebum, the theory being that the fats taken into the body determine the quality of fat in the blood and used in the sebum. Some say that if it is sticky, it creates a sticking of red blood cells, causing a decrease in their ability to bind and transport oxygen to the cells in the body. It can cause the sebaceous gland to have a stickier sebum that cannot get through the hair follicles and causes blockages. When the oil is sticky, it cannot flow freely, and the cells can plug the movement of oil to the surface, therefore causing an eruption.

Infections

We know that acne is caused by infections, and we know that the deep scarring acne, which we really want to avoid, is an infection, and we know that antibiotics will temporarily help clear up acne. But is there a natural equivalent? Many believe garlic and vinegar help. Topically, tea tree oil and lavender are the answer.

To control the potential infections that can take place after a breakout, take "herbal antibiotics" such as garlic, purple coneflower, and wild indigo. Daily dosages of vitamin C can also aid your body in fighting infections.

The part stress can play

Stress, of course, can create or aggravate any health problem. This is where you need to take a good look at your life. Are you happy? Why? Why not? What is causing you stress? Can you begin taking steps to improve or change the situation? Maybe you can start to take small steps to improve the situation today. (See chapter on Happiness.)

Acne and hormones

Frankly, from my nearly thirty-year struggle with acne, this is where I think 90% of all women get their adult acne. My deduction comes from the breakouts and their consistent predictability in a woman's cycle.

The most serious and painful kind of acne has as its source a glandular imbalance. There are two different kinds, which happen at different times of life. The first is adolescence. Of course, this is normal, occurs often, usually stabilizes, and the blemishes go away. The second kind is more serious and occurs in adults. To ascertain if you have hormonal adult acne, answer these questions:

❋ Is it hereditary? That is, did your parents or siblings have acne?

❋ Do topical applications have very little positive effect?

❋ If female, are your periods painful and/or irregular?

❋ Can you predict acne breakouts within your cycle?

❋ Do you have acne that is large and painful?

❋ Is your skin always oily?

If your answer to most of these is "yes," then my considered guess is you probably have acne that is hormonal-related.

Among the many hormones secreted by the body, androgens, including testosterone, a male hormone (which naturally occurs in various amounts in women as well as men), activate the oil glands. These effects usually are balanced by estrogen and other female hormones, but if they are not, this can cause a problem. It is said that testosterone has a contracting and stimulating influence; it can cause fatty acids and other materials to collect in the bloodstream, then around the sebaceous glands where they become sebum and are discharged. Many believe the production of testosterone is speeded up by over-consumption of saturated fats.

Estrogen has the counter-balancing effect; it slows down the speed of fatty acids and other materials moving toward the sebaceous glands. This is why high-estrogen birth control pills are sometimes recommended to women with severe acne. This is also why wild yam root can be valuable.

Side effects and dangers of treatment

Topical antibiotics can also be effective but can have some side effects such as diarrhea and bacterial resistance. Antibiotics are suspected of causing immune deficiencies and being responsible for such conditions as chronic fatigue syndrome. Accutane, a prescription drug, does work for a lot of people. Dermatologists tell me a woman would have to have a pregnancy test once a week while on it, because accutane causes birth defects. My thought? If it has the power to deform a fetus, what else could it be doing to a person's body? I wouldn't recommend taking a risk, but if you decided to use it, I would understand. I'd recommend you try all the natural remedies first.

Remedies

* Primrose and wheat germ oil taken internally to balance hormone production

* Vitamin E oil mixed with the herbs lily and comfrey and applied to heal scarring after inflammation is gone

* Herb teas believed to purify the blood: cleavers is pleasant; also try nettle, yellow dock, Oregon grape root, and dandelion

* "Herbal antibiotics" to control the infections, such as garlic, purple coneflower, and wild indigo

* Many women say their acne gets worse just prior to their period; if this is the case, it is probably because their estrogen levels drop and their progesterone hormones are in excess. To control acne that appears right before your period, try teas made of sage, wild yam, Chinese angelica, and false unicorn root. (Never use during pregnancy.)

* Cleaning your skin with milk and yogurt

* Taking bee propolis internally and externally

* Boiling an onion and applying the water to the face three times a day

* Taking a tea of cleavers, burdock, and dandelion; use as a steam and then apply to skin, and drink a cup daily.

* Using other herbs for female hormone regulation such as black cohosh, dong quai, saw palmetto, and blessed thistle

* Taking B-complex vitamins, a great help in rebalancing the body secretions

* Many people swear by lecithin, taking two tablespoons of the granules in apple juice or five capsules per day. It is said to emulsify and help break down fatty globules in the body.

* Drinking eight to ten glasses of water a day makes for a constant kidney flush and facilitates waste removal. Drinking plenty of water will really help.

* Acne sufferers often need additional supplements of chromium, selenium, magnesium, and zinc.

* Some find iron and iodine helpful, but test both carefully, as they can be helpful or hurtful.

* Blackheads and whiteheads can occur when vitamin A is needed.

* Overactive sebaceous glands have sometimes been linked to GLA insufficiency. GLA is in primrose and borage oil.

* Mega GLA has helped some people to reduce inflammation and help calm overactive glands.

Diet

* One to two apples every day (eat alone, not with other food)

* One salad a day with a high-quality olive oil dressing

* Whole grains such as rye and brown rice

* One high-quality yogurt three times a week

* Seeds

* Fresh fish

* Only free-range eggs and poultry

* Fresh juices daily

Also try

* Applying diluted lemon juice, which is antiseptic, cleansing, and has a high acid pH.

* Adding lemon juice to water or distilled witch hazel; it's a great degreaser.

* Applying fennel essential oil.

* Simmering garlic in olive oil and applying to the pimples–an old Himalayan remedy.

* Taking brewer's yeast.

* Taking acidophilus.

Herbs found throughout history to be beneficial for acne include burdock, clover, horsetail, iris, lavender, lemon balm, white birch bark, Oregon grape, and aloe.

Other Possibilities:

* Honey, as outlined in this book, is wonderful on the skin. You can mix it with wheat germ, papaya, lemon, or any of the above powdered herbs to make a nourishing and beneficial acne-healing mask.

* An Epsom salt and juniper berry bath is highly detoxifying. (See bathing and detoxifying section of this book.)

* Potatoes, tomatoes, apples, grapes, and cucumbers, full-strength or diluted, are all perfect to supply relief to blemished skin. Just apply the fruit, fresh, blended, or mashed, as a mask.

* An acne herbal milk can be made by putting one ounce of herb into eight ounces cold milk and soaking overnight before applying to the skin. Lily, chamomile, yarrow, comfrey, horsetail, coltsfoot, parsley, or watermelon juice can be used.

* For fruit-acid treatments, apply the juice of fresh cucumber, pineapple, papaya, apple, and/or grapes. Rub the cut slices all over the face to cleanse the skin.

My theory is this: Eat impeccably well because your body needs to be functioning properly to operate effectively. Fresh fruit will cleanse the intestinal tract, vitamins will help fight infections, minerals will strengthen your hair, bones, and nails. You will feel better and look wonderful, and you are also taking control and empowering yourself.

Take Lily's apple cider vinegar drink, acidophilus, dandelion root tea, and your choice of the wonderful supplements listed in this book to fight infections and release toxins.

Knowledge and gentleness

Give yourself a break. If you have been doing everything right and you still have acne, you obviously have a predisposition for it through heredity. You can do everything perfectly and still have acne. Some cases of acne can be drastically reduced by your food intake, supplements, herbs, steams, deep-breathing exercises, and great products, but there are going to be a few of you who may have stubborn acne that must be accepted for periods of time throughout your life.

Cleansing acne skin

There are two different schools of thought concerning this and both make sense. I think, like so many things, it is a matter of preference.

Oil and oil-based cleansers can be very effective in cleansing oily skin. Like attracts like. Dirt, oil, and grime stick to the oil base and are cleansed away. Water-based astringents are also effective used with a cotton ball to remove oil and dirt. Soaps reduce the surface tension and allow dirt and oil to be removed.

Water and soap can be drying, and one school of thought is that their usage will encourage the body to produce more oil to replace that which was removed.

Proper and appropriate skin care using fresh, clean, healthful ingredients is fundamentally important to good and long-lasting skin care. Regular use of quality cleansers, toners, lotions, oils, steams, and gentle exfoliating masks is crucial.

Having severe acne can color your entire life, having a dramatic effect that is very difficult to treat. You just can't use this cleanser, astringent, and tonic and it's gone, and I really resent companies that try to sell us that bill of goods. It's insulting to our intelligence and that is why Lily of Colorado doesn't make a lot of wild claims about our products. I remember buying products that never worked, and I felt cheated, fooled, and scammed.

Essential oils application

A small amount of the following oils blended and diluted in a high-quality almond, kukui, primrose, sunflower, or rosehip seed oil and applied directly to the erupted area is helpful: bergamot, camphor, cedarwood, juniper, lavender, and sandalwood.

You can also use the essential oils of bergamot, lemon, lemon verbena, palmarosa, spearmint, tea tree, and wintergreen.

A blend of palmarosa, yarrow, myrrh, and lavender with a light base oil such as evening primrose is a good daily application for a breakout or use a cider vinegar toner. You can make your own by mixing two tablespoons of organic cider vinegar in pure water. Make a clay mask with juniper berry and bergamot essential oils.

Herbal steam facials

Steam is both very cleansing and detoxifying. It is very beneficial to the overall health and condition of your skin. Use the simple method of the towel tent/hood I have described previously in this book. Steaming with plain water is beneficial. Even better is to add essential oils and/or herbs, allowing the steam to penetrate your skin for fifteen minutes, while you are mindful of the scent and benefits of the herbs, breathing in slowly and deeply. Herbs you can include are lily, nettle, fennel, comfrey, and houseleek (a member of the lily family).

My recommended regime for acne

At least daily or twice a day:

Cleanse

Use an oil and soap-based cleanser or a seaweed cleanser. Rinse your skin with cold water to bring warm blood to the capillaries at the skin's surface, helping to increase the circulation.

Astringent

Put a high-quality astringent on a cotton ball and remove any excess soap or dirt. Make sure it includes ingredients like witch hazel, lily, lavender, horsetail, sage, yarrow, and comfrey.

Moisturize

Use an oil-free herbal moisturizer sparingly around your mouth or forehead or wherever you are dry. You do not need to moisturize where you have breakouts.

At least twice a week:

Exfoliate

Use a non-abrasive, botanical mask. Papayas, pineapple, and honey are all perfect ingredients. You may also make an herbal mask of your own using a high-quality yogurt, with ground herbs of lily, lavender, rose, chamomile, and calendula.

Steam

Use a single mixture of the above herbs to deeply cleanse the pores and release pus or to open them up as a preventive measure. To tighten and stimulate the skin, use peppermint, lavender, anise, comfrey leaves, and rose.

Acne Steam

Steep lavender, licorice, comfrey root, lemon, chamomile, and witch hazel in boiling water.

Make-at-home recipes

Cleansing grains:

1 cup finely ground oats

2 cups facial or cosmetic clay

1/4 cup finely ground almonds

Grind all the ingredients. To use, mix one to two teaspoons of the cleansing grains with water. Stir into a paste and gently massage onto face. Allow to dry, and rinse off with warm water. If you have cyst acne and sores, be careful not to aggravate them.

You can add salt or sugar to any cleanser to provide a "scrub" feel, if you prefer.

Any Fruit Revitalizing Mask:

1/2 ripe avocado, peeled apple, peach, tomato, or other fruit

1 tablespoon fresh tomato juice

1 tablespoon lemon juice

Tie your hair back well away from your face, then cleanse your face and throat.

Mash the fruit and add the tomato and lemon juices. Using a fork or potato masher, mix thoroughly. Spread the paste over your face and neck, avoiding the areas around the eyes. Lie back and relax for fifteen to twenty minutes. Rinse off with water, pat dry, tone, and moisturize.

Yogurt and Clay Packs for Oily and Acne Skins:

3 tablespoons Fuller's earth

2 teaspoons natural yogurt

2 teaspoons potato water

Blend the Fuller's earth, yogurt, and potato water into a smooth paste. Apply the mixture to your face for fifteen to twenty minutes. Rinse off with water, pat dry, tone, and moisturize. Because this has a drying effect on the skin, it should never be used more than twice a week.

Good luck!

Scarring

The best herb to use for scarring is lily. Get fresh lilies and soak them in almond oil. After two weeks, squeeze the flower essence from the oil and do the process again. Apply regularly to reduce scarring.

For further information see sections on:

❋ Aloe vera

❋ Rosehip seed oil

❋ Immortelle essential oil (see under Essential Oils)

❋ Lily (see under Herbs)

Skin Resurfacing: Laser and Dermabrasion

Lasers seem to have replaced dermabrasion as the latest technique for smoothing scarred or severely wrinkled skin. Dermabrasion attempts to plane the surface of the skin to remove deep lines and/or acne scars. It employs the use of a small, fast-rotating, abrasive wire brush that rubs off the top layers of the skin.

Laser skin resurfacing is a highly effective surgical procedure to reduce severe acne scars. This is a high-tech dermabrasion of the 1990s. It works through laser beams. Light energy is stimulated by an electric current or radio waves and amplified by mirrors that are placed in a small gas-filled tube. The mirrors create an intense beam of light. The laser is a precise instrument and much more proficient than other procedures such as dermabrasion and chemical peels. It is the newest and probably the most effective surgery available for acne scars. You may guess that the reason I include this in my book is because I have had it done.

The most often asked questions I get are: "What was it like?" and "Do you recommend it?"

What is the laser like?

It is very expensive: $3000 to $8000 for the full face. It takes two weeks to heal enough even to return to work or your regular routine. (I found it difficult to hang around the house to heal.)

Like the dermabrasion, it's not that painful, per se; it's just very uncomfortable.

You really need someone who can help take care of you for that entire two weeks. There are lots of secretions and scabs, cleaning and several-times-a-day treatments that need tending. You have to take pain pills to get through the immense discomfort, not terrible pain, but your face swells up to twice its size and is full of scabs and goo. It must be cleaned and prepped several times a day and that takes time.

I had already had three dermabrasions before I had the laser, so I cannot say I got my money's worth. But these days you could probably just get the laser done first. It is a lot like the dermabrasion, and my first dermabrasion really helped improve the texture of my skin and diminish the scarring. So I would say if you really are unhappy with the scars on your skin and find them very disturbing, and if you can afford the procedure and the time off work, go for it.

If you really want it done, you will find the money. I didn't have any money when I had the first dermabrasion done. But I put my mind to the task. I had my priorities in order. I drove an old car. (I still do; I am against monthly payments of any kind.) I skimped and saved and came up with the money. You will too, if it is really important to you.

Do I recommend dermabrasion?

Yes. I am for anything that will help you feel better about yourself and does not involve taking a health risk. I have always been so desperate for clear skin that it has ruled my life in so many ways, many of them positive, like learning about herbs and starting my company.

Dermabrasion is a desperate measure. It's a serious step to take and you need to tread slowly. You need to interview many dermatologists. The dermatologist who performed my dermabrasion procedures did not offer laser surgery, so I had to search for another doctor.

The best way to check out doctors is to get recommendations from others. Go meet with the doctors. Talk to them. Ask them what they think. Also: What percent improvement can you expect? How many of these surgeries have they performed? How much it will cost? Do they think this is the best course of action for you to improve your skin? Do they have any other recommendations for you? How long have they been doing this particular surgery? Ask them to show you before-and-after pictures. Make a clear list of what you want to know before you go in and talk to them, and stick to it. Do not be intimidated; you are the customer and they work for you. Be clear in your mind about that.

Confidence essential

It is very important that you have complete confidence in the doctor you choose, as a healer and as a human being. It is essential that you like him or her, his or her office staff, your treatment while there, the vibrations you pick up while in the office.

I think it is frightening whenever you deliberately go and ask someone to perform a surgery on you that is not absolutely necessary. Dermabrasion and laser surgery are considered optional or cosmetic surgeries.

I met my doctor's wife at Alfalfa's about three years before I went to him. She had just had the laser procedure done and her face looked terribly sunburned, but she couldn't wipe the smile off her face. She was so pleased that she grinned the entire time I was talking to her. She told me all about the terrific results, the wonderful outcome, and really made me think about it. However, it took me three years to act.

My experience

The day before I was going in to have the laser scar-diminishing done, I was cleaning my house when the *Sally Jessy Raphael Show* came on my television. "Plastic Surgery Nightmares" was the subject. It was all about how all these different surgeries from laser to nose jobs went wrong. People's faces were disfigured and lives were ruined. Two people on the show had the work done by a man who was not even a doctor and had maimed them for life.

This was definitely not good pre-op programming. But it does underscore the importance of investigating thoroughly. After you do all your in-person investigations, call the state board of medical examiners for whatever particular state the doctor is in to make sure he or she is in good standing.

For Colorado, the address is 1560 Broadway, Suite 1300, Denver, Colorado 80202-5140, or phone (303) 894-7690 or fax (303) 894-7692. You can check board certification by calling (800) 776-CERT (800) 776-2378, or check surgeons certified by the American Board of Medical Specialties at www.certifieddoctor.org. Other sources of information are the American Medical Association at (800) 621-8335, ext. 6201; the American Association for Plastic Surgeons, 888 Glen Brook Avenue, Bryn Mawr, PA 19010, phone (610) 527-4833; or the American Board of Plastic Surgery, 7 Penn Center, Suite #400, 1635 Market Street, Philadelphia, PA 19103, phone (215) 587-9322.

Agreement in healing recommendation

One interesting thing is that the doctors all recommend for the most important part of post-treatment a wonderful vinegar soak several times a day. It's a great way to treat your skin, no matter what you have been through, whether surgery, burns, or acne. (See the section on Vinegar for more information on this beauty treatment that is recommended even by the mainstream medical profession.)

Their specific recommendation is one tablespoon of vinegar to one cup of warm purified water on a washcloth placed on the healing face. They did recommend white vinegar, I am sure because it is distilled and because it is placed on open wounds on the skin. While I certainly understand that reasoning, I used organic cider vinegar, and it worked wonderfully.

I enjoyed my vinegar soaks so much, I vowed to keep it as part of my regular regimen. I may have a product out using this as a base by the time you read this.

Any kind of surgery like this is a big step, a large expense, a great commitment, and takes up a lot of time. So it's a big decision that you have to weigh for yourself. I felt sort of overindulgent and vain with the laser, more so than with the dermabrasion, possibly because a plastic surgeon did the surgery. It was expensive. It took a total of almost a month's time off work. It was a little uncomfortable telling certain people I was getting it done because I was worried I would appear too concerned about my looks.

What is really interesting (if your experience is like mine), when you have had this kind of work done, you discover that the people closest to you, the people who really love and appreciate you, don't really notice. They always thought you were beautiful!

So, as far as my advice to you goes, you need to look deep into your heart and see if you think it is right for you. If you have really worked on yourself in every other way, if you have given up most of your bad habits, if you think it will add to your life, if you have the money and the time, then go for it—without guilt!

Cellulite

Cellulite is pockets of fat that often give the skin a cottage cheese appearance. Some people may be more susceptible to cellulite than others. Women are especially plagued with cellulite because they generally are more fatty and less muscular in the buttocks, hips, and thighs than men. A friend of mine studying nursing said that women have cellulite because it helps provide the pliability and flexibility in the abdomen needed for the changes that occur during pregnancy.

Other people claim cellulite is caused by toxins, fats, and waste matter contained in the connective tissue.

Some activities that may help:

* Exercise, walk, swim
* Work out with weights to gain muscle in the thighs and buttocks
* Steam and sauna with sage oil
* Bathe with juniper oil
* Bathe with sea salt and Epsom salts
* Dry brush your limbs and body daily
* Drink detox teas
* Drink fresh juice daily
* Eat fresh foods
* Meditate
* Do yoga to increase circulation and tone
* Get enough sleep
* Eat high fiber foods to encourage frequent bowel movements
* Drink lots of water
* Breathe deeply and mindfully
* Apply essential oils of cypress and sage and massage into skin (dilute with almond oil or sunflower oil)
* Put your feet up high above your waist as often as you can daily
* Take lecithin tablets to help cleanse the fatty deposits
* Eat sunflower seeds, which contain lecithin

Cellulite can be treated with a comprehensive program:

Proper elimination

Make sure the kidneys, intestines, and skin are stimulated and functioning as optimally as possible. When these organs work effectively, the breakdown of fat and cellulite is speeded up. For example, drink cleansing herbal teas and eat high fiber foods.

Breathing and oxygenation
Deep breathing helps purify the blood and rid the system of toxins. It's also an excellent way to help burn up cellulite and help move waste out of the connective tissue.

Exercise
Regular exercise aids in circulation and breathing while stimulating organs. It helps create muscle tone and firm tissue. Many yoga postures are a perfect form of exercise to stimulate the body's vital organs.

Cook with or take herbs that help stimulate circulation
Cayenne helps to get your blood flowing, cinnamon helps to keep your digestive fires going, and ginger warms your extremities by stimulating your circulation.

Beneficial essential oils:

- Cypress
- Fennel
- Juniper

- Lavender
- Rosemary
- Orange

Eczema

Eczema appears as elevated, very parched, crusty, usually discolored patches on the skin. It is a puzzling skin ailment, caused by stress, diet, allergies, or from using highly chemicalized body care and household products, including dish detergents. Another theory is that eczema is an elimination of toxins of hard proteins and fats. From a natural healing standpoint, an internal detoxification program would seem helpful along with external applications.

Skin problems can be your body's way of getting your attention. It is said almost 60% of eczema is caused by emotional stress, and the percentage is even higher for psoriasis. There are several products on the market that are made with healing, skin-relaxing, and anti-inflammatory herbs such as chamomile, calendula, ivy, St. John's wort, lily, comfrey, and feverfew. Apply these to the affected areas.

Recommendations:

* Many studies have demonstrated that the topical use of primrose oil is excellent for treating eczema and psoriasis. The oils appear to loosen hard scales and, used daily, reduce itching significantly.

* Take parsley internally in food or capsules, and apply a parsley tea or a tonic topically.

* Try raw cucumber and potato applied topically.

* Cut down on all non-vegetable proteins, sugars, oils, white flour products, and dairy products.

* Use only fresh body-care products free of any synthetic chemicals.

* Try the homeopathic remedies available at your health food store.

* Take an oatmeal bath; place oatmeal in a muslin bag and tie to the hot water faucet.

* Apply aloe vera gel to affected area.

* Eat foods and take supplements high in the B vitamins.

* Take evening primrose capsules and also apply topically.

* Drink teas of burdock and dandelion.

* Take vitamin A.

* Try vitamin E treatments both internally and externally.

* Take two tablespoons of brewer's yeast daily, as well as applying a paste of it externally.

* Take black-strap molasses, two teaspoons a day; also apply it externally.

* Take two tablespoons of high-quality safflower oil internally daily and also apply externally.

* Steam, using pansy, violet, comfrey root, and white willow bark. (See steaming instructions.)

Other remedies to try:

* Increase your intake of natural grains, greens, and all vegetables.

* Try to relax and recreate more.

* Try journal writing to decrease frustration and find solutions to your daily stress.

* Try meditation to settle your mind and thoughts.

* Try walking to relax and de-stress.

* Take time to look into your relationships and see if they are the best they can be.

* Apply poultices of chamomile; drink chamomile tea.

* Apply creams and lotions with comfrey, lily, and calendula.

* Apply and inhale essential oils of lavender and hyssop.

Psoriasis

The root problem causing psoriasis has not been proven, but it is said to be diet, chemical household and body care products, the body eliminating hard proteins and fats, or an overabundance of activity in one's life. The new cells are occurring at a very fast rate, much faster than the body needs.

Therefore, it is said these new cells become scaly and begin collecting under the skin and cause the dermis underneath to be hard, resulting in dry, scaly, and itchy skin in patches, which bleed when one scratches them. Psoriasis is often hereditary and almost always irritating.

The first cure to reach for is to decrease the amount of stress in your life. Accomplish this by getting daily exercise and relaxing through hobbies, exercise, meditation, yoga, sunshine, or other healthful activities you enjoy. Also:

* Fill your diet with an abundance of fresh and cooked vegetables, and fresh fruit along with natural grains.

* Enjoy more time outdoors. Psoriasis can be helped through intelligent sunbathing, since it usually appears on areas protected from the sun. Also, it seems to get worse in the winter.

* Many psoriasis sufferers have very high cholesterol and can help the condition by eating sunflower oil containing lecithin, which helps emulsify fat in the body.

* Increase your general vitality to help your body's own efforts to combat psoriasis and other conditions. Nutrients are lost because your skin constantly has to renew itself, so taking extra vitamins,

especially vitamin A, vitamin C, the Bs, and folic acid, as well as kelp, have been found to help.

* Drink herbal teas that have relaxing effects on the nervous system such as chamomile, hops, and wild oats, and then apply to affected area.

* Many find taking lecithin tablets of value, three tablets after every meal and applying externally, while others take vitamin E and apply it to the area with good results.

* Drink burdock tea and apply it topically.

* Apply comfrey root poultice.

* Take avocado oil and apply it topically.

* Take evening primrose oil and apply topically.

* Apply essential oils of lavender and bergamot, with almond oil or sunflower oil.

* Try "clean" body care products such as Lily of Colorado herbal moisturizer, kukui oil with lily and lavender, high quality mists with lavender and lily, and dry skin creams with lily and shea butter.

* Take a vacation at the ocean and swim daily, or put sea salts in your bath.

Puffy Eyes/Skin and Dark Circles under Eyes

Water retention not only makes you feel uncomfortable, it can also make you look less attractive. At its worst, water retention can cause an overall bloated appearance including facial puffiness and bags under the eyes. However, there are several simple, natural ways to reduce water retention so you look and feel better.

To improve facial puffiness due to water retention, you need to take care of your overall health, especially the process that helps cleanse your body: the kidney filtration system. According to one of the health evaluation methods created in ancient Asia—the art of diagnosing the condition of your health by studying the face—the region below the eye corresponds to the kidneys, the organs that filter toxins from your bloodstream. Therefore, this ancient approach to health attributes eye bags to stagnation or sluggishness in the kidneys. To address water retention problems, you need to help the kidneys cleanse your body by changing your diet and drinking plenty of fluids such as juice or herbal teas and pure water.

Dietary changes

Causes of water retention are numerous, and poor diet can be a major contributor. To help release excess fluids from your body and enhance your overall health, reduce or cut out fatty foods, especially meats, simple refined sugars, and table salt. Replace these with vegetables, fresh fruits, and herbal seasonings.

Another dietary way to get rid of unwanted fluids from your body is to change your intake of liquids. Eliminate or cut down on coffee, carbonated drinks, and alcohol, and cut out diet soda because it's high in sodium. Replace these beverages with pure water. In addition to adding or eliminating certain foods and liquids from your diet, you could include herbs, juices, and teas to help you get rid of excess fluids.

Cleansing herbs

Parsley has long been added to herbal medicines for its ability to help cure many ills including kidney dysfunction. Combine parsley with foods such as salads or try a parsley salad (stems removed) all by itself. It's delicious with a vinaigrette or lemon dressing.

Horseradish, believed to be one of the more potent herbal diuretics, is another food used to eliminate excess water from the kidneys. A traditional preparation consists of one ounce of fresh chopped horseradish root, one-half ounce of bruised mustard seed, and one pint of boiling water. Let the horseradish and mustard seed soak in the water in a covered dish for four hours, strain, and take three tablespoons three times a day. You can also grate fresh horseradish into your favorite sauces.

Healthy juices

Try celery and lemon juice to cleanse impurities from the bloodstream. Peach juice promotes urination, which helps eliminate stored waste, whereas pear juice cleanses the bowels and kidneys; cranberry juice contains a natural fruit acid which can also aid elimination.

Herbal teas

Adding herbal teas to your diet can also help purge your body of excess fluids. Make your own by purchasing bulk herbs or buy one of the many packaged herbal teas formulated specifically for detoxification and cleansing. Check the labels.

Beauty rest

Like diet, sleep habits can affect fluid retention in your body. In fact, sleeping positions help determine where fluids settle on your face. To help this problem, you may find it useful to sleep on your back with your head and upper body slightly elevated. Otherwise, fluids can pool in your face, creating facial puffiness and eye bags.

Facial masks

As an added measure to help release fluids from your body, facial masks help reduce facial puffiness. Look for anti-inflammatory and anti-puffiness products that contain seaweed in your natural products store. Seaweeds are cool and soothing, help reduce inflammation, and are high in tannic acids, natural astringents that won't dry your skin; or use chamomile, calendula, or rosemary.

Try the following to reduce puffiness:

* Placing an ice pack over the eyes for five to ten minutes can help reduce puffiness. A bag of frozen vegetables wrapped in a towel or piece of cloth over the eyes, works really well.

* Get lots of fresh air and adequate sunshine.

* Drink lots of cranberry juice.

* Use eye masks high in tannic acid; apply wet, black-tea bags to closed eyes.

* Go to a steam room regularly.

* Bathe with juniper, rosemary, essential oil, and Epsom salts.

* Do an internal detox.

* Do yoga to stimulate the vital organs and increase circulation.

* For a quick fix in the morning, open the freezer door and stick your head in momentarily; cold contracts tissues.

* Soak a cloth in a weak solution of juniper berry oil and lavender, or cypress and water; do not get in eyes.

* Other essential oils that can decrease puffiness are rose geranium or fennel, used very diluted with water, as above.

* Apply a poultice of chamomile flowers.

* Dissolve one teaspoon of sea salt in one cup of hot water and then refrigerate the water; after it is very cold, check that the sea salt is dissolved and apply to the eye area with cotton balls or a compress for twenty minutes. Rinse with very cool water and apply a light, oil-free herbal moisturizer.

* Eyebright herb steeped as a tea, one teaspoon per one cup of water, and applied with cotton balls or as a compress will go a long way to refresh eyes from redness, dust, tiredness, or overwork.

* Lily's vinegar tonic really helps cleanse, tone, and stimulate the fluids in the body. (See section on Internal Cleansing and Detoxifying.)

* For dark circles, try strawberries; they are very bleaching.

* To treat puffy or dark circles under the eyes, try a potato compress. You can cut the potato and apply or grate the potato and put in gauze; leave on for one-half hour while lying down, relaxing, and thinking positive thoughts.

* Use a cucumber the same way as potatoes for great results.

* Eating a lot of steamed asparagus is also helpful in increasing the flow of urine.

* Apply cut apples.

Skin Discolorations (also called Liver Spots and Age Spots)

Brown spots on the skin, some say, may be due to vitamin deficiencies in the diet. Others say that it is just a part of aging. Many skin discolorations can be from the sun, birth control pills, or chemicals applied to the skin. Brown spots that begin appearing when one is in his or her 40s or 50s, it is said, are from many years of poor nutrition; therefore, you must be patient to cure the problem.

Marie Antoinette is said to have applied and bathed in buttermilk, which was said to undo the negative effects of the sun and lighten brown spots. Try her method, applying plain, raw certified buttermilk.

There are many effective folk remedies; try the following:

* Apply cooked oatmeal.

* Apply fresh lemon juice for bleaching.

* Grate fresh horseradish in yogurt and apply.

259

* Mix onion juice with vinegar and rub on the age spot.

* Apply feverfew topically in oil or water.

* Apply cranberry juice directly to the skin and allow the juice to dry; drink lots of it at the same time.

* Apply dried apricots heated with a small amount of water to the affected area.

* Apply vinegar poultices to help fade the spots.

* Make a plain mask of yogurt or mix it with herbs of elder and mint.

* Apply castor oil daily to the affected area.

* Make a mixture of horseradish, cider vinegar, and cornmeal and apply as a mask.

* Mix parsley juice with vitamin C powder, apply, and leave on for 45 minutes.

* Mix cucumber, whole and blended, with fresh buttermilk, and use as a skin bleach.

* Improve your circulation through daily brushing with a complexion brush.

* Try applying the sap of a birch tree in the spring.

* Make a mask with vitamin C powder and mashed cucumbers or cucumber juice.

* Try a mask of one-fourth cup buttermilk, one-half teaspoon of fresh horseradish, and one tablespoon of cornmeal. Mix together. Place on the area you want to lighten. *Do not get into the eyes.* Leave on for 40 minutes; reapply every other day until the spots lighten.

* Soak horseradish in milk for twelve hours without refrigeration and apply to the spots several times a day.

* Mix one-half cup of milk with one-half cup organic cider vinegar; stir well before applying; put on your skin every night before bed. Leave on, rinsing in the morning.

* Apply essential oils of lemon or rub onions on freckles to reduce.

* Buy almond butter and apply with lemon juice as a mask, leaving on for one hour.

* Eat fresh fruits and fresh salads.

* Blend one lemon and one cucumber in a blender and apply to area you want to bleach.

* Take folate supplements.

* Take vitamins A and D.

* Take all the vitamin Bs, and E and C.

* Some have found taking selenium is helpful.

* Take wheat germ oil and also apply topically.

* Apply a tea of elder flower and chickweed.

* Apply raw potato.

* Apply mashed strawberries.

For people who just want to cure blotchy and uneven skin tone, try an equal mixture of water, organic vinegar, and milk; apply nightly and wash off in the morning.

Stretch Marks

Skin should be elastic. To maintain elasticity, the connective tissue must contain adequate amounts of collagen for softness. If your diet is full of animal fats and simple carbohydrates, as in refined and processed foods, the skin doesn't maintain that natural elasticity, and then if it is stretched due to weight gain or pregnancy, it doesn't go back to normal and stretch marks result.

One of my best friends swears by daily application of cocoa butter during pregnancy, as it helps the skin allow more flexibility. And stretch marks can even be diminished after they appear by applying nutritive skin care such as cocoa butter and by eating a healthful diet. Try taking wheat germ oil internally and applying it externally. Rub castor oil on the reddened area.

Sunburn

If you get sunburned, here are some remedies:

* Get in a bath of cool water with one-quarter cup of baking soda, or apply it with compresses.

* Apply aloe vera.

* Make a compress of skim milk and oatmeal and apply.

* Apply witch hazel with a cotton ball.

* Apply diluted essential oil of lavender.

* Make a paste of cornstarch and yogurt and apply.

* Put slices of potato or cucumber on the area.

* Put your moisturizer in the refrigerator before applying.

* Drink lots of water to counteract the drying effects.

If it's a serious sunburn, see your doctor.

Varicose Veins

Varicose veins usually appear in the legs when the veins on the surface become blocked and inflamed. They are often from a predisposition inherited from a parent. It is said that they are caused from an excess intake of fluids, sugar, and animal fats. The fats can cause blockages in the veins, and the fluids put pressure on the circulatory system, particularly the veins. When these surface veins of the legs become blocked and swollen, it can be quite painful and unsightly.

Put your feet up. I always do whenever I can. Sometimes it just seems to annoy people that you look so comfortable at work, but I love it. It feels good. And anytime you can get your body out of the normal position, I say do it. This is an essential concept of yoga, to put your body in different physical positions to move the blood, getting it circulating properly throughout your body.

Many yoga poses get the blood going in the opposite direction, especially any that get your legs above your body, such as the headstand, shoulder stand, and the plow. If you can't do head- and handstands unassisted, buy a body lift. This invention allows you to do them effortlessly. You can order one from (888) AGE-EASY [(888) 243-3279]. Until you become expert at these more strenuous yoga poses, don't do them alone. Begin with lessons to learn to do yoga poses properly.

Other suggestions:

* Alternately applying hot and cold compresses can be helpful. Apply a towel wrung out in cold water and then a towel wrung out in hot water, leaving each on for at least fifteen minutes.

* Standing and sitting in one place can pool the blood. Move around. Change positions. Go for a walk.

* "The pill," with the hormonal imbalances it creates, can cause varicose veins, as can smoking.

* Trim your weight. The extra weight adds additional pressure to the veins.

* Avoid negative fluids (e.g., pop, caffeine, alcohol).

* Cut down on animal foods.

* Get plenty of fresh air outside.

* Walk, swim.

* Use lotions that contain chamomile, calendula, and lily.

* Drink teas made of chamomile, Oregon grape, or red clover.

* Apply essential oil of juniper diluted with almond oil.

* Apply herbal poultices of chamomile and calendula.

* Apply vinegar or take a bath with a pint of vinegar added to the water.

Warts

Warts are the second biggest skin care problem after acne that people ask me about. They are benign skin tumors caused by a virus, which you can easily pick up from the air. Warts like a moist environment. They spread easily, so don't touch them. Like so many things, people seem more apt to get warts when they are run-down and not taking proper care of themselves. One remedy is to improve your overall constitution so your body can naturally fight off warts.

Remedies to try:

* Make a paste of vitamin C and apply externally.

* Cover the wart with a Band-Aid; keep covered for at least a month, changing as needed.

* Rub the inside of a banana skin on the wart and cover with a Band-Aid.

* Grate a potato, wrap it in gauze, and apply to the wart.

* Apply vitamin E oil.

* Apply essential oil of clove.

* Apply aloe vera juice.

* Apply fresh garlic juice and take garlic internally.

* Place lemon slices in apple cider and let sit for two weeks; then apply directly to the wart with a little salt daily.

* Dilute the following essential oils in vinegar: lemon, cypress, and lavender and apply.

* Use dandelion juice.

* Mix vinegar and onion juice and apply to the wart.

* Apply dandelion sap to the wart for twelve days.

* Crush a clove of garlic and tape it to the wart.

* Scrub the wart gently twice a day with soap and a nail brush.

New Choices in Natural Healing states: "In the morning crush a vitamin A capsule, mix it with just enough water to make a paste, and apply it directly to the wart. In the afternoon, apply a drop of castor oil, in the evening, apply a drop of lemon juice. This should help dissolve the wart."[*]

---

[*] Bill Gottlieb, ed., *New Choices in Natural Healing*. Emmaus, PA: Rodale Press, 1995, p. 556.

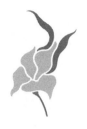

PART FOUR

Rejuvenation Therapies for Health and Beauty

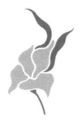

Alternative Practices and Diagnostic Tools for Health

Introduction

If you're like me, you believe there's a whole new world out there for you to discover. For many of you, this world is on the misty fringes of your awareness. I'd like to bring it into clearer focus for you, so you can make the best choices for yourself in the areas of beauty, health, and happiness.

This is my attempt to glean the best of both worlds—modern medicine and traditional healing methods. I figure you're familiar enough with modern medicine, so let me introduce you to therapies beyond conventional medicine. You can relax as this is an exploration only, and a limited one at that, as I am covering only those therapies I have personally experienced.

This voyage of discovery requires only that you bring an open mind. We'll see how the ancients, tribal peoples, and different cultures, answered the age-old problems of improving beauty and health. Alternative diagnostic tools for health, health practitioners, and health practices—herbalists and pendulums, iridology, Oriental medical doctors, Oriental facial diagnosis, hair analysis and nutrition—are fun to explore and interesting, as well as informative.

The route I have used the most is the herbalist one. I must have half of the books ever written on the subject. I have also consulted other herbalists, which is easy in Colorado. I am sure someone in your area is a practicing herbalist; ask at your local health food store if you don't know anyone. An herbalist can help you take responsibility for your own health. You could also just go buy books on the subject and work from there. However, I don't think you can underestimate the power and fun of relating to a real person on these matters.

Hanna Kroeger

The first herbalist I ever went to was Hanna Kroeger in Boulder in the 1970s. My sister dragged me in there. I had no interest in checking out this pendulum-waving senior citizen at the time. There was a long line to see her even back then. I was feeling a little run-down and I had to wait with my sister anyway so I figured, what the heck, I'd let her swing that little pendulum around me, just for grins. We waited for what seemed like forever before we finally got to the head of the line. Gnome-like Hanna swiftly whisked her pendulum around me, asked how I was feeling, and quickly announced I had mono and needed to take some particular herbs. Before I could even resist her assessment, she was on to the next person.

A legend in her own time

Hanna was a legend throughout the healing world. Born in Turkey of German missionaries, she came to the United States in 1952 after studying nursing at the University of Freiburg, and natural healing at a hospital in Dresden.

In the 1950s, Hanna started the first health food store in Boulder. Many well-known alternative health product entrepreneurs have had a start there, even one tea mogul, I have been told. Her New Age Health Foods is one of the first stores where I sold my products.

Hanna's Chapel of Miracles

I attended Hanna's famous "Chapel of Miracles," located just east of Boulder a few years ago on a glorious, bright, warm Sunday in February. My mom and I hopped in my car and followed the directions to an unpaved rural road between scattered homes. Turning into a dirt drive, we saw before us an L-shaped, two-story building, with one main section clearly added on recently.

The service, which is still held, was upstairs in a room complete with church pews and a colorful altar you might see in a church in Tijuana. The overflowing congregation sang several inter-denominational hymns and listened to a brief sermon about peace in the world and the importance of prayer. Hanna stressed, like so many, that the angelic beings only come when asked.

Cake and coffee were available after the service. A massage therapist was on hand who kindly offered me and others his complimentary treatment, which I found very beneficial.

We waited patiently in the crowd for Hanna's personal, free psychic reading of our health. Donations were accepted but not asked for. She did the same thing she had done twenty-five years ago. She whisked her pendulum around me and asked how I was feeling. I told her I was feeling tired a lot, and she quickly announced I had Epstein-Barr (which is caused by the same virus as mononucleosis). Her assistant wrote down what I should take as Hanna turned to the next person waiting.

Mom and I took off down the street to Hanna's new building where we purchased her recommended herbs. Her herbal store has an Epstein-Barr kit, which for about $24 has herbs and homeopathics you take in combination. It took almost two months for me to take all the herbs, and I really did feel better.

Hanna used the pendulum widely, as do many people around here. She wrote a book called *The Pendulum and the Bible*. According to her book, the pendulum was widely used historically and is often mentioned in the Bible for healing purposes. The basic premise, as I interpreted it, is that your superconcious knows what is best for you and the pendulum is a method for gaining access to that information.

Hanna also did Psychometric Aura reading, according to her flyer, using a saliva sample to "measure the aura energies of the body psychometrically. From these readings, she can make recommendations to help you increase the aura vitality of your organs. Please understand that this is a spiritual reading and is not intended to replace or discourage a regular visit to your physician." Her ministry for this reading was passed on to her granddaughters before her death in May 1998. The cost is $20 and you send in your saliva on a cotton ball. Please call her store to get more information:

Hanna's Herb Shop
5684 Valmont Road
Boulder, Colorado 80301
(303) 443-0755 or (800) 206-6722
fax (303) 938-9021
e-mail hshop@aol.com

Bush doctors

While I have studied under and been diagnosed by many herbalists, I have to say some of the most interesting I have met have been bush doctors. I met two in Belize, Central America. My brother, mom, and I went to see one recommended by some Belizean friends we had made. Of course, I wanted to ask them about my blemished skin and seek what cures they employed. My mom wanted to talk to him about her chronic fatigue syndrome, and even my brother wanted to ask about his hip that has ailed him since an accident he had back in the 1970s.

We pulled up in front of the doctor's modest house and parked. He came right out and took us out in back to what looked like one step above a converted outhouse. One by one, he took us into a private space with room enough for only two to stand in, and looked us over. He gave me some herbs to cleanse the blood. He gave my mom some herbs to aid in digestion, stating that the chronic fatigue was because her digestive system was not retaining any nutrients from the food she ate. He did "body work," a kind of energy/hands-on treatment on my brother, who said he really did feel better afterwards.

Iridology

Iridology is the study of the eyes for information on your overall health. Iridologists analyze the structure of the iris. They say that it reveals the basic constitutional health of a person, and gives details about specific organs. Iridology works closely with nutrition to come up with solutions to problems and weaknesses. It is said that these problems can show up in the iris long before they would show up in more obvious ways.

Many people are shocked at how accurate these diagnoses can be. I have had it done twice but was not impressed either time. It may just have been the practitioners or where I was at the time.

Oriental medical doctors

I went to an Oriental medical doctor about my acne. He recommended some Chinese herbs that I did not find helpful, although I liked him and his methodology. He took my pulse and had me lie on the table to assess my overall general health. He gave me a clean bill of health and sent me on my way. I liked the holistic approach and think they can be a great alternative to a western M.D.

Oriental facial diagnosis

The traditional Oriental diagnosis or health evaluation is based on the premise that the location on the face of pimples, blemishes, or wrinkles corresponds to the internal organs that are affected. This is an ancient art that has merit for speculation and consideration. This technique, primarily practiced in China and Japan, is part of a system that includes massage therapy and acupuncture. I first heard about it from the first acupuncturist I ever went to, a practitioner in Placentia Village, Belize. I told him I was writing this book, and he asked me if I had heard of this method.

I find this diagnostic system interesting. If you continuously get blemishes in a certain area of your face, you may want to investigate further and take herbal teas, supplements, or tinctures to help heal that area. For example, if you have deep vertical lines in between your eyebrows, you may want to take dandelion root to help cleanse your liver.

The theory is that there is a relationship between the face and the total body. For example, problems with organs in the lower body, such as the bladder and intestines, show blemishes or wrinkles in the upper part of the face. Correspondingly, organs in the upper part of the body such as the heart and lungs appear in the lower part of the face. Organs located in the middle part of the body such as the liver and pancreas show up in the middle region of the face.

Blemishes or wrinkles in the forehead or on the hairline are connected to the bladder. The theory states that if you perspire from that area of the face, it is a sign that your bladder may be suffering from too much liquid. Blemishes in this area may also indicate too much fat in the bladder.

In Oriental diagnosis, the middle part of the forehead represents the intestines. Many horizontal lines here can indicate an overdoing of fats, sugars, and liquids. Pimples in this area can show an excess of fat.

Above the nose corresponds to the pancreas. The belief is that this is caused by an excessive intake of hard fats, including animal foods and seafood. It can also be a sign of low blood sugar.

The region below the eyes correlates to the kidneys. Bags under your eyes are a potential sign of excess fluid in the kidneys and can also be aggravated by fatty foods. Dark circles under the eyes can be indicative of fat and mucus accumulation.

Pimples on the nose can be a sign that fats are being released and may be building up in the bloodstream. The cheeks represent the lungs.

This system may seem totally mysterious to us Westerners; however, as you seek to find ways to benefit your life, Oriental diagnosis may be worth trying. Check out all the options available and choose what helps you.

Hair Analysis

Even though I found out later that my dad had his hair analyzed before his death (of course, my sister's influence), I heard about hair analysis from a Lily of Colorado rep we had in Aspen. I was visiting her and our stores up there, and she told me all about it. I thought the concept sounded like a good idea.

She gave me the phone number of the Analytical Research Labs, Inc. They sent me the packet of information with all the details of how to send your hair sample in for analysis. After receiving it and your check, they send you back a complete analysis.

The Analytical Research Labs describes the standard introduction Plan II in the following way: "Tissue mineral analysis is a screening test analyzing nineteen minerals which play a vital role in human health. Mineral function is an essential component for enzyme systems, which regulate virtually every body function. Through the correlation of pertinent data, a properly performed tissue mineral test can assist in identifying mineral patterns which may be associated with stress patterns, blood sugar imbalance, glandular imbalances, abnormalities in biochemical energy production, toxic metal poisoning and other important health information."

The company gives you an easy-to-read analysis of your minerals and dietary principles to follow, broken down by each body type: the slow oxidizer, the fast oxidizer, and the fast-mixed oxidizer.

My analysis stated: "Your current mineral chart indicates acute stress associated with fast oxidation together with a sodium/potassium inversion." It continued that I might be suffering from a sugar and simple carbohydrate sensitivity. It also stated that "many individuals with a high tissue iron level suffer from occasional chronic skin conditions such as acne. If toxins and heavy toxic metals cannot be eliminated from the blood, they will be stored in the liver, until such a time they can be removed. If the liver cannot adequately detoxify or eliminate the poisons, any extra burden will be transferred to the kidneys. If the kidneys cannot adequately eliminate the poisons, they will be eliminated through the skin. A reduction in your high iron level may well contribute significantly to an improvement of your current acne condition."

It also said, "You are exhibiting a mineral pattern often associated with acute stress, which is indicated by your high sodium levels and your high potassium level. It would be helpful, health-wise, for you to realize this and attempt to resolve some of your current frustrations and/or indecisions."

A happy result that came out of this test was the "Dietary Analysis," which stated that "while 85% of our population benefit from a low fat diet, because of your fast rate of metabolism, you require some fats and oils in your diet. Have a serving of one of the following foods with each meal: blue cheese dressing, full-fat dairy foods, olive oil, butter, avocado, meat, cream cheese, or sour cream."

The report was very detailed and insightful in terms of both the mineral deficiencies and the dietary needs, along with a complete list of their supplements that they recommend.

I didn't want to get my supplements from them so I called them and they told me what was in each one. I also had a lot of questions, which they answered, but not enthusiastically. Overall, I recommend it; it provides another diagnostic tool for fun and health. Contact:

The Analytical Research Labs
8650 North 22nd Avenue
Phoenix, AZ 85021
(602) 995-1581

Raw Foods

Raw fruits and vegetables have powerful health effects on the body. Their nutritive energy is transferred to us when we eat them. Plants get their energy from the sun during photosynthesis, and when we eat the plants, they pass this nutritive energy into us. Raw fruits and vegetables are Mother Nature's gift of life.

It is well-documented that in many people a diet high in raw foods can drastically reduce body degeneration and slow down the way you age, give you energy, and make you feel better emotionally.

Food influences the skin by changing the quality of energy that flows throughout the body. It affects the skin in other ways, by changing the quality of blood that nourishes new skin cells and producing the secretion of the sweat and oil glands. The skin receives about a third of the body's blood supply.

Nutrients provided by food are absorbed into the bloodstream, which supplies the skin cells. Therefore, the health of the skin and its connective tissues depends on the quality of nutrients they receive from the bloodstream.

The same is true with body care products applied to the skin. They also affect the quality of energy that flows through the skin. These products are absorbed through the skin into the bloodstream through the cells in the skin.

Blood Analysis

Wild Oats and Alfalfa's, two Colorado-based health food stores, often have nutritional blood-screening tests available that can be helpful in your analysis.

When you find out what blood type you are, you can get the book *Eat Right 4 Your Type: The Individualized Diet Solution to Staying Healthy, Living Longer & Achieving Your Ideal Weight* by Dr. Peter J. D'Adamo with Catherine Whitney. This book explains how and where the four blood types developed and breaks down the different foods best suited for each blood type and why.

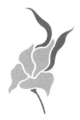

Cleansing and Detoxifying for Beauty and Health

Internal cleansing and detoxifying

Many Americans seem to spend more time and money on their cars than their bodies. My mother suspects it's because cars come with manuals and our bodies don't. Your car and your body do work a lot alike. They both are combustible engines, taking in fuel to produce energy. Each has a system of waste removal. These systems must function properly for optimum performance.

Waste elimination is crucially important. This is done through the skin, kidneys, intestines, and the lungs. The kidneys filter approximately twenty gallons of liquid per day. We need to drink lots of water daily. This will keep the kidneys flushed from the toxins they have taken in as the body's fluid filtering system.

A vast array of foods, water, metals, chemicals, bacteria or other organisms—even emotional turmoil—can cause toxins, substances that are harmful to us. Your susceptibility and your basic immunity to such toxins are very individual. Your body was designed to detoxify itself, but many people either do not have the constitutional strength or the nutrients available for the body to do so. The toxins can inhibit your body's natural regenerative ability. According to the Federal Food and Drug Administration (FDA), approximately 500,000 chemicals are used today. Harmful chemicals and toxins can enter the body via penetration of the skin just as easily as healthy substances can.

Herbal skin cleansing

- Burdock
- Chicory
- Dandelion
- Red clover
- Yellow dock
- Garlic
- Licorice root
- Goldenseal
- Siberian ginseng

Herbs have a long reputation for cleansing the system. The yellow dock, red clover, and burdock root have been used as blood cleansers. Often recommended for acne, they aid in the removal of toxins from the liver and kidneys. Dandelion and milk thistles are the traditional liver stimulators. Dandelion is said to stimulate the elimination of toxins from all cells, and milk thistle stimulates the regeneration of new cells. Licorice root is also famous for its liver cleansing properties and is historically a great detoxifier. Siberian ginseng is a known detoxifier and is often taken to help the liver cleanse the body from drug overuse.

These herbs can be taken alone, as a mixture, in a supplement, or bought in bulk and taken as teas. You can make tea by experimenting with the herbs alone or in combination with each other, or putting them with chamomile or spearmint. There are many more herbs that can benefit your skin by benefiting an internal organ or function.

There are also many products for sale at health food stores to clear up your skin with specific herbs or to do different kinds of internal cleansing. Talk to the folks at your health food store for a wealth of information on different cleansing herbs and methods.

Juicing and fasting

Mae West, the sex goddess of the 1930s, not only drank carrot juice daily, she started every day with an enema. At 62, she looked more like 40. Maybe she was on to something. You decide.

I have been drinking carrot juice every morning for years now. It is a delightful and refreshing way to start the day. Carrot juice is jam-packed with vitamins and nutrients. It helps keep the digestive system and colon in tiptop condition. It also is a breakfast replacement for me. It ruins my appetite and lets me skip the mess and fuss of eating a meal in the morning. Sometimes in mid-morning, instead of a snack I put apple juice (a great cleanser), brewer's yeast, wheat grass, alfalfa powder, and spirulina in a blender. I drink this instead of eating solid food. At lunch, I often eat an apple and banana with an oat bran muffin. For dinner, I eat whatever I want, maybe a burrito, pasta, or a salad.

You can juice vegetables and fruits alone or in combination. Fix your juice according to what you need. For example, cranberry is beneficial for urinary tract function; pineapple juice helps to dissolve mucus in your body. Celery juice and grapefruit juice help cleanse the liver. Everybody can benefit from carrot juice, for it provides vitamins A, beta-carotene, vitamin C, and fiber. Any of the follwing are great for juicing:

- carrot
- beet
- celery
- wheat grass
- cranberry
- apple

How beneficial is juice? Listen to Carlson Wade who says in his book, *Inner Cleansing: How to Free Yourself from Joint-Muscle-Artery-Circulation Sludge*: "Fresh fruit and vegetable juices are powerhouses of enzymes that revitalize and regenerate your entire body. These refreshing juices send forth cleansing catalysts that penetrate the innermost recesses of your body and dislodge the accumulated grit and pollutants from your cells and organs." [*]

A good way to get introduced to juicing is hanging out at your favorite full-service health food store. I try to make it a habit to do a shot of wheat grass whenever I come near a juice bar. Going to health food stores as often as possible and doing at least some of your shopping there is the beginning. It's easy, educational, healthy, and fun. So once a week, say, every Wednesday after work, stop by your health food store, try a different juice every time, and get started.

---

* Carlson Wade, *Inner Cleansing: How to Free Yourself from Joint-Muscle-Artery-Circulation Sludge*, West Nyack, NY: Parker Publishing Company, 1983.

Happy-hour option

Many of the Wild Oats stores here in Colorado hold a happy hour offering two-for-one prices on coffees and juices. They even offer live entertainment for the alternative happy-hour crowd.

After you are convinced that you want to make juicing a permanent part of your life, invest in a juicer. They start around $100 and can be bought at Kmart or Wal-Mart, or if you want a better quality one, check out the ones at your health food store. Like most of the healthful practices I outline in this book, you can get rather addicted to juicing. But it's a good thing.

Nutritional detoxifying

In addition to fruit and vegetable juices, other foods can be helpful in detoxifying your body. These include:

- fiber
- acidophilus
- garlic
- algae, spirulina, and blue-green algae
- green tea
- wheat grass

If you are eating a lot of rice, beans, fruits and vegetable, and emptying your bowels regularly, you are probably getting adequate fiber. Judge for yourself what your individual needs require.

I have taken acidophilus over the years off and on. I took a lot after being immunized before I left for India, and then I took it daily in India, continuing for months after my return. I took it again after a root canal to combat the antibiotic the dentist told me I absolutely had to take. Against my better judgment, I took that antibiotic for the week, which was the prescribed time. It is important if you are going to take antibiotics that you take the complete dose. Otherwise you can create more problems by killing only enough of the strain to make it stronger.

Garlic cleansing

Because garlic is so beneficial, I did a garlic cleanse once; I thought it was a good idea. I ate six raw garlic cloves, chewing them thoroughly. The problem: I couldn't get rid of the smell, and I had tickets to the ballet that night! I brushed my teeth twenty times, gargled repeatedly, and chewed gum. The scent refused to leave. It was coming out of every pore of my body. I could tell that everybody at the ballet could smell it on me. The lesson: Plan on staying home for at least that day if you do a garlic cleanse. And don't expect anyone you live with to come close to you either.

Algae

I have taken various kinds of algae off and on for years; it started with a friend doing a trade out with a famous multi-level algae company for my products. Now another friend of mine represents a spirulina line here in Colorado whose product I use. I am now a pretty big proponent of these products because they are packed with nutrients we need to stay healthy.

Cleanliness from the inside out

For optimum skin beauty, it's important to be clean both inside and out. Several methods are available including colonics.

Colonics, lower bowel cleansing, colonic irrigation, or colon hydrotherapy are all terms describing the process of cleansing the large intestine or colon with water from an external source. The purpose is to remove toxic materials, to release old physical matter, to provide relief of intestinal stress, and to enhance appropriate function by stimulation of the intestinal muscles. Other benefits can include weight loss, relief of bloatedness, improvement of general wellbeing, and sometimes release of emotional stress.

People have long believed that health and sickness have their roots in the colon. My chiropractor told me his office performed colonics in their building until the 1980s, when it became illegal for chiropractors to do them. Like many subjects we discuss in this book, colonic irrigation is controversial, so study and decide for yourself.

I had mine done when I was going through a period of heavy stress and searching. I didn't have a particular health problem, but I was doing research for this book. I had already made some serious healthful changes in my life, and I was looking for more ways to bring great health and improved good looks into my life.

The woman who did my colonic was in her 70s, bright, educated, in the health food business for a long time, but a little dogmatic. Her colonic detox program was over a six-week period and included taking acidophilus, green foods, and probiotics (a supplement) that she said would clear up any skin blemishes I had, as well as cancer, infertility, emotional problems, or virtually any other negative human condition.

The only other thing I had to do to adhere to her program was to give up coffee, sugar, all wheat products, all dairy products, and all meat. I told her flat out that the coffee wasn't going anywhere. I enjoy my coffee; I *love* my coffee! It's something to look forward to every morning; it's something you can depend on in your life, and it is always there for you. Warm, wet, and beautiful—that's coffee. Interestingly, the next day, I only had one cup of coffee and decided to cut down.

So what about wheat, dairy, sugar, and all meat? I didn't eat much meat of any kind; I used milk only in my coffee, although I did enjoy yogurt and cheese. I thought whole wheat bread was OK. And sugar, well, I did have a tiny addiction going off and on with these very small peppermint patties.

The colonics practitioner just threw all this information at me like it was carved in stone. There was no leeway, no excuses, no other modality, no other cure. The fact is that her emphatic listing of "do's and don'ts" made me feel like a loser for the few things I enjoyed. So instead of feeling good about giving up smoking, walking four miles a day, doing my vinegar, green drink, and brewer's yeast drink, taking supplements, oils, and herbs daily, drinking my carrot juice, doing my yoga— all that went unrecognized as I guess I had been mean to my colon. And if I wouldn't give up coffee, I must have had a real desire for my own imminent demise.

Frankly, I thought her telling any person born and raised in America to suddenly one day give up sugar, wheat, dairy, and meat was ridiculous. This just reinforced in my mind a very important point, namely the need to recognize where people are, to accept and appreciate them, and to let them know that where they are is perfect for now. Being rigid is boring, and we all need to watch out for it. Any of us can become a know-it-all. The trick is to discover if we have become one so we can change it.

The Colonic

The colonic itself was a little scary. The whole concept of deliberately asking someone to insert a rather large tube in your anus, well, it's a little frightening. As usual, when I'm a little fearful, I try not to give the thought a lot of energy. I was busy at work that day and really didn't think much about it—until at her office she gave me little booties to put on my feet when I took off my shoes. I was thinking, "Oh, no."

"Is this really a good idea?" I asked myself. "Do I really need this?" It reminded me of skydiving. I was perfectly cool until at 80 miles an hour at 3,000 feet up, the instructor said, "Put your feet out of the plane and hang from the struts."

The treatment went smoothly, although it was mildly uncomfortable the entire time. I can't say I enjoyed it, but I'm glad I had it done. I think if you are regularly eating sufficient fiber, this procedure shouldn't be routinely necessary. However, I do agree that it is important to keep the colon and the rest of the digestive system in optimum working condition.

The worst part of the colonics treatment for me was the day before. The instructions included no solid food except steamed vegetables at dinner and to take three tablespoons of virgin olive oil, one in the morning with my green drink, one with my carrot juice for lunch, and one atop the steamed vegetables for dinner. The day of the treatment I was instructed to eat a large breakfast. My appointment was at 2:00 P.M.

I was more antsy the day of fasting than the day of the procedure. Just knowing I couldn't eat got on my nerves. I felt deprived, hungry, and irritated. I was cranky and tired. A lot of frustration and just plain ugliness were coming out.

I didn't eat the day of the colonic. I just couldn't. I guess I lost my desire to eat because of the fasting. I went to my appointment without following the instructions to eat. Fortunately, the practitioner didn't seem to think it was that big of a deal and I was glad of that. I was concerned that I might have spoiled the whole process.

I didn't feel like eating right away after the procedure either, but I think it's worth doing. Colonics make you feel clean and light. I would recommend it if you are going to make big, healthful changes and you want to jump start the process.

Nutrition

Many people recommend a diet made up of whole grains, vegetables, and fruits, eaten in certain combinations, and only eating foods for the purpose of nourishment. No meat, no sugars, no processed foods, no white flour. On this type of diet, as in fasting, the body does not need to expend so much of its energy on digestion, and it can spend its energy on healing.

There are so many great books on the subject of nutrition and on macrobiotic diets that I am not going to expound. Visit your library, health food store, or bookstore and enjoy a smorgasbord of helpful information.

Saunas, steams, and baths

These treatments are often used in conjunction with many of the other methods and are also considered a cornerstone to an overall detox program. Dry saunas are often recommended for up to three hours per day in many detox programs. However, the temperature is lower than in most saunas in health clubs and the sweat slow, consistent, and gradual. These treatments are done under close supervision with set times for the patient to come out, cool down, and have her temperature taken. I mention this treatment to underscore the value of dry saunas, not to recommend this type of sauna to the reader. It is not to be tried on one's own.

I personally prefer steam to dry heat. I like to sit in the steam room as long as I can comfortably stand it and then get out and jump into a cool pool. I then just do the process over and over again. *Please note*: It is very important to replace your fluids by drinking lots of water or you may faint. Some people carry a cup or plastic bottle of water to sip in the steam room and sauna. Check with your doctor for any health problems before trying either a steam or a sauna.

When we were in high school, my sister had a Latvian friend whose family had a sauna in their house. My sister described how the family used to sit in the sauna naked, then go roll around in the snow and return to the sauna again. I always thought they sounded like a fun bunch. My father had friends in Michigan's Upper Peninsula who had a separate building for their sauna. In the winter, these northerners would sit in the sauna, then dash outdoors, break through the ice in a nearby stream and enter the frigid water before returning to the sauna. The basic benefits behind this hydrotherapy are said to be increased circulation and accelerated detoxification, providing an overall healthy tone to your body and clarification to your mind.

Baths

Baths are another great detox method and they can be taken at home. Hot water brings the blood closer to the skin, opens the pores, helping in the release and elimination of toxins. I love baths and try to take at least one a day. My favorite detox bath has juniper berry oil added. I like to take baths as hot as I can. Many people recommend you shower before and after a detox bath to remove residues.

Epsom salts baths are also very popular and help remove toxins by aiding in perspiration. I really like putting vinegar in my baths to help reduce irritation and itching that often occurs from hot baths. It also aids the skin in regaining its natural acidic balance.

Herbal tea baths are enjoyable and beneficial. I like to bathe in my herbal astringent; I add one-half cup of Lily of Colorado Herbal Astringent to my bath water for a healing and relaxing bath. Or make a tea of any or all of the following herbs, used in conjunction with each other or alone: lily, lavender, peppermint, chamomile, calendula, or horsetail. (See sections on Baths and Essential Oils.)

Emotional components

I believe many toxins in the body are caused by our emotional turmoil. Stress causes portions of the body to contract; muscles become tight, moods become vile. I think our negative emotions can cause great chemical imbalances in our body. It is important to avoid creating these toxins to begin with by being mindful about our thoughts and dealing with our emotional traumas of the present or past. This can be greatly aided by counseling, psychotherapy, attending The Landmark Forum, journal writing, meditation, having faith in yourself, and in God.

There is even a method of psychiatry that concerns itself with removing toxins from the body for improved mental and emotional health; it is called Orthomolecular Psychiatry, a method of treating the mind by treating the body. It claims to be able to treat people whose problems are caused more by biochemistry, by reducing toxins rather than experiential type problems.

Environmental help from the space age

According to information from the Northwest Healing Arts Center, the National Aeronautics and Space Administration (NASA) has done studies over the past two decades to find out, for use in space stations, which plants could remove toxic chemicals from the air. The plants that topped their list are:

- Mass cane (*dracaena massangeana*)
- Pot mum (*chrysanthemum morifolium*)
- Gerbera daisy (*gerbera jamesonii*)
- Wamecki or Wameckei (*dracaena deremensis*)
- Ficus (*ficus benjamina*)

The above five plants were particularly effective at clearing the air of formaldehyde, benzene, and trichloroethylene. The other plants that have been shown to be effective in purification are:

- ❧ English ivy (*hedera helix*)
- ❧ Marginata (*dracaena marginata*)
- ❧ Mother-in-law's tongue (*sansevieria laurentii*)
- ❧ Peace lily (*spathiphyllum* "Mauna Loa")
- ❧ Chinese evergreen (*algona* "Silver Queen")
- ❧ Banana (*musa oriana*)
- ❧ Bamboo palm (*chamaedorea seifrizii*)

Be aware

Remember, the release of toxins through a detox program can make you feel worse before feeling better. This is especially so if the liver is loaded up and cannot take the increased load of newly released toxins.

Cleansing the body of physical toxins can also stir up old emotional toxins. If this happens, many naturopaths recommend you seek counseling or at least a support mechanism or book or two to help you deal with these issues. As emotional toxins surface, they have to be dealt with for us to achieve optimum health.

Detox programs

A few health facilities around the country offer detoxification programs. I spoke to the Northwest Healing Arts Center in Bellevue, Washington. They can be reached at (425) 747-9200. For approximately $1000 a week you can go through their four- to six-week tissue-cleansing program. Living expenses are extra, as this is an outpatient program, not a residential facility. The treatment includes blood work and physicals and a prescription for a diet and supplements. Their program also includes hydrotherapy of alternating hot and cold packs on the chest and back, weekly colonics, and three hours of sauna a day.

This would be wonderful for those who could afford it. For the rest, you can make a start at home over a long weekend. If this sounds beneficial to you, check with your doctor and see if an at-home program would work for you.

Juice Diet

You could choose to start on a juice and vegetable diet on Friday. Have a friend or family member accompany you. Rest. Keep your juices and water nearby. Saturday morning, take an enema. Rest. Treat yourself to our Homespa (also known as our Goddess Kit).

If you're lucky like me, you have a beautiful recreation center with both a steam room and sauna by your house. Go sit in the sauna or steam room. Sip pure water. Have a friend drive you home; go to sleep. After resting, take some liquid, either water or juice. Go walking or exercise mildly for an hour and then go back to the sauna for more detoxing. Return home, sip more liquid, and relax, meditate, read inspirational books, sleep, and then do the same thing on Sunday.

In addition, you could incorporate the following into your cleansing program:

* Flower essences

* Massage

* Acupressure

* Chiropractic treatments

* A diet of only fruits and vegetables

* Lots of fluids

* A tablespoon of olive or flaxseed oil (can be in salad dressing)

* Lecithin

* Evening primrose oil

* Detox baths with Epsom salts or juniper berry oil

* Gentle skin brushing

* Skin care products that are free from harmful preservatives

* Daily relaxation and meditation

* Milk thistle (improves liver function)

* Exercise to help the body eliminate toxins

* Steam

* Avoiding all harsh, chemical body care and household products

* Avoiding mainstream hairdyes that contain toxins
* Dandelion supplements
* Niacin once a day
* Vitamin A
* Vitamin B complete complex tablets
* Vitamin C
* Calcium-magnesium tablet daily
* Multi-mineral tablet daily

Essential oils to detoxify

Simply place ten drops of one of the following essential oils in your bath:

* Fennel
* Geranium
* Juniper
* Lemon

My favorite daily pick-me-up

Lily's Vinegar Tonic™:

1 quart pure, unrefined apple cider vinegar (I like Bragg's brand)

½ cup garlic chopped finely

½ cup horseradish

½ cup onions cut and chopped finely

1 apple, cut and chopped

2 tablespoons ground ginseng

Place all ingredients in the vinegar and let sit for three to four weeks in a dark place. Shake daily. Strain. Take half a shot every morning with a glass of water.

This is just a brief introduction into the myriad of methods of detoxification and cleansing. Please visit your health food store and talk to the many educated people there and check out all the great books on juicing, power foods, green foods, and detoxing. One of my favorites is *The Whole Way to Natural Detoxification: The Complete Guide to Clearing*

Your Body of Toxins by Jacqueline Krohn, M.D., Frances A. Taylor, M. A., and Jinger Prosser, L.M.T.

A Daily Checklist for Health

No matter how you plan to obtain optimum health or what positive things you plan to bring into your life, fundamentally you really have to remember one thing: it's all about each day, everyday. It's all about developing a habit. It's all about making positive things happen over and over again.

Taking charge

If you're just beginning to take charge of your health, beauty, and happiness, start slowly. Don't try too much and then get discouraged. Begin gently, and work up to what's comfortable and beneficial for you. Here's my checklist. Pick and choose what's good for you, then make it a habit.

My daily checklist for health, beauty and happiness:

Morning

* Yoga

* Exercise; determine for yourself how mild or strenuous. I do 100 sit-ups or crunches. I also stand on my head for at least one minute. Let me repeat: Start an exercise program slowly and gently. Develop one that fits *you*.

* Meditate

* Bathe with essential oils

* Commit to being positive and calm all day

* Repeat positive affirmations

* Keep a daily journal

* Use day planning

* Drink green breakfast drink

* Take vitamins/supplements

* Take vinegar and tonics, determining which are most helpful to you

Mid-morning

* Drink carrot juice
* Drink a large glass of water

Noon

* Drink green drink with spirulina and brewer's yeast for lunch

Afternoon

* Eat an apple and a banana with a large glass of water
* Walk (I do three miles) or work out, or use Stairmaster in office
* Take my afternoon herbs with a tall glass of water

Evening

* Work out at the recreation center
* Eat an average small dinner (e.g., spinach salad with dressing, or pasta)
* Brush hair with kukui oil and rosemary
* Take one tablespoon of aloe vera juice
* Drink two cups of a beneficial herbal tea
* Take night herbs
* Read uplifting and relaxing text
* Pray and give thanks for all my blessings

Once or twice a week

* Steam and use whirlpool
* Swim
* Ride bicycle or exercycle
* Homespa (also known as my Goddess Kit)
* Herbal steam facial

Make your own list, one which is right for you. Remember, start slowly and be gentle with yourself. After determining what's best for you, make it a habit. Be flexible—an occasional change is okay.

Emotional Detoxifying

Our task in developing a lifestyle which promotes beauty, health, and happiness goes beyond detoxifying the body, the physical. Our task involves detoxifying our emotions as well.

What seems to happen is this: The more positive changes you make in your life, the more changes you find you're eager to make in your life. Once you get started with these rejuvenation therapies, you want to know more. Your mind becomes more open to more and more ideas. Things that you would have laughed about five years ago, you're now doing, undergoing, and enjoying. The wonder of it all!

Another thing that seems to happen is this: When you stop your addictions (smoking, drinking, and overeating), you can go through withdrawal. As you detox, a lot of junk that you have been covering up with the busy-ness of smoking, drinking, and eating too much often comes to light. Problems surface that were always there, but you never even knew you had.

Avoidance

There is a reason people always like to have something to do by smoking, drinking, and eating. We are often avoiding other issues in our lives. We keep ourselves too busy by these activities to notice our own patterns, neuroses, anxieties, reactions, and dysfunctional relationships.

These emotional toxins need to be dealt with as well as the physical toxins. The physical side is a little easier to deal with and less complicated. I think the important thing is to get started in some really definite, small way and relish feeling good about it. Relish feeling good about yourself. Make a list and do the things on the list that are going to help you feel good about being you. Break the list down to bite-size pieces.

Happy to be you

A friend of mine said to me the other day, "You just seem so happy to be you." And of course, that day I did. He was comparing the time before when I visited him. He made mention of the earlier visit because then I was all upset due to negative events happening to people I love. I had given him Joko Beck's *Everyday Zen Book,* and he had mirrored it back to me saying, "That is just the way it is. They made their choices. There is nothing you can do about it—let it go." Sometimes, some days, it is just so difficult, you want to kick something. You want to rant and rave. I think we want someone to say, "Wow, how awful for you; that *is* awful; I'm sorry that happened to you."

The truth is that you are going to die and so is everyone you love. Bad things will happen to you and to the people you love, but beautiful things will happen, too, daily. Pay attention to them. Don't let your mind spin too much; catch yourself, correct it. Read books that bring you solace. Spend lots of time alone. You are not just your mind. You are something much deeper, much more important. As a guru in Eldorado Springs says, "All your thoughts are just a nuisance."

A *teacher*

If you're ready and if you're interested, at some point during these transformations, these detoxifications, these rejuvenation therapies, you may want to seek a teacher, a spiritual path or psychotherapy, a safe, loving, accepting environment where you can really spill your guts. Just say whatever comes to your mind, speak to someone objectively about your deepest feelings, resentments, frustrations, relationships, and go through your past, present, and future.

Living in Colorado really helps in all these areas because Boulder is the capital for therapies. Check the therapies available to you in your area. You can also find therapists that are of particular religions who understand where you are coming from and may help you discover where you want to go.

A *journey*

See this search as a journey. There will be steep mountains and deep valleys, to be sure, but beautiful meadows and broad scenic vistas, too. Embrace them all as you emotionally detox, lighten your load, and free yourself. Enjoy the trip.

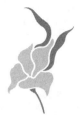

Specific Beauty Treatments

Cleansing

Physical beauty begins with a well-cleansed face. We must clean up all dead skin debris and aid in the process of new cellular growth. The simple purpose of a cleanser is to remove dirt, oil, and grime from your skin. This is the foundation of any skin care regime, because you must start with fresh skin for the rest of the program to function properly. A quality cleanser helps the skin to breathe better by helping remove debris, without removing moisture and disrupting the skin's acid balance.

There are several different kinds of cleansers, soaps, milks, and gels. Bar soaps are more typically for young or oily skin. All skin types can use cleansers, milks, and gels. Pure vegetarian soaps are the only ones I use. So read your labels carefully and look for vegetable oils. Many of the gels are formulated by using seaweeds.

If you use an alkaline cleanser, a soap, you may want to be sure to rinse well with a little acidic vinegar in a lot of rinse water, or use a toner to preserve the natural acid mantle of the skin.

You should have the wisdom to pick an ideal cleanser for your skin. Evaluate first by ingredients, and then by how it cleans your skin and the feeling it leaves. The right cleanser should contain all the ingredients you want and leave your skin tingling and prepared for a mask, steam, or moisturizer. If after using the cleanser your skin appears better, then you can continue using it.

I think the best cleansers are made from almond oil soap, lily, vegetable glycerin, and essential oils of lavender, rosemary, sage, and lemon juice. A good cleanser should go on easily and be a pleasure to wash with. They work best if followed by a fine scented, refreshing toner or astringent.

A make-it-yourself cleanser

Baking soda used as a gentle cleanser helps detoxify the skin from the outside by removing the grit, grime, and pollution. A simple cleansing formula is:

2 tablespoons baking powder

1 teaspoon almond oil

2 drops lavender essential oil

1 cup water

1 tablespoon honey

On low heat, combine all ingredients except honey. Remove from heat and let cool. Add honey. It will separate, so stir before using. Apply to the skin like a soap and rinse off with tepid water.

Cleansing creams and lotions that are made with beneficial herbs and oil are great for dry skin. They remove dirt and debris on the skin but don't dehydrate or strip the skin of too much oil.

Scrubbing grains were popular a few years back before the enzyme masks became the rage. They do a good job of removing debris from the top layer of skin. Many people, however, don't like their abrasive quality.

According to Jessica B. Harris in the *World Beauty Book*, "The first soaps came from a mixture of the fats of sacrificial animals and the ashes of the fires in which they had been sacrificed." [*] Native Americans used plants like yucca and soapwort.

Facial steam

I love steam, and I love to do facials. The wonderful fragrance of the herbs penetrating your skin and the warm, wet mist just makes you feel good, and you feel good knowing you are doing something so beneficial for yourself and your skin. The best thing of all is the way it so effectively deep cleans the pores and allows for any blocked ducts in the skin to be freed of debris, thus allowing the skin to breathe and perform its functions efficiently. Steaming is probably the best way to really cleanse the skin. You can change the type of steam by the kind of herbs you use.

---

[*] Jessica B. Harris, *The World Beauty Book*, San Francisco, CA: Harper Collins, 1995.

If you suffer from acne, you may be able to really clear your skin if you steam daily for ten minutes before bed. For blemished skin, try lavender for its antiseptic and cleansing properties, comfrey for its skin healing properties, and rose for its astringent properties. (See the individual herbs in the Herb section for more ideas on mixtures.) For normal skin, you may want to keep your skin looking fresh by doing a steam twice a month.

For serious, all-over-body deep cleaning, try steaming your skin in a steam room; it is not only a relaxing experience, it helps purify your entire body. Be sure to drink plenty of water before, during, and after. Steaming regularly once a week and doing a full body brush and then bathing in Epsom salts and juniper oil will keep your skin squeaky clean. Body brushing dry skin helps remove dead skin so your new skin can breathe.

Exfoliating

Purpose and methods

Exfoliants are designed to remove dead cells from the skin. This can be done chemically, botanically, or mechanically. Chemically, it is achieved through glycolic acids or alpha hydroxys, which were once natural ingredients but which now have often been chemically synthesized to strengthen the effect of the acids. Botanical exfoliation of dead skin can be done by applying pineapple juice directly to your skin, or mashing fresh papaya and applying alone or mixed with honey or yogurt. Mechanically, you can exfoliate by placing sugar, sea salt, or cornmeal with a cleanser and scrubbing the face, or any part of the body.

As you get older, a nice purely botanical™, gentle exfoliation is a wonderful addition to any skin care regimen. If you use the products made with pure ingredients of papaya, pineapple, comfrey, lily, mint, and honey, you can't overuse. Papaya, pineapple, and comfrey all have necrotic properties, which means they have protein digestive enzymes that literally eat the dead skin off your face. And these do not irritate or harm live skin.

Your skin has an inherent wisdom, and while its natural ability to renew cells slows down, it still is not wise to use abrasive products that will irritate and inflame your skin. I have met so many women in the health food stores with skin reddened and burned after using the glycolic acids and alpha hydroxys; like so many other fads and trends, I think this one should be ignored.

Making your own exfoliant

Mix equal parts of mayonnaise and cornmeal. Rub all over the body in a circular motion and then shower off. Another way to exfoliate the entire body is to mix salt with almond or olive oil, with a few drops of juniper oil dispersed in the olive oil. Start with your feet and go up over your whole body, rubbing gently. Shower off.

You can easily make other exfoliants by applying fresh papaya or pineapple, blended or mashed, to your face, or you can apply the juice of either fruit alone or mixed with honey, clay, or both. Experiment, come up with your own recipe, and have fun!

I make a wonderful Botanical Enzyme Exfoliant Mask. It has a base of honey and papaya. In addition, it contains comfrey, horsetail, lily, and vitamins A, C, and E with grapefruit seed extract.

Mists

Mists are a relatively new concept in the commercial marketplace. I love them! I like to have one in my car, one in my bath, one in my office, one in my living room, one by my nightstand, and one in my purse. I don't leave home without one! I particularly love the blend of lavender and ylang ylang in our Lily Moisturizing Mist. It is moisturizing and hydrating to your skin, while it is joyful and uplifting to your spirits.

What to look for in a mist

Look for mists with pure essential oils that are wonderful for your skin, like lavender and ylang ylang. Look also for other ingredients like comfrey for its cell proliferating properties, vegetable glycerin for its humectant value (its ability to pull moisture from the air to your skin), seaweeds because most of them can hold twenty times their weight in water, lily for its calming and healing action on the skin, and chamomile and calendula because they are soothing.

These mists, like herbs themselves, are so versatile that I use the same mist as a perfume before going out and spray it onto my pillow before going to sleep. I find the essential oil of lavender especially nice. I use it as a light moisturizer alone or with one of our creams before applying makeup. It is a perfect light summer moisturizer for oily skin and a nice addition to a cream for dry skin. I use it to set my makeup after application. I keep one in my refrigerator and use it after a bath to cool me from the heat of the water. For those lucky enough to have a hot tub, a mist is a perfect accompaniment.

I am constantly using the mist in my car, not only to hydrate and tone my skin, but also to calm down during stressful moments on the highway. I often use the one in my office while typing, talking on the phone, if I need a break, or if I need a pick-me-up.

These mists are one of life's little pleasures. Get one at your health food store or simply make your own by adding five to ten drops of your favorite essential oil or oils to eight ounces distilled or herbal water, and put in a spray bottle.

Moisturizers

"What kind of moisturizer is best for me to use?" This question is one I'm most frequently asked. My reply is usually, "What kind of moisturizer do you prefer?" Fundamentally, this is what it is all about. If you have oily skin, you most likely are not going to feel comfortable slathering a heavy almond oil all over your face. It just doesn't seem natural.

Amazingly, there are lots of people who advocate just that. They say you should put oil on oil, because your oil glands are not stripped of oils as they are with soap. Therefore, the theory is to trick your skin into thinking it already has enough oil so it doesn't produce any more. Not a bad theory; try it for yourself.

Keeping your skin moisturized is just as much about water as oil. A good moisturizer needs to help your skin retain moisture. You can look in the mirror and see if it is doing its job. You can also feel it.

Making choices

I know you would prefer me to be definitive in my theories and instructions, but I am here to present the information; you have to make the ultimate decision about what is best for you. American consumers have been brainwashed not to have to think. Many want to be told what to buy in ten seconds or less. I am saying break away from that mind set. Truly ask yourself, "What do I think is best for me? What feels right? What are the ingredients? Does this make sense to me? Do I like the feel, the scent, the texture, the consistency, the viscosity? Does it soak into my skin? Does my skin look better after using it? Does it feel right?"

With that said, people with dry skin usually love oils and thick, rich creams, and at the risk of bragging, I do make one of the best creams available. But there are many others. You need to buy or try samples, read the labels for ingredients, and see which one works best for you.

People with normal skin tend to prefer a light cream or lotion. Again, this all makes perfect sense.

People with oily skin are often scared of an oil or very rich cream. They are not sure if they want to use any product with any kind of oil in it at all. They prefer "oil-free" moisturizers. I admit I did not come up with any of this on my own. You, as consumers, told me. After doing approximately a thousand demos in stores all over the country, this is what I have learned from you.

Why moisturize?

Let's discuss why to use a moisturizer at all. First of all, if you are 18 and have blemishes, you probably do not need a moisturizer, but if you still have blemishes at 25, it does not necessarily mean you do not need a moisturizer. You probably do if you live in anything but a humid, balmy climate. In that case, you may want to use just a light lotion or herbal oil-free moisturizer around your eyes, mouth, and possibly your forehead if it is dry, or a simple moisturizing mist might be perfect for you.

Moisturizers are essential for most women over 25, especially those who live in a dry climate or have dry skin. A lack of humidity in the air, an increase in "transepidermal" water loss, a nutritional essential fatty acid deficiency in the food you ingest, or use of household chemicals can cause dry skin. So can certain home-heating systems.

Applying a lubricant with penetrating ability creates a barrier that can protect the skin from further drying. Essentially, it is like applying oils to old furniture. It stops the drying process with a layer of oil to protect it from the harsh air.

Moisturizing is like a mechanical process. Oil is put into your car engine to reduce friction. Friction produces heat which in turn produces wear. It is similar with the skin on your face; changing expressions, dryness, and harsh chemical products can be compared to engine friction. The oils and moisturizers create a lubrication process to make your skin glide easily into its many expressions.

Men can also benefit

I have seen people look as old and dried out as a prune, especially men. During a particular demo, I cleansed the skin of some men with our herbal astringent applied on a cotton ball to remove the dirt and dried dead skin. Then, I applied a thin layer of our herbal moisturizer and for an added bonus a couple drops of our Seven Exotic Oils topped with a quick spray of our mist. They looked ten years younger just because we had removed the dead skin cells and debris and applied lubrication and hydration.

Climates and seasons

The climate you live in has a great effect on your skin. Not many people talk about this, and I haven't seen anything about it in any other skin care book; but I feel this is often more important than what kind of skin you have. The climate you live in and the season are going to determine what kind of skin you have at that time of year.

And what about seasons? Come on, we all know how important the changes of the seasons are to our skin, but nobody I'm aware of really has ever seriously addressed it or even talks about it. In the hundreds of books I have poured over in the last twenty years, I don't think I have ever seen anyone give this serious consideration, except you, my customers. You have told me, especially the women in the Midwest. It's a much more dramatic change there. Colorado and New Mexico are always dry, but the Midwest is humid and moist in the summer and then brutally cold and harsh in the winter.

Even though most cosmetic companies don't address this issue, you do. Most women change their skin care regimen with the seasons, and you are right to do so. Especially in places like Michigan, you are probably not going to be able to use the same cream in the summer as you do in the winter. In hot weather, you probably couldn't even get it on your constantly perspiring face. This is what is important. Many women may have oily skin in the summer and severely dry skin in the winter. So you really need to adjust your skin care program.

If you have dry skin in the winter, use the heavy oils, the exotic blends of thick oils, and the heavy, rich creams. You can still cleanse and tone the same, but the skin's loss of moisture is going to be much greater in the winter. Most of you inherently know this; you have been listening to your skin, a wise thing to do.

You can change the climate by purchasing a humidifier and running it in your bedroom while you sleep. This can give your skin a humid climate when it needs it. Constantly misting your skin can also bring humidity to it.

When I travel around the country, I really notice the difference in women's skin. Here in Colorado, people's skin looks pretty dry, even more so in New Mexico. When I travel to the Midwest, women's skin looks better, moister, with less obvious dryness.

When I travel to all the health food stores, I put cream on women's hands, so I get a really good look at not only their faces but their hands. I used to think women in Boulder had the worst-looking hands in terms of dryness, cracking, and peeling; and still to this day the worst hands I have ever seen were on a construction worker from Aurora, Colorado, but I have seen hands as rough in Santa Fe, New Mexico.

It may have to do with what activities women from Boulder and Santa Fe engage themselves in—hiking, skiing, gardening—very much outdoors people, constantly exposed to the elements maybe up to twelve hours a day, oftentimes on a daily basis.

In the Midwest, women's hands seem to look much better, especially in the summer. For obvious reasons I try not to travel in that direction in the winter, so I don't get a chance to see them when the snow flies and the freezing winds blow.

Winter can be hard on skin, but there is no reason to suffer with dry, flaky skin. Not only is the colder weather creating hardship, but the sun is intensified by the snow, and indoors is drier from heating sources. A furnace can dry up any humidity in the air. For this reason, I will often leave my bathwater in the tub to add moisture to the air in my house.

In harsh climates, even oily skin can become flaky. Flaky skin can in fact make you look older while smooth skin can make you look younger. The first thing to do, if this is the case, is to use a mild cleanser and astringent/toner twice a day. Second, find a botanically derived enzyme exfoliant mask to remove the flaky dead skin while encouraging the formation of new skin. I prefer the non-abrasive, honey based, with pineapple and papaya, which are well-known for their protein digestive enzymes that literally eat dead skin. I also like a mask with a stimulant such as mint.

Be sure to use a line of skin care products with pure and gentle ingredients without any drying chemicals. Or make your own. Use products with humectants like vegetable glycerin and honey. Replenish moisture frequently. Use a mist or spritzer with all natural ingredients.

"Kitchen cosmetics"

You can use many "kitchen cosmetics" on your skin in the winter to combat dry skin. I believe pure vegetable oil is much cleaner and more beneficial than many cosmetic products on the market. Pure almond or olive oil is great to apply for extra moisture. For extra benefit, you can soak your favorite herbs in the oil for two weeks and then strain them out or leave them in.

Calendula and lily skin oil

This recipe can use any herbs you desire. (See chapter on Herbs for specific skin types.) Calendula and lily are mild, so they are wonderful for very sensitive skin. You can use this oil for massage, in a bath, after a bath, for babies, dry cuticles, elbows, as a facial moisturizer, under-eye oil, hot-oil hair treatment, or just about anything else.

$^1/_2$ cup fresh calendula petals

$^1/_2$ cup fresh lily flowers

2 cups oil (almond or olive for dry skin, grape seed or kukui for normal to oily skin)

Several drops of essential oils as desired (see chapter on Essential Oils for skin type)

Combine all the ingredients except the essential oils in a large glass bottle or jar, cover and set in a sunny window for two weeks, shaking every other day. Strain out the herbs, add the essential oil, and keep refrigerated.

Steams and Masks

I always cleanse my skin impeccably before steaming, whether it be at home with herbs in a pan or at the recreation center. I like to take a bottle of herbal astringent with me. First, I shower with soap, then I cleanse all over my face and neck with our herbal astringent. Next, I spray the astringent all over my body. I take it in the steam room with me. It is especially pleasant if it has been chilled first. I spray it on as the steam overheats me. Everybody wants to know what smells so wonderful. It adds an extra bonus to the steam room's cleansing process.

Enjoy the process

Please remember: Have fun! This is not an exact science. It is an art. So be creative! Just look in your kitchen cupboards and see if you have any of these or similar ingredients you'll find later in this chapter. Experiment! Or get a list together of what you think you would like to try, go to the health food store and gather those items. Set the time aside to pamper yourself. If you find you don't have an ingredient, or you're allergic, or you just don't feel like using it, substitute something else. This is not making a soufflé; this is more like making a stew or pizza.

So many people ask me to give them such explicit and easily quantifiable directions with specific instructions, but it's not necessary. You know oatmeal and brewer's yeast are good for you and you know they are safe. You have done a mask before and you know you need a certain consistency to apply it to your skin. If you have oily skin, make a mask with some honey and lavender, oatmeal, and brewer's yeast.

It is just as important to enjoy the process and the knowledge that you are taking the time to do something good for yourself as it is for the herbal properties to penetrate your skin while you steam.

Steams

Any kind of skin can benefit from an herbal steam. The heat helps boost circulation and open the pores. This helps bring the dirt and toxins to the surface. The aromatherapeutic benefits include relaxing the tensions and improving the spirits.

Steaming is a deep pore cleansing and helps the body cleanse itself from deeper impurities. Unlike most cleansing programs, it works on a level that aids in removing blockages below the skin's surface. It helps bring blood to the skin's surface, rids the body of toxins and actually can prevent pimples and blemishes. Blemished and oily skin can derive the greatest benefit.

My method of steaming my skin at home is simply to boil one quart purified water in a non-aluminum pan with an ounce or two of my favorite herbs. As soon as you put the herbs in, wait thirty seconds and then remove the pan from the source of heat. Place a towel over your head, making a tent over your head and the pan. Let your skin soak in all the valuable properties of the herbs and the beneficial moist heat. Do this for ten minutes or until the water cools.

If you have dry skin you only need to steam a couple times a month; if you have normal skin, once a week will be beneficial. Blemished skin can benefit from daily to every other day short steams.

Steaming makes the skin more receptive to the next phases of your skin care regimen. The vapor action also can help reduce the appearance of lines and wrinkles because the water helps plump up the skin.

There are no set rules on what ingredients to put in any herbal facial steam. Melanie Sachs states in her book, *Ayurvedic Beauty Care,* that "every steam needs four types of ingredients: those that increase circulation, those that bring out impurities, those that soothe and heal, and some for the therapeutic quality of their aroma . . . Bay leaf draws circulation towards the skin's surface. Licorice pulls out impurities."*

For acne, experiment with yarrow, lavender, witch hazel, lemon grass, dandelion root, burdock root, lemon peel, horsetail, sage, and nettles to discover which work best and are most pleasing to you. You

---

* Melanie Sachs, *Ayurvedic Beauty Care: Ageless Techniques to Invoke Natural Beauty,* Twin Lakes, WI: Lotus Press, 1994, p. 167.

can also steam with several drops of the following essential oils in the hot water: oil of rosemary, sandalwood, juniper, or cypress. You can also make a large quantity of the steam mixture of dandelion and burdock root. Mix enough to steam your skin with it and to drink two cups of the tea with a little honey to sweeten. Put the remainder in your bath adding several drops of juniper oil.

For normal skin, add chamomile, spearmint, comfrey, lavender, rose, or a few drops of essential oils of sandalwood, fennel, bergamot, or geranium to your steaming water.

For dry skin or to use in the winter for normal skin, red clover, comfrey, dandelion, orange peel, chamomile, calendula, elder flower, yarrow, or essential oils of rose, sandalwood, lavender, or rosemary are beneficial and enjoyable. Gel- or honey-type masks are great for dry skin, especially ones made with Irish moss or other seaweeds. For dry skin, I recommend a base of honey, for oily skin yogurt is useful, but both skin types can benefit from using either.

To cleanse, add rosemary, sage, nettles, chamomile, or lavender to the boiling water. To stimulate and close pores, try peppermint, horsetail, coltsfoot, and elder flower. To heal, use lily, fennel, or comfrey. You can use any combination of any of these herbs.

I love steaming my face and doing masks. There is something so self-indulgent, almost decadent about it! Do try it. Indulge yourself!

Masks

Masks are very beneficial. Because a mask forms a solid film on the face, the skin accumulates a large supply of water, which hydrates it. Masks that dry on the skin promote a rosy glow in the complexion due to three things: tightening, stimulation, and increased circulation, each promoting skin quality. When a mask is washed off, it takes the dry dead skin with it, giving the skin a deep cleansing as well as a smooth healthy look.

Masks are a great body care aid. Everything you need to make a mask can be found in your kitchen. Nothing is more fun than experimenting with concoctions for your skin to improve your complexion.

Masks are designed to remove dead skin cells, stimulate new skin, deeply cleanse the skin, refine and tighten the pores, and provide nourishment to the skin.

The most beneficial kind of mask has botanical ingredients with necrotic properties, properties with protein digestive enzymes, usually papaya, pineapple, and comfrey. All three of these ingredients literally eat dead skin off your face without having any effect on new healthy skin, other than removing the dead skin cells so the new skin cells can shine through. I like a mask that is purely botanical™, has in it all three plants with necrotic properties, and in addition, is in a honey base with other herbs such as lily to heal and soothe the skin, as well as mint that is a stimulant. Vitamins A, C, and E provide an antioxidant effect and further nourish and protect the skin.

To deeply cleanse the skin, to remove deep dirt and impurities, clay is a good ingredient. Most people use a green or white clay. This can be mixed with many of the different powdered herbs, such as mint, comfrey, lily, and then mixed with honey, aloe vera, yogurt, or water. Make into a paste and apply. Leave on for twenty minutes, then rinse off.

To refine and tighten the pores, it is advantageous to use ingredients that contract, such as mucilage found in seaweeds like kelp or Irish moss. Aloe vera and herbs that are astringent in nature, such as witch hazel, yarrow, elderberries, agrimony, cucumber, or rose, are helpful. All citrus fruits are toning and astringent.

There are so many ingredients you can use right in your kitchen to nourish your skin. The simplest and easiest way to start is with a base of yogurt, honey, or aloe. Brewer's yeast, grapes, and apples are moisturizing and nourishing. You can make a tomato mask by putting two tomatoes in the blender and adding brewer's yeast and comfrey leaves. Apply to the skin, keeping away from the eye area; leave on for fifteen minutes. Relax in the awareness that these commonplace ingredients from your kitchen are cleaning, stimulating, toning, and refining your skin. Rinse.

In her book, *Kitty Little's Book of Herbal Beauty*, the author gives a recipe to tone the skin with juice from the houseleek, a member of the lily family. Like many lilies, it is known to be outstanding for healing skin. She recommends "liquidizing twelve houseleek leaves" with 200ml (seven fluid ounces) of water, and straining the mixture through a coffee filter. "Houseleek was one of the most cherished cosmetic herbs of Ninon de l'Enclose who up to her death at the age of ninety-one was still called 'the woman who never grew old' and who even in her eighties was still managing to attract ardent young lovers. She almost committed incest with her grandson at the age of seventy and by all accounts led an exciting and scandalous life as a courtesan, gourmand, and friend to Moliere, Voltaire, and Scarron."[*]

---

[*] Kitty Little, *Kitty Little's Book of Herbal Beauty*, Harmondsworth, Middlesex, England: Penguin Books Ltd., 1986, p. 67.

Mask ingredients according to skin types

Dry skin

- honey
- comfrey
- apples
- pears
- peaches
- shea or karite butter
- rosehip seed oil
- primrose oil
- almond oil
- olive oil
- beeswax
- myrrh
- lily
- ylang ylang essential oil
- cocoa butter
- elder
- yarrow

Normal skin

- yogurt
- spearmint
- cherries
- rose
- kosher vegetable glycerin

Combination skin

- mayonnaise
- vinegar
- citrus fruits
- brewer's yeast
- strawberries

Sensitive skin

- lily
- calendula
- comfrey
- yarrow
- elder flowers
- rose
- chamomile
- jasmine
- frankincense
- apricots
- vitamin E

Oily and/or blemished skin

- tomatoes
- bee propolis
- sage
- pumpkin
- clays
- Fuller's earth
- raspberries
- buttermilk
- carrots
- marshmallow eucalyptus
- fennel
- cucumber
- witch hazel
- rose
- calendula
- lavender
- yogurt
- vinegar
- brewer's yeast
- lemon
- lemon grass
- all citrus fruits
- clay
- rose geranium
- niaouli
- sage
- patchouli

* To refine pores and tone, blend equal parts chamomile and honey.

* To soothe skin, blend equal parts mashed comfrey leaves with honey.

* For irritated skin, blend equal parts of powdered lavender, comfrey, and calendula with enough honey to make a paste.

* For oily skin, mix equal parts of powdered lavender and rose in yogurt to make a paste.

* For blemished skin, mix equal parts of chamomile and comfrey with enough yogurt to make a paste.

* For dry skin, blend equal parts of chamomile and comfrey with yogurt and honey to make a paste. Rinse thoroughly after the mask has dried.

Have fun indulging yourself in masks and steams. Both are relaxing and beneficial. Best of all, they can be done right in your own home using ingredients right from your own kitchen!

Toners and Astringents

Common misunderstandings

Astringent is a name given to products for their contracting effect upon tissues. This is why astringents are valuable for closing pores. Astringent does not mean drying; it does not mean containing alcohol; it does not mean for oily skin, even though that is what the marketers have drilled into our heads. Astringents should just feel slightly tightening without drying.

The other common misunderstanding is that witch hazel, a popular astringent, contains alcohol. The bark and leaves of the witch hazel tree are only extracted in alcohol. Although the best extraction process for witch hazel is an alcohol tincture, this does not automatically mean that an astringent with witch hazel contains alcohol. Witch hazel can also be extracted from a hydroglycolic, slow-heat process in water. Read your labels. (Grain alcohol tinctures are okay in a product, but high levels of alcohol can be drying.)

I make a wonderful astringent that I use twice daily and adore. It is made with essential oils of lavender and sage, which when blended give a perfect, classic, clean scent. I also use witch hazel, aloe vera, lily, comfrey root, calendula, ginseng, kelp, nettles, coltsfoot, and horsetail. Look for products that contain these ingredients, or make your own with all or some of these ingredients.

After cleansing, tone your skin by applying a slightly astringent substance to tighten the freshly cleaned pores. Toners and astringents can make your face seem a little firmer and your pores seem a little smaller.

You can easily make these recipes at home:

* Put several strawberries in the blender, then apply to your face. This will help your circulation and remove oil and dirt.

* Add one tablespoon of organic apple cider vinegar to one cup of purified water. Keep in a jar with a tight lid in the refrigerator. This should last more than a few weeks. Apply as needed.

* Add the juice of one fresh lemon to one cup of purified water and splash on your face.

* Add one cup of purified water to ten drops of the following essential oils. Try misting the following essential oils mixed with water:

- cedarwood
- cypress
- immortelle
- bergamot
- sandalwood
- rosemary

- frankincense
- geranium
- juniper
- lemon
- myrrh

* Make a tomato puree mask by simply blending a fresh tomato and applying the pulp to your face.

* Try blending the following ingredients: buttermilk, salt, and cornmeal. Mix to a consistency conducive to application. The salt and cornmeal act as scrubbers.

As a final step, always rinse thoroughly.

To refine large pores

Camphor is great to help refine large pores and heal and tighten the skin. For a quick mask, try mixing two tablespoons of honey with one-half teaspoon of spirits of camphor. Apply all over the face and leave on for twenty minutes. Avoid getting it in the eyes and patch test first.

When purchasing astringents and toners, look for astringents with horsetail, lily, benzoin gum, elder flower, yarrow, lavender, and sage. Putting these herbs in a facial steam can really benefit large-pore skin.

Homemade and healthy

You can use fresh or dried herbs. To make your own astringent, try:

2 cups purified water

1 tablespoon of lily flowers

1 tablespoon of lavender flowers

1 tablespoon of eucalyptus leaves

1 tablespoon coltsfoot

1 tablespoon comfrey

2 drops sage oil

4 drops lavender oil

Bring the water to a boil in a non-aluminum pan. Add the herbs. As soon as you bring the water to a second boil, remove from heat and let it sit until cool. Strain out the herbs with a thin cloth or cheesecloth. Place the astringent in a glass jar with a tightly fitting lid. Add the essential oils and refrigerate. Apply several times daily with a cotton ball or mister.

This recipe can be altered in as many ways as you can think of. You can add witch hazel, aloe vera gel, vegetable glycerin, any of the different herbs listed in the Ingredients section of this book, or any of the essential oils.

Balancing lavender/rose skin toner

Since lavender is so balancing, it is appropriate for all skin types. Everyone can use this toner. You may also just substitute another herb (found in the individual herbal section) as it suits you and your skin type.

3 cups purified water

$1/2$ cup fresh or dried lavender flowers

4 drops essential oil of rose

Combine water and lavender flowers in a glass bottle or jar and place on a sunny shelf for five days. Shake it every other day. Strain and add the essential oil of rose. Keep refrigerated and splash on your face after cleansing twice a day.

You can also add a tablespoon of aloe vera gel or vinegar for oily skin. This should last about a week.

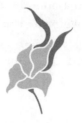

Aging

We ask ourselves, who am I to be brilliant, gorgeous, talented and fabulous? Actually, who are you not to be? You are a child of God.

—Nelson Mandela

Things are beautiful when you love them.
—Jean Anouilh

Anything in any way beautiful derives its beauty from itself, and asks nothing beyond itself.

—Marcus Aurelius

It appears that what accounts most for successful aging is simply a good attitude, a lust for living, resilience, an optimistic outlook, and an active lifestyle.

I have been lucky to have some really good role models in this area. My mother paid so little attention to how old she was that when she was asked her age, she always had to calculate back from the year she was born. Hence, the message was that it wasn't important enough to walk around with it in your head, and it wasn't anything to hide or be ashamed of. I've always thought if you lie about your age, then people may think you look really bad for the age you claim to be.

We are very fortunate in this day and age to know that we can look and be terrific until the day we die.

There are so many fantastic role models out there for us. Examples are Katharine Hepburn, Margaret Thatcher, and Georgia O'Keeffe.

How it used to be

According to Den Dychtwald, the author of *Age Wave*, "Throughout 99 percent of all the years that humans have walked this planet, the life expectancy was under 18 years. We have never before had a mass population of older people. Until very recently, most people didn't age, they died."*

He continues, "How drastic an effect this will have on our lives and the traditional or middle-class values and mentalities. Life used to be so linear. You graduated from school; you maybe lost a few years dating, going to Europe, or tripping around in jobs; then you settled down and got married, bought a house, had a baby, spent 20-30 years raising them; and then if you were really lucky, you had a pension and you retired."

More options today

Life for all of us can be much more promising, much more interesting, and much more flexible than that scenario. Many baby boomers have lived a 20 to 30-year adolescence, not really committing to jobs, children, or spouses. No generation before us has ever had such an extended youth and the opportunities available to enjoy true health and wealth. We have been offered so many options by this extended life span.

Aging really is all in your perception. Think you're old and you are. Think you're young and you are. I have seen so many people hit 40 and you can almost see them age and collapse before your very eyes in the length of time it takes them to tell you the sad story of how awful it is. And the entire time I'm thinking, "Hmm, two months ago you weren't that much younger, but you sure were a lot more interesting, a lot more fun. I don't get it; you're only two months older than you were last time I saw you, and your life didn't look so bleak then."

It's just getting stuck in your own negative and small universe. Open up! Smile! Do what makes you happy! Take excellent care of yourself, love yourself, and treat yourself to what you know will make you look and feel better. Take control, quit whining, get busy, and help someone less fortunate than yourself.

Whining about your age should be one of the mortal sins; forbidding it should be the eleventh commandment. After Buddha said, "Be a lamp unto yourself," I think he should have added, "Thank God every morning for the continued gift of life."

---

* Den Dychtwald, *Age Wave*, Los Angeles, CA, and New York, NY: J. P. Tarcher Publisher, 1989.

Whining about your age is spitting in the Creator's face; it's saying, "Hey, I'm sad you let me continue to live." I mean, if death is sad, then shouldn't life be good? Isn't that why we celebrate birthdays? Hey, one more year. Thank you, God. I am going to get with my close friends and celebrate my good fortune of continued life.

Complaining about age doesn't make sense. It is not even a problem, therefore it cannot have a solution.

Now, I am not saying people can't whine about not feeling good, health problems, and life's frustrations. But to complain only because you haven't died yet is ridiculous.

Another theory

My theory on age is that since we have a life expectancy of at least ten more years than when we did when we were born, we can employ this: If you are 50, well, then you are really only 40, and if you are 40, 30, and if you are 30, you are only 20. It's all in your head, so employ my theory and feel ten years younger. It's the truth, you really do have ten more years, so start enjoying your windfall now, today! Why wait until the ten years between 80 and 90? Get your extra ten years in now.

Baby boomers are the luckiest generation ever. Up until the early 1970s, turning 30 was a drastic sign of aging for a woman, and God forbid if you hadn't snagged a husband yet. You were too old to have children. I escaped the dreaded aging game, which is demonstrated by the old saying, "A beautiful woman dies twice, once when she loses her looks and again when they bury her."

Perhaps I never thought of myself as the least bit attractive; I knew "my good looks" were not going to open doors for me. Good looks do open doors, and they get you invited in, but I don't think they get you invited back for the important events. So I figured I had to develop my brains. I had the good fortune of teachers, counselors, and tests telling me I had brains. (An interesting caveat to all this is if you ask my high school chums, they would not confirm I was that unattractive, and if you ask my family, they would not confirm anyone told me I was that smart—but don't ever underestimate the power of perception. My perception was that I was not attractive, and so maybe I had to cling to the fact I was smart, because I had to have something going for me.)

We are the luckiest generation of women in the history of the world. Look at how drastically better our lives are than our mothers. This is not to say that a lot of our mothers weren't really happy with their lives, but you had better have wanted children and a husband, and you better have landed yourself a good one.

Women my age are even more lucky. We had so many role models, so many women around who were 10 to 40 or more years older than us, beautiful, brainy, and sexy, letting us know that we too could look good at their ages.

So let's get up each morning and before we start our busy days, let's take a moment to thank God for this precious gift of life. Let's thank God that we as American women have it better than any other women on the planet, and better than any other women in history.

If all this doesn't help, here are some cold facts: About 80% of Americans live normal active lives until the end of their lives. Disease, incontinence, cataracts, depression, and senility are *not* a normal part of aging among most Americans.

If, for one minute, you think you are too old to accomplish your dreams, consider the following from *The Speaker's Sourcebook* by Glenn Van Ekeren:

✳ George Burns did not receive his first Oscar until he was 80.

✳ Golda Meir did not become prime minister of Israel until she was 71.

✳ Michelangelo was 71 when he painted the Sistine Chapel.

✳ Grandma Moses did not start painting until she was 80; she completed over 1500 paintings and over 300 of those were done after she was 100.

✳ At 58, Doc Counsilman became the oldest person to swim the English Channel.[*]

Jack London had it right

"I would rather be ashes than dust! I would rather that my spark should burn out in a brilliant blaze than it should be stifled by dry rot. I would rather be a superb meteor, every atom of me in magnificent glow, than a sleepy and permanent planet. The proper function of man is to live, not to exist. I shall not spend my days trying to prolong them. I shall use my time."

---

[*] Glenn Van Ekeren, *The Speaker's Sourcebook*, Englewood Cliffs, NJ: Prentice-Hall, 1998.

The trick, I think, is to live fully in beauty, health, and happiness your entire life, from beginning to end, thanking your Maker for each and every moment you are given life on earth.

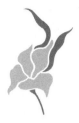

Questions I Am Most Often Asked

Q: I know I should avoid synthetic chemicals, but which ones and why?

A: Say "yes" to Mother Nature. That is what I am saying. That is more important than saying "no" to petroleum and synthesized chemicals. My motto is: "Mother Nature is the best cure for Father Time."

Synthetic chemicals are the ingredients in most skin care products that cause rashes and bad reactions and create all sorts of problems. There is serious documentation about many cosmetic preservatives widely used that are potentially harmful. For further reading, you may want to pick up a copy of Aubrey Hampton's book, *Natural Organic Hair and Skin Care.*

Remember your skin has a powerful ability to absorb. If you rub garlic on your feet, it can later be detected on your breath, so whatever you put on your skin is important.

In addition, we prefer to support agriculture, which is a renewable resource.

Q: I'm 40 and I've always had perfect skin. Now I break out all the time with acne. Why?

A: I think that most adult acne is hormonal. Improving your diet and exercising is going to improve your overall health, but not necessarily have a great impact on clearing up your long-term, stubborn, recurring acne. A program of balancing hormones by taking internally the herbs dong quai and vitex or inhaling the scent of essential oil of fennel can be helpful.

Many benefit from eating lots of fresh fruit, drinking lots of water, and steaming the skin daily with lavender, rose, lily, and chamomile. Others drink teas of burdock root, yellow dock, and chicory. Many experience improvement by taking supplements of lecithin and B vitamins. Consider seeing a highly qualified acupuncturist or herbalist. (See section on Acne.)

Q: What is the best thing to use to wash my face—soap?

A: I think the skin care business has to get away from answering a blanket question like this with a canned answer. They do so because this is what the consumer seems to want: "Just tell me in ten seconds or less what I should use."

There is no perfect answer. It depends mostly on you and your preferences, what you think is right for your skin. What are you using now? Why? Are you happy with the results? Do you find soap drying? Are you 13 with severe acne or 45 with wrinkles?

Like everything else, soap has its place on the planet. I personally like soap. I like the feeling that all the makeup, dirt, and grime has been removed. Look for soaps that have essential oils of lavender or sage and herbs of lily, chamomile, and sage. I personally also like to use a pure herbal astringent on a cotton ball to doubly insure all the makeup and soap residue is gone.

To remove all makeup, tone your skin, and to tighten large pores, look for products with lily, lavender, and sage.

Q: What's wrong with using my body lotion on my face? It is a lot cheaper.

A: Nothing, if that's what you want to use and you are happy with the ingredients, comfortable putting them on your face, and like the way the product performs.

Q: I use Retin A for acne/wrinkles. Are natural products compatible with it?

A: Yes, I think natural products are really perfect for people using Retin A, because they are so soothing and balancing. However, I would not recommend Retin A for wrinkles. I feel it is just too hard on your skin. You must stay out of the sun. It sloughs your skin too quickly. I also think the same about alpha hydroxy products; for most people, they are just too harsh.

It is, in my opinion, much better to use a pure botanical application. I like the honey and papaya blends. You can make them yourself. Just mix or blend fresh papaya with honey and apply to your skin for twenty minutes and rinse off. Another great way to stimulate and rejuvenate skin is to apply diluted pineapple juice, allow to sit on your skin, and then rinse. Diluted vinegar applied with a washcloth is another excellent peel.

Other excellent products to use when your skin is so sensitive due to the harmful effects of synthetic chemicals is a nice rich cream with lily, almond oil, and comfrey. Look for products that contain lots of healing herbs such as the ones outlined in this book. (See sections on Herbs and Essential Oils.) I make an herbal moisturizer with nineteen different healing herbs, plus aloe and vegetable glycerin.

Q: I use a petroleum jelly on my hands and face. Should I change?

A: Use what suits you. Again, if you are happy with the way the product performs and you understand the ingredients and that is what you want to use, that is your choice. You may find using olive oil, or almond or sunflower oil is more desirable. I like to use ingredients grown by Mother Nature, but that is my preference. I like to use products that have a life force.

Q: What will make me look younger?

A: Being happy!

After that, frequent moisturizing and misting your skin to keep it moist, lubricated, and hydrated. This will not only help your appearance, making your skin look more supple, but it will also aid in the long-term care of the skin.

Some people simply look old. During store demos, I will cleanse their skin with our herbal astringent on a cotton ball to remove the dirt and dead skin, and then apply a thin layer of our herbal moisturizer. For an added bonus, I add a couple drops of my Seven Exotic Oils, and they look ten years younger just because we have removed the dead skin cells and dirt and lubricated and hydrated their skin.

This is not just because our products are so great; it's because physically their skin is so dry it almost cracks when they smile. This not only causes long-lasting lines and loss of elasticity but makes them look a lot older. Never let your skin look or feel dry. I carry our herbal moisturizer and mist with me wherever I go to lubricate my skin constantly.

Exercise and get lots of fresh air and sunshine. Walk, run, skip, hike, inhale deep breaths of fresh air, and feel the sunshine on your body. Get your circulation going; get your cheeks naturally rosy.

You can also:

* Use steam masks to open your pores and let the essence of the herbs in.

* Use a botanical enzyme mask frequently (a commercial one or make your own).

* Reverse everything for a few minutes a day; stand on your head if you've been properly instructed, or lie on a slant board with your feet elevated.

* Eat your fruits and veggies.

* Juice, juice, juice—fresh juice to accompany or to replace meals: breakfast, lunch, or both.

* Do yoga, gentle postures or strenuous ones; you decide.

* Drink herbal teas to meet your needs.

* Learn about vitamin therapies and herbal supplements.

* Take Lily vinegar (see index).

* Be positive.

* Think kind thoughts.

* Be open.

* Eat an apple a day.

* Make a morning drink of spirulina, apple juice, brewer's yeast, alfalfa, and wheat grass; start with small amounts.

Q: What reverses sun damage?

A: If you have sun damage from decades of overexposing and daily sun-bathing, an exfoliant mask may help. I have had lots of customers tell me that botanical enzyme exfoliant masks can really help diminish some signs of damage. Use products with papaya and pineapple, lily, vitamin E, and comfrey.

Q: What products will firm up the skin on my face?
A: Horsetail and coltsfoot are very high in silica, which is said to help rebuild the collagen in your skin. Look for products made with them.

Q: I'm busy and I'm broke; what is one really good product I could buy that is simple and not too expensive?
A: If you are really busy, with normal skin, I'd say a mist. Mist after cleansing, mist again before bed. Use products with lavender. It is very balancing. Look for comfrey, which is very healing. If you are really dry, I'd say a rich cream containing comfrey root, lily, rosehip seed oil, primrose oil, and rosemary. Another option for dry skin is to use just a high-quality oil, preferably with calendula, chamomile, and rose.

As a matter of fact, the reason I came up with my face and body flower oil is to provide a product for people who demand quality but don't have a lot of money. About ten years ago, I did product demonstrations at Wild Oats on East Colfax Street in Denver. It is located by the Hare Krishna temple, so many Krishnas come in to shop. They'd come up to me and say, "Oh, Lily of Colorado, I love your products. They are so fresh and clean." I would beam to receive such generous compliments. Finally, after many compliments but no sales from them, I had to ask, "So, do you want to buy any?" And they would chant, "I wish I could, but I'm a 'renunciate,' and I don't have any money for any extras." So, of course, I had to give them free samples!

My sister is the same way. She buys little but only has the finest quality things. She's extremely particular and has only a few skin care products. "I need to come up with a product that anyone can afford," I decided. Thus the Lily of Colorado Face and Body Flower Oil was born. I made it to be versatile and multi-purpose. You can cleanse your face with this oil and a soft, wet cloth. You can then moisturize with it. You can put it in your bath and on your hair as a hot-oil treatment.

If you suffer from acne and blemishes and were to buy only one product, I would recommend either buying a blend of herbs to steam daily or an astringent that contained lavender, lily, witch hazel, and calendula. You can cleanse your face with it and a cotton ball throughout the day if you don't wear makeup. You can put a little in your bath. And you can put two tablespoons in water to rinse your hair. Happily, you *can* be on a strict budget and still take beautiful care of your skin.

Q: I'm just getting started in all this health and herb lifestyle. Where do I begin?

A: Start at your nearest health food store. I find the health food stores I've been to across the country are like libraries, full to the brim with knowledge and information. The employees at the average health food store are about the highest caliber, most educated bunch of people you'll come across. It's amazing how bright and intelligent these people are everywhere in the country. Health food stores just naturally attract this special breed of up-beat people. I dare say that virtually every health food store strives to serve each customer to its utmost. The workers are trained and there to help you solve your problems and satisfy your needs.

Q: What are the best products for a teenager with breakouts?

A: If the teenager has only a few pimples, a good topical ointment with tea tree oil, calendula, and/or essential oil of lavender is generally beneficial. If the youngster has serious breakouts or acne, I would try to balance the hormones and boost self-esteem.

The bigger problem here can be the self-image, not the acne. As we all well remember, adolescence is a very important, yet frustrating and confusing time in one's life. It's a time when looking good is everything. So a parent has to be aware of how devastating this time can be. You must be sensitive and supportive and help clear up the breakouts.

Try one or more of the following: applying topically the vinegar wash we talked about and drinking Lily's vinegar drink, green drinks, steaming the face and the body, and taking dong quai and vitex for a female. Try to get them to eat lots of roughage and fresh apples. You may want to consult an acupuncturist, or try homeopathy. If the acne persists, see a dermatologist but be very careful regarding what is prescribed and whether your child should participate in the treatment.

For example, in the 1970s, tetracycline was often prescribed. Luckily for me, my parents could never afford the medication, so I hardly ever took it. Why was I lucky? Because tetracycline yellowed your teeth; okay, so now your skin is clear but all your teeth are the color of the lines down the middle of the road.

Accutane is another potentially dangerous cure. A mandatory pregnancy test must be given each week, because it is that potentially harmful to a fetus. We must consider then what else it might be negatively affecting.

It is valuable for parents to try to shift some of the focus of attention to other positive attributes of the child. Maybe they have a gift for art or excel in math or history. Be active about this. Help them understand that while this condition is unpleasant, it's not what is fundamental. Point out that you understand this may seem paramount in their own world, but that many other teenagers on the planet are suffering in much more fundamental ways.

Teach your kid to focus on the positive. Nobody gets all the breaks. My mother used to say all the time, "What makes you think life is fair?"

Focus on their other physical attributes, telling them how lovely a smile or engaging laugh they have. Encourage them to do interesting and exciting things, take ski trips, hike, learn Spanish, for instance. While good looks are great to have, they are not what really makes our life worth living. Substance is—and knowing what is important in life.

Q: The skin around my eyes is constantly flaky and makes me look older. What can I do?

A: There are far fewer oil glands around the eyes, so the delicate skin there is likely to be dry in anyone over eighteen. It is important for people with this condition to use high-quality creams, lotions, or herbal moisturizers that contain ingredients like primrose oil, rosehip seed oil, chamomile, calendula, comfrey, and almond, which all greatly benefit the skin.

Never apply a product, any product, close enough for it to get in the eye. The very best idea is to treat this area yourself with fresh kitchen cosmetics, where you control all the ingredients and know they are free of harsh chemicals and bacteria. Exfoliate with a natural botanical mask with ingredients like papaya, pineapple, and comfrey. Or make your own mixing fresh papaya and pineapple with honey or yogurt. Then moisturize with a rich cream or use oils and an herbal moisturizer. You can also simply apply a light oil of kukui or almond, or mix the oil with an essential oil.

Q: Why is it better to buy products at a health food store, rather than a grocery or department store?

A: The likelihood of finding superior products in the health food store is greater than anywhere else. So I buy my body care products only there. I would not buy them anywhere else, except maybe directly from a manufacturer who makes them up fresh in small batches.

You, as a consumer, need to be able to determine a pure, clean product for yourself. Some of you may have much more critical standards than others. For me, I only want purely botanical™, agriculturally derived ingredients for my skin.

The "green" fad with the large companies is just that, a fad. Next year they will be on to the next trend, but the health food store will continue to provide you with clean products whether they are in mainstream fashion or not.

Q: What is wrong with petroleum products?
A: Nothing. I put them in my car every week.

A lot of people have problems with the oil companies. I, however, have a hard time bad-mouthing companies from which I buy products. I do think it would be a good idea for the world, particularly America, to implement some serious incentives to decrease our dependency on crude oils, or anything else we as a nation can't seem to live without.

I personally have always valued being as removed from the grid as far as I feasibly can be. That value must be hereditary because my Mom has four sources of power at her house: wood, propane, electricity, and, for emergencies, a diesel generator that could be converted to waste oil. My sister only has wood heat in her house. I lived eleven years without any source of heat other than wood and a blow dryer.

Q: Do I want to put petro products on my skin?
A: I would answer this question "no," for me. But you have to answer this question for yourself. This is not a philosophical or political question. This is a simple ingredient question. "Which do I think would benefit my skin best, lavender, calendula, lily, and essential oil of ylang ylang, or mineral oil and parabens?"

I feel similarly about synthetics. I use synthetic products everyday, but I wouldn't want to ingest or put them on my skin.

Q: Is your company political?
A: No. Like most people in the world, I want children to have childhoods free of abuse, famine, and psychological hardship that will inhibit them from being loving, responsible, productive, happy adults. I want people to have opportunities to be able to make their life the best they can be, to be able to think for themselves, be financially independent from the government, and to be educated enough to make their own decisions. I want us to be able to pass down a clean and healthy planet to our children, and I want to work hard to support people and companies that are trying to make the world a better place.

I want to be a positive force on the planet. My company has already helped me do that. It is the best thing that ever happened to me as a person. I have learned so much, in every way—personally, profession-ally, about business, skin care, health, life, herbs, and ingredients. I have made so many dear and wonderful friends; I am twice as happy and ten times as healthy. If the company went belly-up tomorrow and all my hard work over the last ten to twelve years went down the drain, I wouldn't trade the experience for anything.

Q: Was your dad an organic farmer?
A: No. My dad was actually a proponent of the productivity of pesti-cides. In addition to farming, he supported our family for many years selling farm chemicals. He truly believed this method was best.

We did for many years have a very large organic garden for the ben-efit of city friends of my parents from a "hippie church" we attended in the late 1960s and early 1970s. They would come to the farm and work the garden.

Q: I have dry patches on my skin. What can help them?
A: Many herbs and oils have been effective to combat all dry skin prob-lems. For example, calendula blossoms have been revered by herbalists for centuries for just about every sort of skin ailment, including dry patches. Long tradition claims comfrey root contains cell-regenerative properties. Herbs high in silica have been found to help dry patches. Most notable are horsetail and coltsfoot. Many oils work wonderfully on dry skin. My favorite blend is rosehip seed, almond, and primrose oils. Vita-min E softens and lubricates, and wheat germ oil is skin nourishing.

Q: What products do you use?
A: I use all of our products, and I go through phases where I will use something a lot and then start using something else. I am very attached to my Lily Herbal Moisturizer, both for sentimental reasons—it was my first product and the one I have used the most over the years— and because I can use it under or over makeup; it's nice and light to wear all day. It is viscous and I like that feel. It feels like it is really staying on, and of course, I love the ingredients.

I use a lot of my herbal astringent. I use it twice a day to clean my face; I also put it in my bath and often times will steam my face with just one-fourth cup of herbal astringent in the water.

I switch off and on between the seaweed cleanser and the Lily cleanser in my bath to cleanse my entire body. I also use the Botanical Enzyme Exfoliant almost daily in the bathtub, too. Nightly, I use the Seven Exotic

Oils in my hair. I brush my hair out and put them in it, and my hair just soaks it right up. If I put a very heavy layer of oil on my hair, I can hit it with the blow dryer, which really increases penetration. When I am feeling really dry, I put the Seven Exotic Oils on my face at night, usually in the winter months. I keep a flower oil in my bathroom to use all over my body sometimes, and because I like the way the oil looks.

The lip moisturizer and the mist are always around me. I have a set of each in my car, at my desk, in my bathroom, living room, and bedroom. I also spray the mist in my hair, use it as a perfume, and spray it on my pillow before I go to bed.

I switch off and on between creams. I will use the original cream for dry skin on my legs; it is too rich for my face. And I will use the lavender cream all over my body and sometimes as a night cream. In the summer months, I sometimes use the lotion instead of the creams.

Q: Do you have any products with sunscreen?

A: No. (See the section on sunscreens.)

Q: What do you think is the best eye cream, day cream, night cream, etc.?

A: I do not subscribe to the theory that you need different products for every separate area of your body. One or two good products should suit you. For example, if you have dry skin and you use my dry skin moisturizing cream at night and are happy with it, you will probably be happy with it during the day. If you find you prefer something rich at night but not during the day, then you could purchase the lotion or the herbal moisturizer, or the lavender cream for during the day. But I want to stress again that you don't need separate products for the eye area, day, night, décolletage, etc. Buy one good product and use it in as many ways as you feel comfortable.

Caution: When using a product around the eye area, do not get it into eyes or let it leach into eyes. Any product can contain bacteria, and many preservatives can be dangerous to the eye area as well.

Q: What are the parabens, and why are they bad?

A: The parabens, or para-hydroxybenzoic acid esters—which include what I refer to as the "paraben sisters"—methyl, butyl, and propyl—are used as preservatives. They are synthetic chemicals. I am not saying they are bad, just undesirable in my opinion, compared to essential oils and to grapefruit seed extract, or a fresh product you just made yourself.

Q: Why don't you make a shampoo?

A: I have made many shampoos for my own use, but I have not yet made one good enough to go to market. It takes me years of trial and error to come up with a clean, high-performance product.

Q: What is best for the eye area in general, under-eye lines, and bags under eyes?

A: The best products for the eye area are ones you make up fresh yourself that day, for a couple of reasons. First, it is best to feed your skin, particularly the delicate eye area, with as nutritious and healthful products as possible and to have the added life force of a product that is fresh off the vine, which will really benefit your skin.

Second, if you make the product yourself, then you not only control all the wonderful ingredients that the product is made of, but you also know it is free from any harsh and damaging chemicals as well as mold or bacteria that arise from a product aging.

I would say the best thing for under-eye puffiness is sliced cucumbers, but you can also apply sliced apples, potatoes, or damp, cold, black tea bags.

Q: I want to move to Colorado and start an herbal business. What do you think?

A: Move to Colorado? Well, lots of people are doing it. I did it in 1975, and there was a big boom going on then, too.

I first moved to Boulder, and it was then a sleepy little hippie town. It's not really like that anymore. It is a very educated town with the average Boulderite possessing a master's degree. It's very expensive and Denver is right behind it, with an average house selling for somewhere around $211,000. Getting to the mountains on the weekends is a very hectic thing to do. The return traffic is especially a mess on Sunday nights.

The sun shines all of the time and I love living here. This is so "home" to me. But to move here now while there is such a boom going on would be difficult.

On the other hand, do what you know is going to be right for you. If you are sure moving to Colorado is for you, then do it. Colorado is a high-profile place between our sports teams, blizzards, and the bizarre.

On starting an herbal business, there's more than meets the eye in going into business. It's a long haul—a long time till it pays its own way—a big investment of time, energy, and money. Government forms and meeting regulations, meeting payroll, meeting deadlines, long hours, and many elements are beyond your control.

There are lots of areas to research: Who's your market? How to reach them? Can you survive till the company makes money? Do you have a back-up plan?

Entrepreneurs are risktakers. Do you have the capacity to take risks, to dare losing what you have? While some people can't handle the uncertainties being in business presents, others love the roller coaster ride. Determine which kind you are before taking this big step.

Don't be fooled into thinking going into business makes you the boss! If you're growing herbs, you're not—Mother Nature is. The market is. Your buyer is.

Lots of books are available at libraries and bookstores, and courses are available at colleges on going into business. Agricultural colleges and county agents hold field days and short courses open to the public. Don't miss a chance to learn.

It's a bit like choosing your skin care products; *you* have to decide what's right for *you*. If, after self-study and research, you decide to go into business, go for it! Good luck!

Q: Do you think any topically applied cosmetic product in a bottle can reverse the aging process?

A: No. Now saying that, I'll expound. Many companies claim that their alpha hydroxy acids do that, but is that the case, or do they expedite the aging process by exfoliating the skin at an extremely accelerated pace? I think that natural acid exfoliation is a good thing, especially if it is from honey or some other extremely soothing substance. However, I think you want to be really careful speeding up the sloughing of your skin to any extreme.

Cleansing, toning, nourishing, and moisturizing your skin is fundamentally important and can make a great difference in the appearance of your skin, especially as the years pass. We all have met people whose skin looks much older than their age. Sometimes, fast-aging skin can be caused by a hereditary factor. Often it can be from physical abuse of one's body. Serious, continuous, heavy drinking and smoking, malnutrition, lack of adequate sleep over a year or decade, and being consistently unhappy seems to give people permanent frown lines.

Just as important is keeping your insides cleansed, toned, nourished, and moisturized. You need to keep your thoughts and food clean and positive. You need to keep your intestines cleansed. "An apple a day" can be a good and easy way to start helping your intestines. Studies proved an apple a day is a beneficial practice. A colonic can be beneficial if you are going to make some serious changes in your life and want to jump on a fresh start.

As I said earlier, Mae West, the glamorous movie star of the 1920s and 1930s, used to do a daily enema and drink fresh carrot juice. She attributed her longevity, good health, and good looks to that. By the way, even though she always portrayed herself as a "party girl," she never smoked, drank, or went to parties offscreen.

Keeping your thoughts clean can demand a lot of discipline. If you are having trouble with the same old "baggage," you may want to consider therapy, rolfing, yoga, meditation, or joining a church or spiritual group.

You need to keep your internal organs toned through herbal teas and supplements, and physical exercise. Yoga especially helps keep your organs toned. Mother Nature has traditionally been relied on to help in this area. Dandelion root tea helps keep your liver toned, cranberry helps your kidneys, burdock root helps cleanse the blood, and red clover helps stimulate the lymphatic system.

You need to nourish your body and give it the proper fuel to operate efficiently. You can start by simply bringing into your life good, enjoyable, and healthful things. If you are just getting started on these lifestyle changes, you may want to start by simply taking vitamins and an herb or two every morning. Now what could be a more simple and easy way to get started? It takes about ten seconds a day, and then you will start feeling better and have more energy to add another helpful and beneficial thing, like starting to drink one cup of an herb tea per day that has something you need in it. For example, if you are over-anxious and stressed, start drinking a cup of chamomile tea every night. Be kind to yourself. Start to love and nourish yourself. (See the The Lily Method chapter for more ideas.)

You also need to moisturize your body two ways. You need to make sure you are getting enough high-quality fats, such as olive oil. Almost everyone needs these high-quality fats to moisturize your body from the inside out, especially if you have dry skin and live in a dry climate and are thin. If you are overweight and have oily skin, it may not be as important.

Q: How do you obtain your essential oils?

A: I purchase my essential oils already distilled; we have over 100 suppliers.

Q: Why is there sometimes a sediment in your products?

A: Since my products are purely botanical™, I make them with herbs and strain them many times by hand; sometimes there will be a residue sediment. Frankly, that is a good sign and indication of a purely natural product.

Q: Do Lily products have shelf life, or do they need to be refrigerated?

A: I guarantee to stores that my products will have a one-year shelf life. That means if they deteriorate, I will replace them for the store. Since my company makes its products fresh every week, I recommend stores only purchase what they can sell in a month or so; that way the consumer will always have a fresh product. We want people to use up our products right away. You can keep them in the refrigerator for extra freshness, but if you just buy them and use them, that should not be necessary.

Q: Where does the marvelous scent of Lily products come from?

A: All of the Lily products are scented only with 100% pure essential oils. Lavender and ylang ylang are my favorites, so therefore you will find many of them with those essential oils. The Oil of Kukui and Herbal Moisturizer are not scented at all; the scent of the Herbal Moisturizer is simply the natural scent of the blended herbs, and the Oil of Kukui is just the natural scent of the oil. The reason many people do not recognize the scents is because most scents these days are synthetic and most companies do not go to the trouble or expense of using pure essential oils.

Q: Are all the herbs in Lily products grown organically?

A: No, I wish. While organically grown herbs are becoming more plentiful, they are still not widely and consistently available. We do not want to put "organically grown" on products and then have trouble keeping that promise. We use organically grown whenever we can. Approximately 80% of our herbs are organic.

Q: What skin types are Lily products formulated for?

A: We have many products that are for specific skin types, but the American consumer does not seem ready for the concept that many natural products do not need to be limited to specific skin types. For example, lavender historically has been used for oily skin and then again for dry skin; it has been used as an aphrodisiac and again to remain chaste. The point is, it is balancing. Herbs and essential oils are composed of the same chemical compounds as your body. Synthetic ingredients are designed by man to do one specific thing. For example, detergents are made to reduce surface tension and do so very effectively, and part of that process is to strip dirt and oils. So maybe you would use a detergent on oily skin, but never, never on dry skin. Botanicals are not like that. Soapwort can be used on any skin type, but it doesn't produce much lather, and we have been conditioned to believe that soaps should lather.

Q: What are the active ingredients in your products?

A: Every ingredient is an active ingredient in any product. Every ingredient you put in a product is going to change the chemical consistency of the product, whether you want it to or not. So this question comes from a person who has bought into a commercialized mindset that doesn't believe every ingredient is already active. My mindset is that a product cannot perform better than its ingredients, all of which are active.

Q: What makes your products different?

A: My company is one of the very few in the world that makes a truly pure and clean line of products. This means, with the exception of a clay ingredient, bee products, and soap ingredients, our products are purely botanical™. Just look on the label. Use our products once, and if you do not see, smell, and feel the difference, don't buy them. How many companies do you know that can make the following statements about their products:

No parabens, propylene glycol, or urea

Nothing synthetic or artificial or petroleum-derived

Only use pure essential oils

Use kukui, primrose oil, and rosehip seed oil

Made fresh weekly

Performance-formulated products

100% guaranteed for consumers

Best customer service around!

Q: How do you do most of your herbal extractions?

A: We do hydroglycolic herbal extractions on most of our herbs, which is a slow-heat process in water. We extract some in oils and resinous materials, like bee propolis, which we extract in alcohol and then use an alcohol evaporation process.

Q: Why do some natural and pure products sometimes feel sticky?

A: When you only use natural ingredients, you only have the natural consistency and viscosity of that ingredient, unless you chemically alter it by adding another ingredient, usually something synthetic like carbomer, which is a man-made substance to perform just the task of reducing stickiness. Or man-made formulations start with something that is synthetic and therefore never have that problem to begin with. There is also value added to a moisturizing product that is viscous, such as honey or vegetable glycerin. They are usually a humectant, and their sticky nature is what makes them effective in drawing moisture from the air to your skin. So, especially for dry skin or people in really dry climates, stickiness is a benefit. But we as a culture have been "chemicalized" and have bought into a mindset that believes moisturizers should be white, creamy, maybe even pearl-colored, and preserved to last well into the next century.

Q: How did you get into this business?

A: My dad was a pomologist and horticulturist, euphemisms for a farmer with a formal education. My sister became a vegetarian at five years old, but the bottom-line reason is I have always had awful skin. I've been to many dermatologists, have had three dermabrasion treatments (and laser skin resurfacing), spent tens of thousands of dollars, and searched the world over to find cures. Finally, I just began believing that all the men, with all their scientific degrees, in all the labs around the world, would never come up with anything to heal skin as perfect as a plant.

Q: Do you have an organic farm?

A: Yes. My company does operate an organic farm. It's more of a "farmette," affectionately referred to as "Rancho Starvo." Last year, we planted chamomile, calendula, lavender, sage, and comfrey. This year we planted many trees. The intention is to be able to grow and control our quality and supply of herbs; however, it hasn't quite happened yet.

Q: What makes products work—the fancy packaging, the big price, the cetyl alcohol, the parabens, the propylene glycol, what?

A: The ingredients make it work—or not. This is how I got started. I wanted to know what the difference was between products from big-name companies. Is this pricey one worth paying five times as much for?

Does it work better? Okay, why does it work better and what ingredient makes it an effective moisturizer, an effective treatment for acne? What specific ingredient in this jar makes it work? Every ingredient we put in every product not only is active but is placed in the preparation for a specific purpose, to function as it has historically. For example, our mist contains seaweeds to soothe and attract moisture, lily because it helps reduce scars, chamomile for its anti-inflammatory action, calendula for its anti-spasmodic and skin-relaxing action, and comfrey for its cell-proliferation properties. The vegetable glycerin helps the product and your skin retain moisture, essential oil of lavender is anti-bacterial and balancing on your skin, ylang ylang is an anti-depressant, and the grapefruit seed extract is high in Vitamin C and is a preservative. Remember: A product cannot perform better than its ingredients.

Q: Does Lily of Colorado test on animals?
A: No. When we come up with a new product, we test it on our present customers, my family, and friends and do lengthy in-house testing. We do long-term incubation at temperatures perfectly conducive to mold and bacterial growth.

Q: Will Lily products keep me from aging?
A: No. Hopefully, if you are lucky, you will age. You will get old, have grandchildren, collect social security, and get wrinkles. But you don't have to rush the process. I believe Mother Nature is the best cure for Father Time. Maybe someone else believes that the chemical companies have more going for them. That's okay. Again, you choose.

Q: Are all of your products pH balanced?
A: We do not routinely do pH testing. We usually do it in the developmental stages and as part of the overall testing in the beginning, before putting a product on the market. When you make a natural and clean product, a purely botanical™ product, you cannot guarantee 100% consistency. You can only do that with synthetics. When you make fresh salsa or green chili or vegetable soup, it is never identical. It depends on where and when the tomatoes are harvested, how much rainfall that year, and how much care they had. Did they have a freeze that season? How much were they watered? What was the consistency of the soil? Were they grown in sunny California or overcast Michigan? Were they grown in a hothouse? What variety are they? When were

they harvested—early, late? Are they ripe? Did they ripen on the vine or in your refrigerator? Have they been in cold storage and for how long? Mother Nature has many variables; the synthetic manufacturers do not. That is also why more companies do not make a pure product.

Q: Are your products non-comedogenic?

A: A product is only its ingredients. Some ingredients may irritate some skins and/or clog pores, while other skins may experience no ill effects at all. So you would need to look down the ingredients list and independently decide which ones you think are safe for you.

Q: Do you do ongoing research about ingredients to use in your products?

A: Yes. I read articles and books in the field to keep up with current research, and I check out places, healers, products wherever I travel. In February 1999, I went to Brazil and the Amazon Basin, where I visited the Amazon Research Center in Manaus. While there, I found two herbs to test as coloring agents in makeup.

Q: Why do natural creams and lotions sometimes just seem to sit on my skin and not penetrate?

A: You are clearly using a product that is too rich for your skin. Try wetting your hands and then applying sparingly and gently rubbing it into your skin.

For more information on Lily of Colorado products or to mail order products, call (800) 333-LILY (5459) or write P.O. Box 12471, Denver, Colorado 80212, or visit us at www.lilyofcolorado.com. Or simply ask for our products at your local health food store.

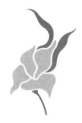

A Skin Care Dictionary

Acetone: Used as a solvent in many skin care products; it is a volatile liquid. Synthetically made, it is often used in nail polish remover, astringents, and toners. Acetone is toxic.

Agrimony: This astringent herb is useful in preparations for oily, acne-prone skin with large pores.

Alcohol: It can be synthetically or petroleum derived, as with isopropyl alcohol, or it can be naturally derived from fermenting carbohydrates, as with grain alcohol or vodka.

Alcohols: A large group of compounds often found in volatile oils. Waxes are a combination of alcohols and fatty acids.[*]

Alginates: Seaweeds that aid waste elimination and dermal circulation.

Alkaloid: Any nitrogenous organic base, especially one of vegetable origin.

Alkanet: A member of the borage family; the root of the plant is a natural red coloring agent.

Allantoin: A crystalline oxidation product of uric acid used to promote healing. It can be synthetically derived; the best natural source of this is the plant comfrey.

Almond oil: See sweet almond oil.

---

[*] Richard Mabey, *The New Age Herbalist*, New York, NY: Macmillan Publishing Company, 1988.

Almond Oil Soft Soap: Lily of Colorado's own homemade, mild, cleansing soap, made with no detergents; gentle for the face.

Aloe vera: An extract from the aloe vera plant that soothes irritated or burned skin. Anti-inflammatory and powerfully healing. A member of the lily family, it has been used through the ages in moisturizers and cell-therapy treatments because it contains biogenic stimulators and wound-healing powers.

Alpha: Of or relating to one of two or more closely related chemical substances. Used somewhat arbitrarily. Used to specify ordinal relationship or to specify a particular physical form.

Amorphous: Without definite form or shape. Formless, like a cloud or dust, not allowing clear classification or analysis.

Apigenin: A yellowish crystalline compound, occurring usually as glycosides in various plants.

Aqua Herbal Complex: Includes seaweed, laminaria, and bladderwrack. These sea botanicals are known as superb moisturizers. Many seaweeds dry easily with much shrinkage, then become firm yet elastic in water. They may be kept for years and will absorb moisture at any time and swell to their original size.

Arnica: Soothes skin externally, relaxes stiff muscles, relieves pain, inflammation, and bruising. Anti-varicose and anti-blotchiness.

Azulene: A liquid hydrocarbon of intense blue color found in some essential oils, such as chamomile.

Balsams: The resins derived from trees, usually oily or gummy. They can have a positive effect in products for the hair and skin.

Bassorin: A substance obtained from certain gums that is insoluble in water but swells to form a gel.

Bee propolis: Healing to open, slow-healing sores, with direct anti-bacterial activity. Inhibits microbe growth. Gathered by bees from trees to coat the opening of the hive for sterilization of all that enters. Good acne treatment.

Beer: A fermented liquor brewed, especially by slow fermentation, from malt or from a mixture of malt and malt substitutes, and flavored with hops or other bitters. Allowed to become stale, it can be used as a setting lotion.

Beeswax: An emollient and thickener in many products, it is obtained from the honeycomb of the bee's hive.

Benzoin tree gum: This tree gum has antiseptic, astringent, and possibly preservative characteristics.

Bladderwrack: A soothing skin treatment, this sea plant has detoxifying capabilities for the skin. See Aqua Herbal Complex.

Borax: a.k.a. sodium borate; a naturally occurring mineral, it stiffens creams and is used as an emulsifier. A popular alkali, it is also called sodium tetraborate. It emulsifies fats, mixing them with water.

Buttermilk: This sour liquid left after the butterfat in milk has been made into butter can be applied as a mask for oily skin. It is also a mild bleach for skin.

Calendula: Also known as marigold, this flower's use dates back thousands of years for the treatment of scorpion bites in ancient Egypt, reducing inflammation almost instantly when the flower is directly applied. Beneficial for soreness and cell regeneration.

Camphor oil: An essential oil very beneficial for acne and inflammation. It stimulates the circulation.

Candelilla: Derived from a shrub, it is a natural wax.

Cantaloupe: A fruit of the melon family that helps control oily hair. One of the least acidic fruits.

Capsules: Herbs are powdered and placed in gelatin capsules. Capsules are a good way to avoid the bitterness of the herb and an easy way to take the herb internally at regular intervals.

Carnauba: A natural wax from a palm tree grown in South America.

Carotene: A precursor of vitamin A, it occurs naturally in plants. It consists of three isomers: about 15% alpha, 85% beta, and 0.1% gamma. Its properties are ruby red crystals, easily oxidized on contact with the air. Insoluble in water; slightly soluble in alcohol, ether, and oils. Occurs as an orange yellow pigment in plant and animal tissue, butter, eggs, sweet potatoes, alfalfa, rye, and wheat. Carotene is produced in comparatively pure form by extraction from carrots and from palm oil concentrates, and by a chromatographic process from alfalfa. Carotene is a hydrocarbon member of a large class of pigments called carotenoids. It has the same basic molecular structure as vitamin A and is transformed into the vitamin in the animal or human liver.

Carotenoid: Any of the several highly unsaturated pigments, most of which are yellow, orange, or red, occurring widely in plants. Crystalline solids; soluble in fats and oils; insoluble in water; high melting; stable to alkali but unstable to acids and to oxidizing agents; color easily destroyed by hydrogenation or by oxidation.

Carrageenan: This usually refers to the mucilage derived from Irish moss; an emulsifier and very healing.

Castor oil: Oil derived from the castor bean, used on dry hair.

Cetyl alcohol: Usually produced synthetically, this is a waxy solid alcohol often used as an emulsifier or thickener.

Chamomile: A remarkable botanical with anti-inflammatory action from azulene. Chamomile is useful to soothe and normalize rough skin, relieve pain, and heal wounds. Antiseptic.

Chestnut: The smooth-shelled, sweet, edible nut of any of a group of trees in the beech family. Extract of chestnut is effective for treatment of blotchy, varicose skin conditions.

Chlorophyll: Derived from the green matter of plants, it is used as an antiseptic, as an odor absorber, and a natural coloring agent. Chlorophyll performs an important function in plant life. Usually extracted from alfalfa, it is great in anti-inflammation products, to reduce pus and heal the skin, and in anti-wrinkle products.

Citric acid: Derived naturally from citrus fruits by a fermenting process. It is used as a pH adjuster, preservative, and sequestering agent.

Citrus seed extract: See grapefruit seed extract.

Cocoa butter: Naturally occurring fat expressed from the seeds of the cacao tree. Cocoa butter melts at body temperature. It is great for stretch marks and is used in many cream formulas to thicken them.

Coconut oil: Expressed from the kernel of the seeds of the coconut palm. It is stable in air and can remain years without refrigeration. Used as an emollient.

Coltsfoot: An herb abundant in silica, essential for connective tissue health.

Comfrey root: Claimed by long-standing tradition to contain a considerable amount of flesh-forming substance, thus used as a cell proliferate. Helps lacerations grow back together. Therefore, a great anti-wrinkle cream ingredient.

Compress: Also known as a fomentation. A compress is usually recommended for swelling, pains, flu, or colds. It is an external treatment, working like an ointment with the added benefit of heat. Many herbalists recommend a compress when the needed herbs are too strong to be taken internally; with the compress, only small amounts will be absorbed into the skin. To prepare a compress or fomentation, bring one to two tablespoons of the needed herbs to a boil in approximately eight ounces of water. After the herbs are strained, dip gauze or cotton cloth into the liquid, drain off the excess liquid, and place the warm cloth on the affected area immediately. Then cover the wet cloth with a dry cloth, preferably wool. When the compress cools, apply another warm one.

Cornmeal: Ground corn used as a light scrub in cleansers and useful as a dry hair cleanser.

Corn oil: From wet milling of the corn grains, a very heavy oil with a high unsaturate content. Not often used in cosmetics.

Cornstarch: From the grains of corn as a water extract, contains amylose and amylopectin. An excellent powder; can also be dissolved in creams or used alone in the bath. Great for itchy or dry skin.

Cucumber: A long, green-skinned vegetable with firm, white flesh, used in salads and preserved as pickles. Cool and soothing to the skin.

Decoction: This is a method often used for extraction of the hard parts of plants, bark, seeds, or roots to obtain the bitter principles of plants. It is best if the herb is cut in small pieces and boiled in four parts water to one part of the herb until one third of the water has evaporated—about 25 minutes. While still hot, strain the herbs. It helps the extraction process if the herb is soaked in cold water first and then brought to a boil. Decoctions are best if used soon after preparation.

Dry skin: Dry skin has small fine pores and tightens upon smiling. It has a tendency to wrinkle much earlier than oilier skin and needs constant moisture by manually applying lotions, creams, and mists so facial expressions don't cause permanent lines.

Elderberries: Small dark berries of the elder plant. A gently firming, astringing herb used topically on the skin.

Elder flowers: See elderberries.

Emollients: The agents in products that lubricate the skin; they soothe, soften, and protect the skin to keep it supple and help it retain moisture, and therefore fight wrinkles.

Emulsifiers: The ingredients that help the product mix or emulsify. Natural emulsifiers are lecithin, carrageenan, and processes such as blending or shaking.

Essential oils: The "blood" or life force of plants, these liquids are distilled in high concentrations and possess potent, aromatherapeutic qualities. Many have historic uses, and they are effective as botanical preservatives, especially when used synergistically.

Esterification: Resulting from the reaction of an alcohol and an acid.

Esters: Organic compounds corresponding in structure to salts in inorganic chemistry. They may be considered as derived from the acids by the exchange of the replaceable hydrogen of the acid for an organic alkyl radical. Esters are not ionic compounds, but salts usually are.

Ethanol: Or called ethyl alcohol, this is the base of common alcoholic ingredients. It is used as a preservative and as a disinfectant.

Eucalyptus leaf: The leaf of the eucalyptus tree. Has antiseptic, wound-healing qualities, with a cooling effect on the skin.

Eyebright: A small European herb of the figwort family with white, yellow, or purple flowers, used in treating diseases of the eye. Traditionally used in preparations for around the eyes, this herb's tannic acids (natural, non-drying astringents) are effective for inflammation around the eyes.

Fennel seeds: Antiseptic botanical known for its varied uses.

Feverfew: Known to relieve swelling, this herb softens and desensitizes the skin.

Flavone: A colorless crystalline ketone found as a dust on the leaves, stems, and seed capsules of many primroses. Also prepared synthetically.

Flavonoid: Of, relating to, or like flavone or isoflavone in chemical structure. Or a flavonoid compound (as a plant pigment).

Flavonoid glycosides: A common group of plant chemicals named from their yellow color and their wide variety of uses, including diuretic, anti-spasmodic, and circulatory stimulants.

Ginseng: An adaptogenic herb that is helpful in strengthening the skin's response to stress.

Glucose: A form of natural crystalline sugar. Occurs in fruits and other foods and reacts chemically with starch. It is often used as a thickener in skin care products.

Glycerine: a.k.a. glycerin or glycerol; an odorless, colorless, syrupy liquid, prepared by the hydrolysis of fats and oils, which can be naturally or animal derived or synthetic. You need to be careful when purchasing, because the synthetic and the natural appear to be identical, so it is best to buy only pure vegetable glycerin that is kosher so you know it is vegetable derived. It is often used as a humectant, emollient, and emulsifier.

Glycols: Are formed by reacting glycerine with alcohol; they can be natural, but most are synthetic.

Glycosides: These plant chemicals consist of molecules made up of two sections, one of which is a sugar.

Grapefruit seed extract: a.k.a. citrus seed extract; natural preservative made from the seeds of the fruit, glycerin, and an UV light process. An anti-microbial solution that, when used in small proportions and sometimes combined with essential oils and vitamins A, C, and E, is a reliable preservative for botanical products.

Gums: Many gums are resins from trees: gum arabic or gum acacia, gum tragacanth, xanthan gum, and gum benzoin. They are used as emulsifiers and thickeners.

Hectorite mineral: A clay usually from volcanic origin. It is used as an emulsifier in natural products and as a natural emulsifying and binding agent in cosmetics.

Honey: This amazing bee product has many uses in healthy skin care. It has powerful, wound-healing abilities is a humectant (draws moisture from the air to the skin).

Hops: This herb possesses several valuable skin-enhancing properties: soothing, toning, anti-inflammatory, and anti-microbial. Important in treating psoriasis and eczema.

Horsetail: An herb with exceptional silica content, it is vital to the elasticity of the skin. It lends its texturizing ability to the silica, which is like a collagen to the skin, except in vegetable form.

Humectant: Humectants are ingredients that are capable of bringing moisture from the air to your skin. They help a product retain moisture and attract moisture. Natural humectants include vegetable glycerin and honey. Often humectants are sticky by nature; they help maintain a product's richness and can aid in the emulsion process. Many companies use synthetic glycols like propylene glycol, butylene glycol, and ethylene glycol, perhaps because they are easier, more available, cheaper, and do have the sticky consistency of the natural humectants.

Hydroglycolic: A slow-heat process.

Hydromel: A liquor, usually unfermented, consisting of honey diluted with water; when fermented, it is called mead.

Hygeia: In Greek mythology, the goddess of health; daughter of Aesculapius, the god of medicine.

Hygro: A combining form from the word *hygros,* meaning wet, denoting relation to moisture.

Imidazolidinyl urea: According to the *Natural Health Handbook 1995,* in their "Retailer's Guide to Natural Products": "Imidazolidinyl urea is a synthetic formaldehyde compound used as a preservative and sequestering agent in baby shampoos, moisturizing creams, eye shadows, and hair tonics."[*] Many skin care companies use it in creams as a preservative.

Inulin: A tasteless, white, non-digestible polysaccharide that occurs usually in place of starch in many composite and other plants.

Irish moss seaweed: A thick sea vegetable that soothes, detoxifies, and heals with its naturally occurring mucilage when used in cosmetics.

---

[*] Mark Bittman, *Natural Health Handbook 1995, Retailer's Guide to Natural Products,* Brookline Village, MA: Boston Common Press Ltd. Partnership, 1995, p. 106.

Isomers: Molecules that contain the same number and kind of atoms but differ in structure.

Isomorphism: The condition in which two or more entirely different substances have closely similar crystal structures, lattice dimensions, and chemical composition.

Isopropyl alcohol: A petro-chemical derivative.

Ivy: An herb that helps improve the appearance of dull skin by stimulating the skin.

Jojoba oil: A wonderful oil for the hair made from the seeds of the jojoba shrub. Like kukui, a good oil for normal or combination skin; it can moisturize without clogging pores.

Kelp: A seaweed with purifying, soothing, and healing abilities.

Kukui oil: An oil derived from the Hawaiian kukui nut. This light, non-greasy emollient is rich in essential fatty acids that produce healthy skin. It is a great facial oil. Kukui smoothes and softens irritated skin and treats superficial burns and chapped skin. It can be used after sunning and as a hot-oil treatment for hair.

Laminaria: See seaweeds.

Lavender: Lavender has an impressive number of uses both as an herb and an essential oil. In aromatherapy, the essential oil is both stimulating and calming as an anti-depressant. The plant is useful in preparations for burns, bites, wounds, and rheumatic conditions, as well as being suitable for any skin type. It is a skin-cell regenerator, normalizes the flow of oil glands, is anti-bacterial, and is an antioxidant. This refreshing herb makes a relaxing bath treatment or sport massage oil.

Lecithin: Found in egg yolks, corn, and soybeans, lecithin is a fatty powder. It is used in creams as a natural phospholipid emulsifier. Wonderfully emollient on the skin and an antioxidant.

Lemon: One of the citrus fruits, lemon is used as an astringent to stimulate and cleanse skin.

Lily: Lily, a fragrant flower, is part of a healing herb family (along with garlic, onions, aloe vera, and tulips). The root of the Madonna lily is used in lotions and creams to heal burns and scars without leaving a scar. The white pond-lily root alleviates inflammation around the eyes. Also useful for bruises and as an anti-wrinkle ingredient.

Linalol: A tertiary alcohol of the formula $C_{10}H_{18}O$, which, with its acetic ester (and traces of other esters), forms the basis of the perfume of bergamot and lavender oils. Through dehydration, linalol is converted into terpenes of which the principles are limonene and dipentene. Linalol converts into acetic ester through esterification. During the development of the plant, the quantity, amount, proportions, and richness can increase and decrease. Acidity often decreases during the development of vegetation. In lavender, the essential oil becomes richer in linalol when the flowers fade, and the ester proportion decreases.

Lye: Used to react with fats to create soaps, originally obtained by leaching wood ashes to extract a highly alkaline material called caustic soda, or sodium hydroxide. *Caution:* Full-strength lye can cause burns.

Mint: A plant that is traditionally used to soothe and cool the skin. It also "wakes up" skin with its antiseptic and stimulating action.

Monocyclic: Arranged in or consisting of one whorl or circle (the floral organs of many plants are monocyclic); or containing one ring in the molecular structure.

Mucilages: Have a soothing effect when applied to inflamed tissues, and their gel is perfect in cosmetic preparations. The gel-like substances have molecules made up of long chains of sugar units.

Myrrh: Infection-fighting myrrh possesses antiseptic, anti-microbial, and anti-inflammatory agents and is able to reduce oiliness and cool the skin.

Natural colors: Chlorophyll creates a blue-green color; saffron or annatto a yellow color; beet juice creates a red; grape-skin a purple; henna creates an orange; and logwood purple.

Nettle: An herb of the genus *Urtica*, with opposite leaves, inconspicuous, greenish, imperfect flowers, and minute stinging hairs. Nourishing nettles are packed with essential nutrients for healthy skin.

Oatmeal: Made from milling the seeds of oats, oatmeal is nourishing, cleansing, and used as a scrub.

Oily skin: Created by over-functioning of the sebaceous glands, demonstrated by large pores.

Ointments: Also called salves, usually prepared with an oil such as almond, olive, or vegetable, a butter or wax, and healing herbs. All ingredients are blended together over low heat for a few hours; it is usually strained and placed in small jars to apply to the skin.

PABA: Or para-aminobenzoic acid; a member of the vitamin B family. It is found naturally in wheatgerm, brewer's yeast, and whole wheat. It is the only natural sunscreen of serious effectiveness.

Papaya: This tropical fruit contains a known protein-digestive enzyme that, when applied externally, softens the skin by eliminating dead cell buildup. Also an effective antioxidant, slowing down free-radical damage to skin. One of the best ingredients for exfoliation of the skin. It literally eats the dead skin that dulls the complexion and revitalizes the new skin underneath. The papaya's enzyme papain, like bromelain, has powerful protein digestive abilities that aid greatly to clear up a sluggish or muddy complexion. Papaya and pineapple are the best exfoliants used directly and freshly.

Parabens: The most widely used preservatives in skin care products, these are synthetic chemicals used to preserve cosmetics and provide long shelf-life.[*]

Peanut oil: a.k.a. arachis oil; a heavy oil and inexpensive; in my opinion, almond oil is superior for cosmetic use.

pH: A measurement of acidity or alkalinity of a product or substance. Neutral pH is 7.0; anything under is acidic, such as orange juice. A pH over 7.0 is alkaline, as with soap. Normal skin has a pH of 5.5.

Pineapple: The proteolytic (protein-digestive) enzyme bromelain, similar to papain, contained in this fruit makes it a superb skin softener, especially in combination with papaya. I use pineapple juice in our Botanical Enzyme Exfoliant mask; it is perfect used with honey and herbs such as mint and comfrey, especially if mixed with vitamins A, C, and E. Can be used alone for oily skin and/or acne. Dilute it with water or an herbal tea or infusion, or use alone and apply directly to the skin, leaving it on for 10 or 20 minutes instead of using a glycolic acid or similar product. It is highly acidic and can be used as an ingredient in many homemade products.

---

[*] Aubrey Hampton, *Natural Organic Hair and Skin Care,* Tampa, FL: Organica Press, 1987, p. 297.

Poultices: Poultices are a remedy used to draw out toxins, relieve pain, or increase circulation. The chosen herb is heated and mashed and either applied directly to the skin, as in other countries, but in the U.S., usually put on a cloth first, then covered with another warm cloth to keep the heat in. In many countries, hot oil is applied to the skin before applying the herbs.

Primrose oil: An expensive, highly revered oil derived from the evening primrose plant's seeds, this substance treats skin with a variety of essential fatty acids. High in essential fatty acids including the rare gamma-linolenic acid (GLA), which occurs only in a few plants and in mother's milk. Can be used alone or added to other oils to moisturize skin and help skin conditions such as eczema. Add to shampoos or apply directly to clean, dry hair to add luster.

Propylene glycol: Often used in cosmetics as an humectant. A petroleum derivative found in antifreeze and brake fluid. [*]

Proteins: The basic building blocks of life forms. They are amino acids stuck together in various sequences and chains.

Rose: The well-known rose has been included in skin care formulations for centuries because of its delightful fragrance and its cleansing and skin-softening abilities.

Rosehip seed oil: a.k.a. Rosa mosqueta; extracted from the tiny amber seed of the rosehip fruit. An expensive oil, rosehip seed is high in essential fatty acids. It helps heal burns, sunburn, and acne scars, reduces wrinkles, and helps skin look smooth and vital. Clinical research in South America has indicated that this oil can be effective in reducing the early signs of aging, wound and scar healing, for overall improvement in the quality of the skin, in normal and oily hair to add luster, or applied to damaged hair as a hot-oil treatment to repair and revitalize.

Rosemary: An antiseptic herb, rosemary purifies and tones the complexion and is helpful in cases of acne.

Safflower oil: An unsaturated oil and one of the richest and most difficult to keep from going bad. Unsaturated oils tend to penetrate the skin better than saturated oils. An emollient.

---

[*] Ibid., p. 301.

Sage: This distinct-smelling herb purifies and tones dull skin and is an antiseptic, a cleanser, and a deodorant.

Scrubs: Used to exfoliate dead skin; make by simply adding salt or sugar to soap or cleanser; make a paste of any of the following with clean spring water, herbal teas, or milk: powdered rose petals, powdered almonds, or oats.

Seaweeds: Sea plants are therapeutic for skin because they bring oxygen to the tissues, thus stimulating circulation and waste elimination. Hydration results from their ability to reabsorb moisture over time from within the skin.

Sebum: A fatty material secreted by the skin's sebaceous glands. Every hair on your head has a sebaceous gland attached to its root, which lubricates the hair as it grows out.

Sequestering agent: An ingredient that prevents changes in the product, such as changes in color, texture, etc.

Sesame oil: A very light, unsaturated oil and one of the best natural sunscreens. A skin softener, it is said to absorb UV light.

Shea butter: a.k.a. karite butter and African butter; a superior skin care ingredient from the nut of an African tree. The same consistency of butter, it melts at body temperature. A mild sunscreen, a perfect replacement for beeswax for vegans. Used as an emollient, wrinkle remover, and skin softener. This African plant butter imparts an exotic, silky feel to skin care products and elasticizes the skin, increasing its suppleness.

Sour cream: A dairy product, great for a dry skin mask; high in lactic acid.

Stearic acid: Gives stiffness to body care products and used as an emulsifier. A waxy ingredient derived from fats.

St. John's wort: A plant used as a general healing agent, St. John's wort smoothes chapped skin and wrinkles.

Sweet almond oil: An emollient and nourishing natural oil, softening to the skin and hair. Widely used for massage and in natural skin care products. Extracted from almond nutmeats. Aids dry skin and used as a makeup remover, massage oil, or bath oil. Use sweet almond oil as a base for homemade herbal oils and skin care products; add to shampoo to aid dry hair.

Tahini: A smooth paste of sesame seeds.

Tea or infusion: Placing the herbs in boiling water to steep for five minutes to give the water a bite of the herb creates a tea or infusion. One teaspoon of herb per eight ounces of water is the preparation for tea and the most common method of taking herbs.

Tea tree oil: This essential oil is a powerful antiseptic and anti-microbial; useful for skin eruptions and wounds.

Tincture: One of the most convenient and economical ways of taking herbs if you prepare the tincture yourself. Tincture usually refers to an alcohol extract but can often be done with vinegar. Alcohol is one of the best methods of extraction for obtaining active ingredients of herbs.

Tocopherol acetate: Vitamin E.

Tomato: The fruit of the tomato plant; helps tone skin and encourages circulation.

Tragacanth gum: See gums. This plant gum is an effective botanical binder and emulsifying agent in natural skin care products.

Unsaturated oils: *The Complete Book of Natural Cosmetics* by Beatrice Travern states that "without even attempting to explain a very complicated part of organic chemistry, it should be noted that unsaturated oils . . . generally tend to disappear quickly when rubbed into the skin. This quality is useful in formulating cosmetics, as the unsaturated oil gives a lighter skin feel and seems to penetrate," although this is not always literally true. Other oils (saturated or hydrogenated oils) stay on the surface more and therefore feel much greasier.

Vegetable glycerin (kosher): Functions as a "moisture-magnet," drawing moisture from the air to the skin. Lily of Colorado uses the kosher grade because it is the pure vegetable form and not synthetic or animal-derived glycerin.

Vitamin A: a.k.a. retinyl and retinol; fat soluble; found in carrots, green vegetables, and yellow fruits. Used as an antioxidant and in a natural preservative system with grapefruit seed extract and vitamins C and E.

Vitamin C: a.k.a. ascorbic acid; water-soluble; found in fresh fruits and vegetables. It is used as a part of a preservation system in body care products and as an ingredient that reputedly enhances the performance of the connective tissue.

Vitamin E: As an antioxidant, vitamin E oil protects skin cells from free radical damage. It can lessen scarring and speed healing when applied to a wound. Vitamin E oil also softens and lubricates the skin.

Wheat germ oil: A vitamin-packed rescue for dry skin, especially for dryness resulting from exposure to harsh elements. Extracted from the heart of the wheat kernel. Nourishes and softens skin and makes it resilient, smoothes wrinkles and softens cuticles. Can be added to facial masks and bath oils to help heal dry skin.

Wild yam: *Dioscorea villosa*; The starchy, tuberous root of various tropical and subtropical vines growing wild, wild yams have been used for years to reduce menstrual cramps and other pain. It is anti-inflammatory. Main constituents: Steroidal saponins, including dioscin and trillin, which provide the diosgenin, phytosterols, dioscorine, and tannins.

Xanthan gum: *Xanthomonas campestris*; a polysaccharide of high molecular weight that is made by fermenting a carbohydrate with a bacterium; often used as a thickener.

Yarrow: A plant that promotes skin circulation and opens skin pores. Used as an astringent; also anti-inflammatory.

Ylang ylang: The sweet smell of this flower's essential oil is effective as a sedative and is calming and euphoric for the nervous system; used in aromatherapy. Soothes the skin, is a well-known aphrodisiac, and helps control oily skin.

Zinc oxide: A white pigment that is soothing and antiseptic.

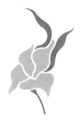

Bibliography

Alexander, Dale. *Dry Skin and Common Sense*. West Hartford, CT: Witkower Press, Inc., 1978.

Angier, Bradford. *Field Guide to Medicinal Wild Plants*. Harrisburg, PA: Stackpole Books, 1978.

Avery, Alexandra. *Aromatherapy and You: A Guide to Natural Skin Care*. Kailua, HI: Blue Heron Hill Press, 1994.

B., Philip, with Lucy Fraser and Wendy Ryerson. *Blended Beauty: Botanical Secrets for Body & Soul*. Berkeley, CA: Ten Speed Press, 1995.

Beck, Charlotte Joko. *Everyday Zen: Love and Work*. New York: Harper San Francisco Publishers, 1989.

Beck, Charlotte Joko. *Nothing Special: Living Zen*. New York: Harper San Francisco Publishers, 1993.

Bittman, Mark. *Natural Health Handbook 1995. Retailer's Guide to Natural Products*. Brookline Village, MA: Boston Common Press Ltd. Partnership, 1995.

Blanche, Cynthia. *The Book of Energy: Invigorating Ways to Revitalize Your Life*. Alexandria, VA: Lansdowne Publishing Pty., Ltd., 1997.

Bland, Jeffrey. *Evaluate Your Own Biochemical Individuality*. New Canaan, CT: Keats Publishing, Inc., 1987.

Bland, Jeffrey, *Intestinal Toxicity and Inner Cleansing*. New Canaan, CT: Keats Publishing, Inc., 1987.

The Book of Calm: Relaxing Ways to Manage Stress. Alexandria, VA: Lansdowne Publishing Pty. Ltd., 1997.

Bragg, Paul C., and Patricia Bragg, *Apple Cider Vinegar Health System*. Santa Barbara, CA: Health Sciences, 1987.

Bricklin, Mark. *Rodale's Encyclopedia of Natural Home Remedies*. Emmaus, PA: Rodale Press, Inc., 1982.

Brown, Donald J., *Introduction to Phytotherapy*. New Canaan, CT: Keats Publishing, Inc., 1995.

Buchman, Dian Dincin. *An ABC of Natural Beauty Recipes*. New Canaan, CT: Keats Publishing, Inc., 1996.

Buchman, Dian Dincin. *The Complete Herbal Guide to Natural Health and Beauty*. New Canaan, CT: Keats Publishing, Inc., 1995.

Butcher, Dana. "Aromatherapy – Its Past and Future." *DCI*, March 1998, p. 22 and 24.

Cameron, Julia. *The Artist's Way*. New York: G. P. Putnam's Sons, 1992.

Campion, Kitty. *Kitty Campion's Handbook of Herbal Health*. London: Leopard Books, 1985.

Castleton, Virginia. *The Handbook of Natural Beauty*. Emmaus, PA: Rodale Press, Inc., 1975.

Ceres. *Herbal Teas for Health and Healing*. New York: Thorsons Publishers, Inc., 1984.

Chodron, Pema. *The Wisdom of No Escape and the Path of Loving Kindness*. Boston, MA: Shambhala Publications, Inc., 1991.

Complementary Healing Guide Denver Edition. Littleton, CO: Kenton Johnson, Publisher, 1997.

The Condensed Chemical Dictionary, Fifth Edition. Revised and enlarged by Arthur and Elizabeth Rose. New York: Reinhold Publishing Corp., 1956.

Conry, Tom with The Science Action Coalition. *Consumer's Guide to Cosmetics*. Garden City, NY: Anchor Press/Doubleday, 1980.

Cosmetic Ingredients Glossary: A Basic Guide to Natural Body Care Products. Petaluma, CA: Feather River Company, 1988.

Crenshaw, Mary Ann. *The Natural Way to Super Beauty*. New York: Dell Publishing Co., Inc., 1974.

Crow, W. B. *Precious Stones: Their Occult Power and Hidden Significance*. Wellingborough, England: The Aquarian Press, 1980.

Culpeper, Nicholas. *Culpeper's Complete Herbal & English Physician Enlarged*. London, 1814; reprint, Glenwood, IL: Meyerbooks, Publisher, 1990.

Dass, Ram, and Hanuman Foundation. *Remember Be Now Here/Be Here Now*. New York: The Crown Publishing Group, 1993.

Dewey, Laurel. *Nature's Miracle Tonics*. Lantana, FL: MicroMags, 1998.

Duke, James A. *Chemical Composition of Belizean Plants Discussed in Rain Forest Remedies: One Hundred Healing Herbs of Belize.* New York: Botanical Garden, 1994.

Dychtwald, Den. *Age Wave.* Los Angeles, CA, and New York, NY: J. P. Tarcher Publisher, 1989.

Firebrace, Peter, and Sandra Hill. *Acupuncture: How It Works, How It Cures.* New Canaan, CT: Keats Publishing, Inc., 1994.

Gaskins, Stephen. *This Season's People: A Book of Spiritual Teaching.* Summertown, TN: The Book Publishing Co., 1976.

Gerard, John. *The Herball or Generall Historie of Plantes.* London, 1597; fac. ed., London: John Norton.

Goldstein, Joseph. *The Experience of Insight: A Simple and Direct Guide to Buddhist Meditation.* Boston & London: Shambhala Publications, Inc., 1987.

Goldstein, Joseph, and Jack Kornfield. *Seeking the Heart of Wisdom: The Path of Insight Meditation.* Boston & London: Shambhala Publications, Inc., 1987.

Gottlieb, Bill, ed. *New Choices in Natural Healing.* Emmaus, PA: Rodale Press, 1995.

Grieve, Mrs. M. *A Modern Herbal: The Medicinal, Culinary, Cosmetic and Economic Properties, Cultivation and Folk-Lore of Herbs, Grasses, Fungi, Shrubs & Trees With All Their Modern Scientific Uses.* 2 vols. New York, 1931; reprint, New York: Dover Publications, Inc., 1982.

Griffith, Joe. *Speaker's Library of Business Stories, Anecdotes, and Humor.* Englewood Cliffs, NJ: Prentice-Hall.

Guyton, Anita. *The Natural Beauty Book: Cruelty-free cosmetics to make at home.* Hammersmith, London, England: Thorsons, 1991.

Hall, Dorothy. *The Herb Tea Book.* New Canaan, CT: Keats Publishing, Inc., 1981.

Hampton, Aubrey. *Natural Organic Hair and Skin Care.* Tampa, FL: Organica Press, 1987.

Hampton, Aubrey. *What's in Your Cosmetics? A Complete Consumer's Guide to Natural and Synthetic Ingredients.* Tucson, AZ: Odonian Press, 1995.

Handa, Parvesh. *Herbal Beauty Care.* Delhi, India: Orient Paperbacks, n.d.

Hanh, Thich Nhat. *The Miracle of Mindfulness: A Manual on Meditation.* Boston, MA: Beacon Press, 1987.

Harris, Jessica B. *The World Beauty Book.* San Francisco, CA: Harper Collins Publishers, 1995.

The Healthview Newsletter, Issue #27–29. 612 Rio Road West, Box 6670, Charlottesville, VA 22906.

Heinerman, John. *Aloe Vera, Jojoba and Yucca: The Amazing Health Benefits They Can Give You.* New Canaan, CT: Keats Publishing, Inc., 1982.

Hepper, Camilla. *Herbal Cosmetics: Simple and Effective Natural Beauty Treatments.* Wellingborough, England: Thorsons Publishers Limited, 1987.

Hill, Ray. *Propolis: The Natural Antibiotic.* Wellingborough, Northamptonshire, England: Thorsons Publishers Limited, 1981.

Hittleman, Richard. *Yoga for Health.* New York: Ballantine Books, 1983.

Housden, Roger. *Retreat: Time Apart for Silence & Solitude.* New York: Harper San Francisco Publishers, 1995.

Hsu, Dr. Hong-yen, and Douglas H. Easer. *Chinese Herbal Formulas for Women Only.* New Canaan, CT: Keats Publishing, Inc., 1995.

Isaacs, Alan, ed. *Dictionary of Physics: Derived from the Concise Science Dictionary.* New York: Warner Books, Inc., 1986.

Jarvis, D.C., *Folk Medicine.* New York: Fawcett Crest Books, 1958.

Jessee, Jill Eva. *Perfume Album.* Huntington, NY: Robert E. Krieger Publishing Co., Inc., 1965.

Kalous, Chris. *Frontier Natural Products Co-op Wholesale Product Catalog, Fall/Winter 97-98.* Norway, IA: Frontier Herbs, 1997.

Kaminski, Patricia, and Richard Katz. *Flower Essence Repertory: A Comprehensive Guide to North American and English Flower Essences for Emotional and Spiritual Well-Being.* Rev. ed. Nevada City, CA: The Flower Essence Society, 1994.

Kaufman, Klaus. *Silica, The Forgotten Nutrient.* Burnaby, British Columbia: Alive Books, 1990.

Kaslof, Leslie J. *The Traditional Flower Remedies of Dr. Edward Bach, A Self-Help Guide: The Famous Drugless Therapeutic System and How You Can Use It.* New Canaan, CT: Keats Publishing, Inc., 1993.

Kowalchik, Claire, and William H. Hylton, eds. *Rodale's Illustrated Encyclopedia of Herbs.* Emmaus, PA: Rodale Press, 1987.

Kroeger, Hanna. *Ageless Remedies from Mothers Kitchen.* 3rd ed., enlarged. Boulder, CO: Hanna Kroeger, 1981.

Kroeger, Hanna. *Instant Herbal Locator.* 3rd ed., enlarged. Boulder, CO: Hanna Kroeger, 1979.

Kroeger, Hanna. *The Seven Spiritual Causes of Ill Health.* Boulder, CO: Hanna Kroeger, 1988.

Kugler, Hans. *The Disease of Aging: How not to grow old before your time.* New Canaan, CT: Keats Publishing, Inc., 1984.

Kushi, Aveline, with Wendy Esko and Maya Tiwari. *Diet for Natural Beauty.* Tokyo and New York: Japan Publications, Inc., 1991.

Lark, Susan M. *Easing Anxiety and Stress Naturally.* New Canaan, CT: Keats Publishing, Inc., 1996.

Lark, Susan M. *Menstrual Cramps Self-Help Book: Effective Solutions for Pain and Discomfort due to Menstrual Cramps and PMS.* Berkeley, CA: Celestial Arts, 1995.

Leyel, Mrs. C. F. *Herbal Delights: Botanical information and recipes for cosmetics, remedies and medicines, condiments and spices, and sweet and savory treats for the table.* 1938; reprint, New York: Gramercy Publishing Company, 1986.

Liberman, Jacob, *Light—Medicine of the Future: How We Can Use It to Heal Ourselves NOW.* Santa Fe, NM: Bear & Company Publishing, 1991.

Liberty Natural Products Wholesale Catalog, Fall 1996. 8120 SE Stark, Portland, OR 97215.

Little, Kitty. *Kitty Little's Book of Herbal Beauty.* Harmondsworth, Middlesex, England: Penguin Books Ltd., 1980.

Lindley, John. *The Treasury of Botany.* Rev. ed. London: Longmans, Green and Co., 1889.

Lust, John B., *The Herb Book.* New York: Bantam Books, Inc., 1974.

Mabey, Richard, ed. *The New Age Herbalist: How to use herbs for healing, nutrition, body care, and relaxation.* New York: Collier Books, Macmillan Publishing Company, 1988.

Majupuria, Trilok C., and D. P. Joshi. *Religious and Useful Plants of Nepal and India.* 2nd ed. Lalitpur Colony, Lashkar, India: M. Gupta, 1989.

McDonald, Kathleen. *How to Meditate: A Practical Guide.* Boston, MA: Wisdom Publications, 1984.

Meyer, David C. *Herbal Recipes for Hair, Salves & Liniments, Medicinal Wines and Vinegars. Plant Ash Uses.* Glenwood, IL: Meyerbooks, 1978.

Mindell, Earl L., with Virginia L. Hopkins. *Dr. Earl Mindell's What You Should Know About Beautiful Hair, Skin and Nails.* New Canaan, CT: Keats Publishing, Inc., 1996.

Moore, Thomas. *Care of the Soul: A Guide for Cultivating Depth and Sacredness in Everyday Life.* New York: Harper Collins, 1992.

Mowrey, Daniel B., *The Scientific Validation of Herbal Medicine.* N. P.: Cormorant Books, 1986.

Muir-Stanley, Heather. *Your Own Little Book of Health.* Denver, CO: Wholistic Practices, 1996.

National Cancer Institute. *Cleaning the Air: How to Quit Smoking . . . and Quit for Keeps.* NIH Publication No. 95-1647. Bethesda, MD: National

Institute of Health, U.S. Dept. of Health and Human Services Public Health Service. Revised Sept. 1993 and reprinted Sept. 1995.

National Cancer Institute. *When Someone in Your Family Has Cancer.* NIH Publication No. 96-2685. Bethesda, MD: National Institute of Health, U. S. Dept. of Health and Human Services Public Health Service. Revised December 1995.

Osho. *The Everyday Meditator.* Rutland, VT: Charles E. Tuttle Company, Inc., 1993.

Parry, Ernest J. *The Chemistry of Essential Oils and Artificial Perfumes.* Vol. II, 4th rev. ed. London, England: Scott, Greenwood and Son, 1922.

Passwater, Richard A. *Evening Primrose Oil: How its amazing nutrients promote health relief from problems including acne, arthritis and heart disease.* New Canaan, CT: Keats Publishing, Inc., 1981.

PETA (People for the Ethical Treatment of Animals). *1998 Shopping Guide for Caring Consumers: A guide to products that are not tested on animals.* Summertown, TN: The Book Publishing Company, 1997.

Quillin, Patrick. *Amazing Honey, Garlic, & Vinegar Home Remedies & Recipes: The people's guide to nature's wonder medicines.* North Canton, OH: The Leader Co., Inc., 1996.

Rector-Page, Linda. *Stress, Headache Relief & Overcoming Addictions.* Sonora, CA: Healthy Healing Publications, Inc., 1993.

Rose, Jeanne. *The Herbal Body Book.* New York: Perigee Books, 1982.

Rose, Jeanne. *Herbs & Things: Jeanne Rose's Herbal.* New York: Perigee Books, 1972.

Rose, Jeanne. *The Aromatherapy Book.* San Francisco, CA: Herbal Studies Course/Jeanne Rose, 1992.

Royal, Penny C. *Herbally Yours: A comprehensive herbal handbook simple enough for the herbal student, complete enough for the herbal practitioner.* Provo, UT: Sound Nutrition, 1982.

Russel, Maggi. *The Complete Book of Natural Beauty.* Feltham, England: Newmes Publishing, 1985.

Sachs, Melanie. *Ayurvedic Beauty Care: Ageless Techniques to Invoke Natural Beauty.* Twin Lakes, WI: Lotus Press, 1994.

Satchidananda, Yogiraj Sri Swami. *Integral Yoga Hatha.* New York: Holt, Rinehart and Winston, 1970.

Shapiro, Eddie. *Inner Conscious Relaxation: A Renaissance in Consciousness.* Rockport, MA: Element, Inc., 1991.

Shapiro, Eddie and Debbie. *Out of Your Mind—The Only Place To Be!* Rockport, MA: Element, Inc., 1992.

Skousen, Max B., *The Aloe Vera Handbook*. Cypress, CA: Aloe Vera Research Institute, 1982.

Smith, Lendon H. *Happiness Is a Healthy Life: Observations, Intuitions, Dicta and Data*. New Canaan, CT: Keats Publishing, Inc., 1992.

Taylor, Dena. *Red Flower: Rethinking Menstruation*. Freedom, CA: The Crossing Press, 1988.

Tisserand, Robert B. *The Art of Aromatherapy: The Healing and Beautifying Properties of the Essential Oils of Flowers and Herbs*. Rochester, VT: Destiny Books, 1977.

Tkac, Debora, ed. *The Doctors Book of Home Remedies: Thousands of Tips and Techniques Anyone Can Use to Heal Everyday Health Problems*. Emmaus, PA: Rodale Press, 1990.

Travern, Beatrice. *The Complete Book of Natural Cosmetics*. New York: Simon and Schuster, 1974.

Treben, Maria. *Health from God's Garden: Herbal Remedies for Glowing Health and Well-Being*. Rochester, VT: Thorsons Publishers, Inc., 1987.

Upton, L. K., and M. M. Kulow, compilers. *Börlind of Germany's Dictionary of Skin Care Product Ingredients: With Reference to Their Natural Sources*. New London, NH: Börlind of Germany, Inc., 1989.

Valnet, Jean. *The Practice of Aromatherapy: A Classic Compendium of Plant Medicines & Their Healing Properties*. Rochester, VT: Healing Arts Press, 1990.

Van Ekeren, Glenn. *The Speaker's Sourcebook*. Englewood Cliffs, NJ: Prentice-Hall, 1988.

Vogel, A. *Swiss Nature Doctor: An encyclopedic collection of helpful hints gathered from the Swiss folklore of natural healing*. 3rd ed. Teufen, Switzerland: Edition A. Vogel, 1980.

Wade, Carlson. *Carlson Wade's Amino Acids Book*. New Canaan, CT: Keats Publishing, Inc., 1985.

Wade, Carlson. *Inner Cleansing: How to Free Yourself from Joint-Muscle-Artery-Circulation Sludge*. West Nyack, NY: Parker Publishing Company, 1983.

Walker, Morton. *How to Stop Baldness and Regrow Hair: Preventing and Successfully Treating Hair Loss for Both Adult Sexes*. Stamford, CT: New Way of Life, Inc., 1995.

Weed, Susan S. *Wise Woman Herbal: Healing Wise*. Woodstock, NY: Ash Tree Publishing, 1989.

Willard, Terry, and James McCormick. *Edible and Medicinal Plants of the Rocky Mountains and Neighbouring Territories.* Calgary, Alberta: Wild Rose College of Natural Healing, Ltd., 1992.

Winter, Ruth. *A Consumer's Dictionary of Cosmetic Ingredients.* Rev. ed. New York: Crown Publishers, Inc., 1976.

Worwood, Valerie Ann. *The Complete Book of Essential Oils & Aromatherapy.* Novato, CA: New World Library. 1991.

Worwood, Valerie Ann. *The Fragrant Mind: Aromatherapy for Personality, Mind, Mood, and Emotion.* Novato, CA: New World Library, 1996.

Yogananda, Paramahansa. *Autobiography of a Yogi.* 8th ed. Los Angeles, CA: Self-Realization Fellowship Publishers, 1959.

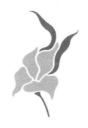

Afterword

One of my favorite remarks is from Albert Einstein, the Nobel Laureate in Physics and one of the greatest scientists of all time. In response to a question, he said that the greatest decision in life that one must make is whether or not one believes the universe is a friendly place.

I'm interested in your comments, reflections, and insights. Please write me at P.O. Box 12471, Denver, CO 80212 or e-mail through our web page, www.lilyofcolorado.com, with your comments, ideas, additions, criticisms, and experiences, or if you would like to be on our mailing list.

Thank you,
Lily

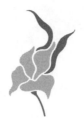

A special thank you to all our customers

Thank you for your loyalty, support and friendship:

Arizona
Grendl—All In The Hands, Green Valley
Meredith—Aqua Vista, Tucson

California
Amy—Cornucopia Community Market, Carmel
Christine—Cosmetics And..., Sacramento
Gwen—Other Avenues, San Francisco
Ashley—Country, Sun, Palo Alto
Ken—Great Earth Vitamins, San Mateo
Johnaleigh—Whole Foods, Monterey
Jim—Great Earth Vitamins, Daly City
Barbara—New Frontier Natural Foods, Solvang

Colorado
Sharon—Alfalfa's, Boulder
Jennifer—Alfalfa's, Lakewood
Erika—Alfalfa's, Littleton

Danielle—Ambrosia Natural Foods, Pueblo
Larry—Clark's Market, Aspen
Deb—Crystal Vegetarian Market, Boulder
Sherri—Great Mother Market, Fraser
Michelle—Lily's Herbery, Denver
Julie—Mountain Mamma, Colorado Springs
Katie—Vitamin Cottage, Boulder
Christina—Alfalfa's, Denver
Tania—Alfalfa's, Ft. Collins
Artimes—Alfalfa's, Westminster
Margie—Back To The Basics, Colorado Springs
Beth—Clark's Natural Foods Market, Carbondale
Debra—Dancing Willow Herbs, Durango
Donna—Heavenly Body, Winter Park
Debbie—Mountain Harvest, Colorado Springs
Blanche—Vitamin Cottage, Arvada
Tena—Vitamin Cottage, Denver
Gail—Alfalfa's, Denver

Nancy—Alfalfa's Glendale, Glendale
Jeff—Ambrosia Health Enterprises,
Wheat Ridge
Marge—Body & Soul, Glenwood
Springs
Melanie—Clark's Market, Steamboat
Springs
Becca—Durango Natural Food,
Durango
Jill—Jubilee He Restoreth, Parker
Debra—Nature's Oasis, Durango
Stacy—Vitamin Cottage, Aurora
Amy—Vitamin Cottage, Denver
Susan—Vitamin Cottage, Englewood
Christine—Vitamin Cottage,
Lakewood
Shari—Wild Oats, Aurora
Teresa—Wild Oats, Denver
Dawn—Vitamin Cottage, Lakewood
Karla—Vitamin Cottage, Littleton
Dawn—Wild Oats, Boulder
Debbie—Wild Oats, Greenwood
Village
Bevin—Vitamin Cottage, Lakewood
Darci—Whole Foods, Boulder
Debbie—Wild Oats, Colorado
Springs
Lynn—Vail Botanicals, Eagle

Connecticut
Amy—Bobbitts Natural Food Store,
New Milford

Florida
Gail—Nutrition World, West Palm
Beach
Nancy—Food Works, West Palm
Beach
Alba—Health Mall, Boca Raton
Frank—Nutrition World, West Palm
Beach
Stacey—Wild Oats FLF, Ft.
Lauderdale

Kat—Wild Oats MBF, Miami Beach
Julianna—Wild Oats PCF, Pine Crest
Barb—Nutrition Cottage, Delray
Beach
Christa—Lake Worth Nutrition
World
Robert—Wild Oats, West Palm
Beach
Susan—Wild Oats, Ft. Lauderdale

Georgia
Annabelle—Mia's Health Food,
Macon

Illinois
Cynthia—Annapurna, Evanston
Diana—Bonne Sante, Chicago
Denise—Fruitful Yield, Lombard
Joann—Sunrise Farm, Lansing
Nicole—Whole Foods, River Forest
Veronica and Annette—Whole
Foods, Wheaton
Joann—Apple Valley, Westmont
Alan—Fruitful Yield, Skokie
Pam—Total Approach, Markham
Chris—Whole Foods, Evanston
Karen—About Face & Body Works,
Hickory Hills
Kim—Aromatic Essentials, Sterling
Peggy—Fruitful Yield, Elmhurst
Mary—Mary's Health Hutch,
Chatham
Wendy and Sher—Whole Foods,
Palatine
Bekla—Whole Foods, Chicago

Indiana
Kathleen—Health & Harmony,
Highland

Kansas
Jackie—Wild Oats, Mission

Maryland
Diana Kay—Terressentials,
  Middletown

Michigan
Suzanne—Arbor Farms, Ann Arbor
Dori—Harvest Health Inc., Grand
  Rapids
Lynn—Whole Foods, Ann Arbor
Jody—Fruit Cellar, Dearborn
Marilyn—Nutri Foods, Royal Oaks
Nicholle—Whole Foods, Troy
Mary—Harvest Health Inc., Grand
  Rapids
Patty—Patty's Kitchen, Montgomery
Jill—Zebro's Health Foods, Livonia

Missouri
Melanie—Wild Oats, Kansas City
Kristen—Wild Oats, Ladue

Nevada
Jordan—Wild Oats, Las Vegas
Gregory—Wild Oats, Las Vegas
Verna—Health Nuts, Boulder
Stephanie—Wild Oats, Las Vegas

New Jersey
Allen—Health Food Mart, Short
  Hills

New Mexico
Sylvia—Alfalfa's SF, Santa Fe
Gaye—Moses Country, Albuquerque

Carol Lee—Wild Oats, Albuquerque
AnnaBel—Wild Oats, Santa Fe
Becky—BK's Health Pantry,
  Albuquerque
Kathi—The Market Place, Santa Fe
Kimberly—Wild Oats, Albuquerque
Sherry and Beth—CLD's Food
  Market, Taos
Chuck—Vitamin Cottage,
  Albuquerque
Roger—Wild Oats, Santa Fe

New York
Michelle—Health Beat Natural
  Foods, Johnson City
Maria—Queens Health Emporium,
  Flushing

North Carolina
Lorraine—French Broad Food Co-op,
  Asheville

Pennsylvannia
Mary—Dewalt's, Pittsburgh

Texas
Carol—Herbs & More, Decatur

West Virginia
Karen—Sunflowers, Morgantown

Utah
K'Lynn—Good Earth, Midvale

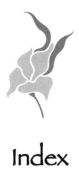

Index